Multiple Sclerosis

The Questions You Have
The Answers You Need

Multiple Sclerosis
The Questions You Have
The Answers You Need

Rosalind C. Kalb, Ph.D., Editor

The development of this book was made possible by an unrestricted educational grant to the Consortium of Multiple Sclerosis Centers by BERLEX LABORATORIES, Inc.

demos vermande

Demos Vermande, 386 Park Avenue South, New York, New York 10016

Library of Congress Cataloging-in-Publication Data

Kalb, Rosalind.
    Multiple sclerosis : the questions you have, the answers you need
/ Rosalind C. Kalb.
      p. cm.
    Includes bibliographical references and index.
    ISBN 1-888799-04-8 (softcover)
    1. Multiple sclerosis—Popular works.   2. Multiple sclerosis-
-Miscellanea.   I. Title
RC377.K35   1996   96-25890
616.8′34—dc20   CIP

Made in the United States of America

To all the individuals and families who live with multiple sclerosis every day, asking questions and searching for answers; and to my mother, who never got to see the finished product.

Contents

Foreword

The most predictable feature of multiple sclerosis is its unpredictability. No two people with the illness follow the same course and each individual experiences variability in the behavior of the malady over time. This uncertainty layers substantial psychological burdens on top of the physical problems caused by MS. The effects of the disease are magnified by the fact that they typically come during a very dynamic phase of life—when families and careers are evolving and critical choices must be made.

Because of the unusual combination of physical and emotional stresses engendered by MS, affected individuals are often best served by a multidisciplinary team of health care professionals. The Consortium of Multiple Sclerosis Centers (CMSC), established in 1986 to support this kind of comprehensive, team approach to MS treatment and related research efforts, is now the premier organization of professionals dedicated to improving the lives of people with the disease. The Consortium's mission is to educate and inform both clinicians and patients, increase resources and opportunities for research, and improve the standard of care and quality of life for people with MS. The organization brings together physicians, rehabilitation specialists, nurses, psychologists, social workers, and many others who contribute to MS patient care and research. This question and answer book reflects the Consortium's commitment to an interdisciplinary approach to the disease. Most of the contributors are affiliated with the CMSC or with the National Multiple Sclerosis Society, a key partner in education with the Consortium.

This book is unique in the growing literature on MS. It is a collaborative effort between people living with MS and their health care professionals to provide answers to the most frequently posed queries about the disease. Although the cause of MS is still unknown, and its cure remains elusive, we have entered an exciting time of therapeutic choice. A variety of new treatments, both to modify the course of the disease and to ameliorate symptoms, have recently become available or are under intensive clinical investigation. This volume provides the best answers we can give today to the questions and riddles prompted by MS. We know that many of the responses will change as we come to understand more about the disease and as better treatments become available. We will welcome the challenge to update and revise our answers, for that increased knowledge can only mean a brighter future for everyone touched by multiple sclerosis.

Aaron Miller, M.D.
Professor of Clinical Neurology
State University of New York - Health Sciences Center
Director, Division of Neurology
Maimonides Medical Center
Brooklyn, New York
Past President, Consortium of MS Centers

Preface

This book was written for everyone living with MS—those who have the disease and those who share life with someone who has it. It covers a wide range of topics in a format that is familiar, accessible, and easily understood. Its question and answer format reflects the collaborative relationship between individuals with MS and their health care professionals; the authors of each chapter answer the questions that they have been asked repeatedly in the course of their work with MS. The format also provides a model and a vocabulary for those who are not certain what questions to ask or how to ask them, and makes it possible for readers to find information about specific topics related to their individual needs.

It is important for someone with a chronic illness to understand its potential impact and become familiar with positive steps that can be taken to manage this major intrusion into daily life. The book can prepare you to talk more comfortably with your health professionals and help you become an informed and active participant in the management of your MS. Factors such as the symptoms you are experiencing, the course of your MS, and career and family plans, all need your thoughtful consideration. This book provides one tool to help in that process.

Concerned professionals will also assist and support you through the difficult aspects of adjusting to MS.

Although many people with MS do not have debilitating symptoms, others experience a more problematic course. Since all of the information in this book will not pertain to everyone, and some material may be upsetting to those who have not experienced the more disabling problems, we recommend that you be selective in your reading. There is no need to read this book "from cover to cover." Each chapter has a short introduction to the particular topic, a series of questions and answers relating to the topic, and a listing of recommended readings for people who wish to pursue the topic in greater depth. Where applicable, the authors have also provided a list of available resources, including organizations, agencies, product manufacturers, and other potential sources of relevant information or goods and services.

The recommended strategy is to use this book for reference purposes, reading first for answers to your immediate questions and for general background information, and again whenever other problems or questions arise. The Neurology and Treatment chapters provide a useful overview of the disease and up-to-date management strategies. The Employment and Insurance chapters highlight important issues for you to think about now in order to safeguard yourself and your family down the road. The Psychosocial chapter deals with the ways in which people with MS and their family members react to the intrusion of MS and learn to cope with the changes that a chronic illness can bring to their lives. The introductions to the other chapters will help identify additional areas you might want to pursue in more detail. The Appendixes provide specific reference materials, including a detailed glossary of terms commonly encountered in reading about MS, information sheets about many of the medications commonly used in its management, a recommended reading list that includes books and other publications that relate to multiple sclerosis and to chronic illness in general, and a resource list that includes government and private agencies and organizations that provide information and/or services to deal with MS-related problems.

Multiple sclerosis is an unwelcome and distressing intruder for everyone involved. One way to manage the discomfort is to become more informed about what to expect and what can be done. Although some people with MS have an easier time than others, this book attempts to deal with the full range of possible problems, even the most disabling ones. Remember to focus on the topics that relate to your own unique situation; try not to become preoccupied with questions and problems which are unrelated to your own. If you continue to have questions or concerns about the information provided here, be sure to contact a member of your health team for further discussion.

Acknowledgments

This book has been a "team" effort in the very best sense of the word; its creation mirrored the collaborative approach that enables people with MS and their families to live comfortably and productively with the disease. With an unrestricted educational grant generously donated by Berlex Laboratories to the Consortium of Multiple Sclerosis Centers, people with MS, their family members, friends, health care providers, and community resources worked together to identify the questions and provide the answers to living with MS. Many people helped to make this book happen, and I am grateful to all of them.

Oscar Dystal came up with the idea for an MS question and answer book and encouraged us to pursue the project. June Halper, in her role as Administrative Director (and President-Elect) of the Consortium of Multiple Sclerosis Centers, presented the idea to Berlex Laboratories with her usual energy and enthusiasm. Ann Palmer, Director of Library, Reference, and Technical Services at the National Multiple Sclerosis Society, provided a computerized tally of the types of questions addressed to the Society over the past several years. Bob Cornelison and Marla Shawaryn-Cornelison, Steve and Harriet Doniger, Debby and Larry Giuliani, Holly and Nick Goebel, Bob

Goldberger, Heidi Knoll, Nicholas LaRocca, John Lufrano, Rob Muller, Debby Pastion, Paula and Tom Revello, Nancy Santoro, Faith Seidman, and Phyllis Wiesel all contributed helpful suggestions and comments about the questions to be included.

I particularly appreciated the efforts of the authors who responded to my persistent prodding with good humor and hard work, even though many were in the throes of serious illness or significant personal loss in addition to their usual heavy workloads.

The Glossary was laboriously reviewed by Drs. Donald Goodkin, Aaron Miller, T.J. Murray, and Steven Reingold, and the Medication Sheets by Dr. Charles Smith. June Halper put her hard work and know-how into creating the Resource List.

Lauren Caruso, Marla Shawaryn-Cornelison, Christine Feil, Nancy Holland, Nicholas LaRocca, Susan Lopez, Charles Smith, Pam Sorensen, Gary Sumner, and Phyllis Wiesel reviewed parts or all of the manuscript, providing invaluable suggestions and creative ideas. Dr. Diana M. Schneider and Joan Wolk of Demos Vermande guided me along, helping to make the parts into a whole.

And thank you to my family—for their help, patience, and good cheer.

1

What Should I Know About This Book?

Nancy J. Holland, Ed.D.

Is this book for me?

Multiple Sclerosis: The Questions You Have, The Answers You Need was written primarily for people with multiple sclerosis. However, if you love someone with MS, work with a person who has MS, or are just curious about the disease, you will find this book helpful and informative. It covers a wide range of topics in a format that is familiar, accessible, and easily understood. The question and answer format was selected for several reasons. First, it reflects the collaborative relationship between individuals with MS and their health care professionals. The authors of each chapter answer the questions that they have been asked repeatedly in the course of their work with MS. Second, the questions included here provide a model and a vocabulary for those who are not certain what questions to ask or how to ask them. Third, the question and answer format makes it possible for readers to zero in on particular topics, and even particular questions, without having to wade through material that may be irrelevant to their individual needs.

What is the purpose of this book?

It is important for someone with a chronic illness to understand its potentially far-reaching impact and to know what positive actions can be taken to manage this unexpected intrusion into daily life. An open dialogue with the physician and other professionals on the health care team is an important part of the adjustment process. This book answers specific questions about living with MS and can help prepare you to interact with health professionals as an informed and active participant in your health promotion plan. Factors such as the symptoms you are experiencing, the course of your MS, and career and family plans all need to be considered in a thoughtful manner. This book provides one tool to help in that process. Concerned professionals will also assist and support you through the difficult aspects of adjusting to MS.

How were people selected to answer the questions in this book?

Recognized experts in the field of multiple sclerosis were invited to participate. Most of the authors are affiliated with a comprehensive MS care center and/or the National Multiple Sclerosis Society and have extensive experience in assisting people to deal with MS-related problems. Others work in related fields that target the medical, psychosocial, and economic challenges faced by those with chronic illness.

How were the questions selected for inclusion?

Each of the contributing authors was asked to provide a list of questions, related to his or her area of expertise, that are commonly asked by individuals with MS and their family members. Authors were also asked to include questions that they felt people should be encouraged to ask even if they were not routinely doing so. Additionally, the Information Resource Center at the National Multiple Sclerosis Society provided a computerized listing of topics most frequently asked about on the telephone information line. The proposed questions for each chapter were then reviewed by a number of people with MS, family members, caregivers, and health professionals in an attempt to ensure that the list of questions was both comprehensive and meaningful.

How should I use this book?

There are a few factors to consider before deciding how to use this book. First, the course of MS and its related symptom picture can vary significantly from one individual to the next, as can the individual's response to treatment. People also vary in the individual characteristics they bring to the situation—their age, sex, family composition, social support network, and occupation, to name a few. Personality characteristics can also influence how a person will deal with MS and how he or she will choose to use this book. For example, some people want to know *everything* about MS, regardless of immediate or long-term relevance to their own medical situation. For most people, however, this is not the case. They want to know answers to specific questions that are pertinent to decisions that they need to make now and in the immediate future. You can use this book in any way that best suits your needs and your style of dealing with information.

The book attempts to answer questions for everyone living with MS—those who have the disease and those who share life with someone who has it. Although many people with MS do not have serious or debilitating symptoms, others have a rougher time. Since all of the information in this book will not pertain to everyone, some material may be upsetting to those not experiencing the more disabling problems. We recommend that you be selective in your reading and not see this as a book you must read from cover to cover. No one person will face all of the problems addressed here, and the full range of circumstances can be overwhelming if not dealt with selectively. Each chapter has a short introduction to the particular topic, a series of questions and answers relating to the topic, and a listing of recommended readings for people who wish to pursue the topic in greater depth. Where applicable, the authors have also provided a list of available resources, including organizations, agencies, product manufacturers, and other potential sources of relevant information or goods and services.

The best strategy is probably to use this book for reference purposes, reading it now for background information and answers to your immediate questions, and in the future as other problems or questions arise. The "Neurology" and "Treatment" chapters provide a useful overview of the disease and its management. The "Employment," "Insurance," and "Life Planning" chapters will alert you to important issues that you need to be thinking about now in order to safeguard yourself and your family down the road. The chapter on "Psychosocial Issues" addresses the ways in which people with MS and their family members react to the intrusion of MS and learn to cope with the changes that a chronic illness can impose on their lives. The introductions to the other chapters will help identify additional areas you might want to pursue in more detail. The Appendixes provide specific reference materials:

◇ **Glossary.** Medical words and phrases that are in bold type in the text are explained in the alphabetized glossary in Appendix A. Also included in the glossary are terms that you might encounter in other MS-related reading materials or in discussions with your health care providers. Multiple sclerosis is surrounded by a new and unfamiliar vocabulary of neurologic terms, anatomical parts, and rehabilitation language. Learning the meaning of these terms will increase your understanding of the complex information and facilitate your efforts to communicate with your health care providers.

◇ **Medication Information Sheets.** Many medications are used to deal with the variety of MS symptoms. A particular medication will likely be of interest only if your physician has recommended it or if you read or hear about it as a suggested therapy for a symptom you are experiencing. Each sheet in Appendix B describes how the particular drug is used in MS and provides important information that you need to know about any drug you are taking, including potential side effects and drug interactions. While the information sheets are designed to help you be a more informed participant in your own care, your physician should always be your primary source of information about the medications that he or she is prescribing for you.

◇ **Recommended Reading List.** Included in this list in Appendix C are books and other publications relating specifically to multiple sclerosis or to chronic illness.

◇ **Resource List.** Your particular needs at any given time will direct your use of the Resource List in Appendix D. Included in this list are government and private agencies and organizations that provide information and/or services to deal with MS-related problems. Since many resources vary according to the state or community in which you live, the Resource List can also guide your efforts to identify local sources of information and assistance. Resources that are specifically relevant to the area covered in a particular chapter are listed at the end of that chapter.

◇ **List of Authors**. Brief professional biographies of the authors are included in Appendix E.

What if I have only recently been diagnosed with MS?

In general, it will not be helpful for someone with a recent diagnosis to read the entire book. If you were only recently diagnosed, you probably have a relatively short history of MS symptoms to look back on and limited experience with the impact of these symptoms on your daily life. People differ in their responses to both the diagnosis and the challenges it poses. Additionally, there is considerable variation in disease course and symptoms in MS. Therefore, much of the material in this book will not be pertinent for you now and may or may not be pertinent for you in the future. If your MS follows a mild or moderate course, some of this information will never be relevant to your situation.

What if some of the answers (and even the questions) upset me?

Multiple sclerosis is an unwelcome and distressing intruder for everyone involved. One way to reduce the discomfort is to have accurate information about what to expect and what can be done. Some people with MS have an easier time than others, but this book attempts to deal with the full range of possible problems, even the very difficult ones. Remember to focus on the topics that relate to your particular and unique situation, and try not to become preoccupied with questions and problems that are unrelated to your own. If you continue to have questions or concerns about the information provided here, be sure to contact a member of your health team for further discussion.

How can I get additional information about topics addressed in this book?

Each chapter includes a list of recommended readings for people who wish to pursue more detailed information about a particular topic. Most of the recommended readings are for lay audiences. Articles from professional journals have been included in some lists, particularly in those areas in which little has been written for nonprofessionals (e.g., speech and swallowing disorders, cognition). Information about articles pertaining directly to multiple sclerosis can be obtained from the Information Resource Center of the National Multiple Sclerosis Society; publications may be available at your public library, through the library's inter-library loan service, or from an on-line computer service.

More general readings are listed in the Recommended Reading List in Appendix C. You can also contact a member of your health care team for additional recommendations. The Information Resource Center at the National Multiple Sclerosis Society (1-800-FIGHT MS) is another valuable source of up-to-date information about MS. Staff will answer questions and send you reading materials on a wide variety of MS-related topics. Obviously, no single book can include every possible question. Each individual is different and will experience MS in his or her own way. You will probably have questions of your own that do not appear in this book. The goal of this book is to help you ask the important questions—and find accurate, meaningful answers—so that you can manage life with MS in the way that best meets your needs.

2

Neurology

Charles R. Smith, M.D.
Randall T. Schapiro, M.D.

Multiple sclerosis (MS) is a **chronic**, neurologic disease that appears most commonly in young adults. Although ninety percent of those diagnosed are between the ages of sixteen and sixty, MS has been known to make its first appearance in early childhood or long after age sixty. The currently estimated **prevalence** of MS in the United States is 250,000–350,000 individuals, which means that more than one in a thousand people have the diagnosis at any given time. While an **incidence** rate of 9,000 new cases per year has been estimated in the United States, the availability of more effective diagnostic tools is gradually resulting in a higher rate of accurate diagnosis than was previously possible. Multiple sclerosis is more common in women than in men, by a ratio of 1.7:1. It appears more frequently in whites than in Hispanics or African-Americans and is relatively rare among Asians and certain other groups.

Multiple sclerosis is more common in temperate areas of the world and is relatively unusual in the tropics. The disease is seen more frequently in individuals from Great Britain, Scandinavia, and Northern Germany than from areas around the Mediterranean Sea; Canadians and individuals from the northern part of the United States seem to be more susceptible than

7

those living in the southern part of the continent. Multiple sclerosis is unknown among the Black peoples of Africa.

Although not directly inherited, the disease seems to appear in genetically predisposed individuals who are apparently more reactive or susceptible to whatever stimulus or agent causes the disease to become active. The general conclusion is that people of Northern and Central European ancestry, as well as those whose ancestry has become mingled with this group, seem to have some genetic predisposition to the disease. While we do not know as yet what factors within the environment cause MS to make its appearance in some of these individuals and not others, most researchers continue to believe that some unidentified virus is the likely culprit.

MS is thought to be an ***autoimmune disease*** in which the body's own immune system attacks a normal tissue or organ of

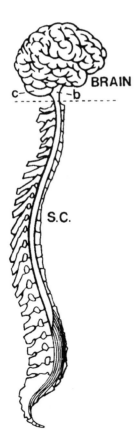

Figure 2–1   Central nervous system. The brain and spinal cord (S.C.) are the principal components of the central nervous system and are separated by a broken line in this schematic diagram. The cerebellum (**c**) and brainstem (**b**) are regions of the brain often affected by multiple sclerosis.

the body. In MS, the immune attack is directed against the *myelin* of the *central nervous system (CNS)*.

The symptoms that occur in MS result from damage to the myelin sheath that surrounds **neurons**, a process termed **demyelination**. Symptoms can include loss of vision, double vision, stiffness, weakness, imbalance, numbness, pain, problems with bladder and bowel control, fatigue, emotional changes, and intellectual impairment. The type and number of symptoms vary tremendously from one individual to the next, depending on where in the CNS the myelin damage occurs. At this time, we do not know why the demyelination occurs or why some people get more or different symptoms than others.

As is clear from this description of MS, there is much that we do not know about its causes or its pattern of symptoms. This uncertainty has been largely responsible for the frustrations faced by scientists searching for a cure. We do know that the disease tends to appear during the highly formative period of a person's life in which career and family growth are at their peak. Fortunately, although MS is a chronic illness, it is not necessarily a progressive one. The majority of people with MS are able to lead healthy and productive lives. For them, the symptoms of MS are more of an episodic inconvenience than a hindrance to their life's ambitions. For those whose MS is more severe and therefore more debilitating, we now have a variety of management strategies available that may help to keep the various neurologic *impairments* that can be caused by the disease, and their resulting *disabilities*, from becoming role-restricting *handicaps*. These distinctions, identified by the World Health Organization, are important to keep in mind as you read the questions and answers in this and other chapters. While we have as yet almost no control over the neurologic changes (impairments) that can interfere with a person's physical abilities such as running or seeing clearly (disabilities), we can do a great deal to reduce or eliminate any disadvantage (handicap) that interferes with that person's ability to lead a full, enjoyable, and productive life at work and at home.

Much can be done to improve quality of life after the diagnosis. Developing a positive attitude and getting educated are half the battle. Finding a health care team that understands and accommodates your needs is an important step. With their help, you can feel more in control and take on the challenges of life with MS with confidence. The following questions and answers highlight the primary concerns of people who are trying to understand this somewhat puzzling and unpredictable disease.

The Disease: Its Diagnosis, Course, and Prognosis

What goes wrong when a person has MS?

The body's actions and reactions to outside stimuli involve a lightning-quick and complicated process in which the body receives those stimuli through its various senses (vision or touch, for example), sends a report to the brain, and then responds to instructions from the brain about what to do next.

This ongoing process depends on the coordinated transmission of nerve impulses from one nerve cell to the next. Nerve impulses pass along nerve fibers, which connect at synapses. A fatty substance called myelin, which forms a sheath around the nerve fibers in the CNS (which is made up of the brain, optic nerves, and spinal cord) makes this conduction of nerve impulses possible. The myelin, which is made and maintained by cells called **oligodendrocytes**, has a whitish appearance, leading to the identification of MS as primarily a **white matter** disease of the CNS.

Any damage to this sheath results in some disruption of the impulse or message that is being transmitted, much as would occur in a damaged telephone wire. In MS, overactive, misguided cells of the immune system enter the CNS and destroy areas of myelin. Wherever myelin is destroyed, a **plaque** (lesion) forms, with a gradual buildup of hardened scar tissue (**sclerosis**) at the site. These sclerotic sites occur in several varied locations throughout the CNS, giving rise to the name *multiple sclerosis*. While many of these scars may be "silent," causing no apparent symptoms, others interfere with whatever sensation or function is controlled in that particular area of the brain or spinal cord. Additionally, demyelination may disrupt communication between different parts of the brain, even if the parts themselves remain intact.

Why is the diagnosis of MS so difficult?

At the present time, there are no specific blood tests, imaging techniques (e.g., **MRI** or **CAT scan**), tests of immune function, or genetic tests that can, by themselves, determine if a person has MS or is likely to have it in the future. The diagnosis is a clinical one, made

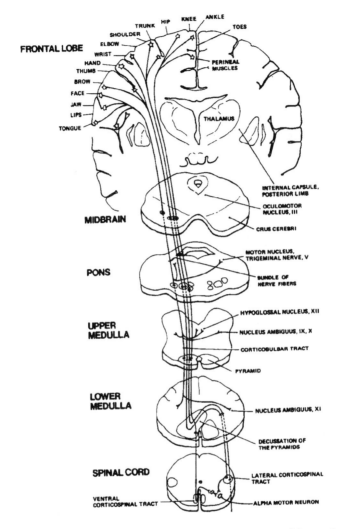

Figure 2-2   Nerve fiber pathway. The pathway depicted from the brain to the spinal cord involves fibers responsible for control of movements. (Adapted with permission from Gilman S, Newman SW: *Manter and Gatz's Essentials of Clinical Neuroanatomy and Neurophysiology*, 8th edition. Philadelphia: F.A. Davis, 1992:77.)

on the basis of a person's medical history, an assessment of the *symptoms* experienced and reported by the person, and the existence of *signs* detected by the physician (but not necessarily noticed by the person) during the neurologic examination. Both symptoms and signs are necessary because symptoms are subjective complaints that can vary tremendously from one individual to

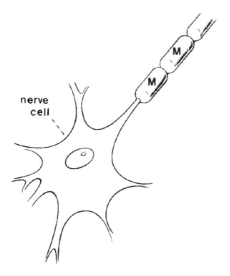

nerve
cell

Figure 2-3 Myelin sheath.
Cuffs of myelin (M) insulate
fibers from the nerve cell that
carries electrical signals.

another, while signs are more measurable, objective observations.
Examples of symptoms that are commonly reported by people with
MS include problems with vision, walking, bladder control,
fatigue, and uncomfortable sensations such as numbness or "pins
and needles." Common signs that can be detected by the doctor
during a physical examination, even if the person has never
noticed or been troubled by these changes, include altered eye
movements and abnormal responses of the pupils, subtle changes
in speech patterns, altered reflex responses, impaired ***coordination***, sensory disturbances, and evidence of ***spasticity*** and/or
weakness in the limbs.

In order to make a definite diagnosis of MS, the physician
must find the following:

◇ plaques or lesions in at least two distinct areas of the CNS
  white matter;
◇ evidence that the plaques have occurred at different points
  in time or have occurred progressively over six months'
  time; and, perhaps most importantly,
◇ that these plaques in the white matter have no other reasonable explanation.

In other words, MS is a diagnosis that can be made only after
every other possible explanation of the signs and symptoms has
been ruled out.

How will the doctor try to determine if I have MS?

The physician will first take a very careful history, including any past and present complaints that you have, any pertinent family history of disease, the places you have lived and visited, substance use (alcohol, drug, and smoking habits), and any medications that you are taking. Through detailed questioning, he or she can determine whether you have ever experienced other symptoms—no matter how slight or transient—that might be indicative of MS-related disease activity.

The physician will do a neurologic examination to check for signs that can explain the symptoms you are experiencing or point to disease activity of which you may have been totally unaware. An eye examination with an **ophthalmoscope** may reveal the presence of **optic neuritis**, which results from damage to the optic nerve. A pale optic nerve in MS is often indicative of earlier damage even if the person reports no past or current visual symptoms. He or she will also test visual acuity and look for evidence of double vision or incoordination of eye movements.

The physician will test for evidence of weakness by asking you to resist efforts to pull or push your arms and legs. You may also be asked to squeeze his hand. Your coordination will be tested in a variety of ways, including the **finger-to-nose test,** in which you are asked to bring the tip of your index finger to your nose rapidly, with your eyes open and then closed, and the **heel-knee-shin test**, in which you are asked to move one heel up and down the shin of the other leg. The physician will evaluate your balance by asking you to perform a variety of tasks, including walking on your heels and then on your toes, performing a **tandem gait** (placing the heel of one foot directly against the toe of the other foot in an alternating fashion), and standing still with your eyes closed.

Sensory changes will also be tested in a variety of ways. Your physician will determine if you can tell, with your eyes closed, where your body parts (e.g., fingers and toes) are in space (**position sense**). **Vibration sense** will be tested with a vibrating tuning fork placed against various places on your body. The physician may also use a (gentle) pinprick to test for changes in skin sensitivity. Unfortunately, many of the sensory changes experienced by people with MS, such as numbness, pain, or tingling, cannot be seen or objectively measured on examination, with the result that some physicians have tended to ignore or dismiss these uncomfortable symptoms as unimportant.

The physician will test the reflexes in various parts of your body. Inequality of reflexes on the two sides of your body is indicative of an abnormal reflex. Absent reflexes, particularly in the abdomen, are also common in MS, although they can have other explanations such as obesity or multiple pregnancies. The **Babinski reflex**, a frequent finding in MS, is clearly indicative of disturbances in major nervous pathways. This neurologic sign is elicited when the physician draws a bluntly pointed object along the outer edge of the sole of the foot from the heel to the little toe. Instead of the normal downward flexion of the toes, it results in an abnormal response in which the big toe extends upward and the other toes fan outward.

For some people, no tests beyond this history and neurologic exam are necessary to make the diagnosis. If the doctor is able to find evidence of multiple lesions in the CNS that have occurred at distinct points in time and have no other reasonable explanation, the diagnosis can be made without any other testing being done. However, most physicians will not rely entirely on this type of evaluation and will do at least one other test to confirm the diagnosis. This is especially true if the history and examination have not been able to provide conclusive evidence of more than one lesion in the brain or spinal cord. The most commonly done test is MRI (**magnetic resonance imaging**) of the brain, which is abnormal in about 90 percent of people with definite MS.

MRI of the spinal cord can also be useful but is not as frequently positive as MRI of the brain. Prior to the development of MRI, a specialized X-ray technique known as the CT scan (**computerized axial tomography**) was used to demonstrate the presence of lesions. However, MRI, which is safer and more accurate than any X-ray technique, provides clear evidence of white matter lesions in the CNS.

Other good tests to help confirm a diagnosis of MS include the **visual evoked potential (VEP)** and the **somatosensory evoked potential (SSEP)**. These tests, which look at the speed and efficiency of myelin conduction, are frequently abnormal in definite MS. VEPs, for example, are abnormal in about 90 percent of people with MS. Evoked potentials are particularly useful in confirming the diagnosis because they can demonstrate a completely asymptomatic lesion that would otherwise go unnoticed. Like MRI, these evoked responses tests are noninvasive and painless.

In some instances, a person will be advised to have a *lumbar puncture* (spinal tap). In this test, *cerebrospinal fluid* (fluid that bathes the spinal cord and brain) is collected for chemical analysis. In performing this test, the physician is looking for (1) elevations in IgG (immunoglobulin G, a protein fraction of gamma globulin), which are indicative of some abnormality in the immune system; and (2) the presence of a specific IgG that appears in the spinal fluid as *oligoclonal bands*. Neither of these is specific to MS, making a lumbar puncture primarily useful for confirming the diagnosis of MS when there is other suggestive evidence. Because this test is somewhat uncomfortable, it is not done as frequently as MRI or evoked potentials. However, one of the most important reasons for doing diagnostic tests is to make sure that some other disease is not masquerading as MS, and a lumbar puncture is an excellent test if there is any doubt about the diagnosis.

Thus, a variety of diagnostic procedures may be used to help *confirm* the diagnosis of MS if the physician believes that one or more are necessary. Keep in mind that the diagnosis cannot be made solely on the basis of these tests because MS is only one of several conditions that can cause them to be positive. Your medical history and the symptoms and signs of CNS demyelination that you and the doctor are able to piece together are the clearest evidence for the diagnosis of MS.

Why did I get MS? Did I do something to make this happen to me?

Because the cause of MS is unknown, why any one person gets the disease remains a mystery. Nothing that you had any control over could in any way have caused your MS. Multiple sclerosis is believed to be an autoimmune disease caused by something in the environment, perhaps a virus. It is also believed that the disease occurs in a person who is genetically predisposed to its development.

What does this mean? Most doctors believe that MS is an autoimmune disease because the plaques or scars in the myelin that are caused by the MS have all the signs of an immune-mediated process. For example, immune cells such as *lymphocytes*, *plasma cells* (white blood cells that make antibodies), and *macrophages* (cells that destroy myelin) can be found at sites being actively damaged. Many plaques start around a small vein, suggesting that these immune cells escape from the blood, pass through the **blood-brain barrier**, and enter the brain and spinal cord to do damage. There is a good animal model for MS, called **experimental allergic encephalomyelitis (EAE)**, which we know is an autoimmune disease. We can cause this disease to occur by injecting animal myelin into laboratory animals, making it an extremely valuable tool in the research efforts to find the cause and treatment of MS (see Chapter 3).

Although no one has yet identified what in the environment causes MS, the fact that the disease is definitely more common in certain parts of the world seems to point to some kind of environmental agent. Additionally, some studies have shown that the chances of getting MS seem to depend in part on where a person lives before the onset of adolescence. There have also been some "epidemics" of MS, which would tend to support the notion of an environmental agent as the cause of the disease. However, no virus or toxin has ever been proven to cause the disease.

Are there different types of MS?

The basic types of MS are now defined in the following way:

◇ **Relapsing-remitting MS** is characterized by attacks that last from days to weeks and then subside. Although there may be a variety of problems during these attacks, there are none or relatively few in the remission stage that comes between them. One subtype of this category is commonly referred to as "benign sensory" MS. Individuals with this type of MS have attacks of numbness or tingling in various parts of the body or visual blurring (caused by optic neuritis) as their only symptoms.

◇ **Primary progressive MS** is characterized by disease showing progression of disability from onset, without any obvious plateaus or remissions, or with only occasional plateaus and temporary, minor improvements.

◇ **Secondary progressive MS** begins initially with a relapsing-remitting course, which later becomes a more consistently progressive course. A physician cannot predict who will remain relapsing-remitting and who might in the future become secondary progressive. This is the reason why it is difficult to give any person a firm **prognosis**.

◇ *Progressive-relapsing MS* shows clear progression in disability level from the onset of the disease, but with clear, *acute* relapses that may or may not have some recovery following the acute episode.

These definitions clearly convey that multiple sclerosis is a disease of unpredictable course that can change its presentation along the way.

I have a neighbor with MS and her symptoms are completely different from mine. How can the same illness cause such different symptoms in people?

Just as there are different courses of MS, there are different kinds of symptoms, even among people of the same sex and age who have had the illness for the same length of time. This results from the fact that the plaques of MS are scattered throughout the white matter of the brain and spinal cord. Although there are areas where the plaques are more likely to occur, the distribution is random. Therefore, one person might experience loss of vision and another might have problems controlling urination. All MS symptoms are caused by damage to the myelin sheath (demyelination); however, the particular areas that become demyelinated vary from person to person.

How is an exacerbation different from a pseudo-exacerbation and what causes each to happen?

An *exacerbation* or "attack" of MS is caused by a new plaque of demyelination or the reactivation of an old plaque. For a symptom to qualify as an exacerbation it must, by definition, last for at least twenty-four hours and be separated from the previous attack by one month. Although these limits are somewhat arbitrary, it is important that they be considered so that symptoms will not be misinterpreted.

A *pseudo-exacerbation* has nothing to do with disease activity. It results from some other problem, such as a fever or pain, that aggravates the neurologic effects of the preexisting plaques. For example, people with MS who develop a fever seem much worse while their temperature is elevated. Once their temperature drops to normal, they return to their baseline neurologic function. Similarly, people with *spasticity* in their lower limbs notice more spasms and stiffness when they have a bladder infection. Once the bladder infection is cured with antibiotics, the spasms and stiffness return to their previous level.

Although there are many identifiable causes for pseudo-exacerbations, nobody knows the cause of true MS exacerbations. There is no convincing evidence for the commonly held belief that stress or trauma can produce exacerbations (see Chapter 11). Some studies have indicated that viral infections such as the common cold or flu can trigger a true exacerbation. This may happen because viral infections trigger the body's immune response.

Is there anything I can do to prevent an exacerbation?

There is no proven way to prevent MS attacks. We know of no medical treatment that always works to prevent an exacerbation or every person with MS would be taking it. There is no convincing evidence that a person can prevent an exacerbation by avoiding or controlling life stresses. However, medications that include Betaseron®, Avonex®, and Copaxone® have now been shown to reduce the frequency and severity of MS attacks in some individuals with relapsing-remitting MS (see Chapter 3).

Because some scientists believe that viral infections might trigger an exacerbation, it makes sense to employ good personal hygiene to reduce the possibility of getting such an infection. For example, washing your hands is known to reduce the chance of getting many contagious viral illnesses such as the common cold.

Is there anything I can do to prolong a remission?

There are medical treatments that may help to prolong remission for some people. For example, Betaseron®, Avonex®, and Copaxone® have been shown to reduce the frequency and severity of attacks in some individuals with relapsing-remitting MS. Although doctors frequently use **corticosteroids** to treat MS flare-ups, there is no proof that these medications prevent exacerbations. Once an exacerbation has begun, however, corticosteroids seem to make it resolve more quickly than if no treatment were given.

How will my MS affect me in the future? Will I end up in a wheelchair or bedridden?

It is not possible for the physician to predict with complete accuracy what the future holds for any particular person with MS because it is such an unpredictable disease. However, many physicians will hazard a guess based on such factors as the frequency of attacks and the types of symptoms that the person has experienced. Individuals who have frequent attacks, especially during the first few years of illness, seem to do less well than those who have infrequent attacks. People whose attacks last for a long time, especially if these attacks are characterized by weakness or incoordination, tend to do less well than those who have brief attacks consisting primarily of numbness or visual loss. Those individuals who have prominent weakness or incoordination that does not go away with time tend to have a worse prognosis.

Many physicians use the "five year rule." According to this rule, how a patient is doing after the first five years of symptoms will predict, with some degree of accuracy, how he or she will fare in the next ten years or so. This means that if someone has had mild MS symptoms during the first five years of illness, the chances are good that the condition will remain mild for the next ten years. If, on the other hand, problems have been more serious, then more severe problems are also likely with time. It must be emphasized, however, that even people who have been well for many years sometimes develop progressive disease. Unfortunately, the converse is not true. Once a person has developed progressive disease, the disease is not expected to change to a milder form, although he or she may have long periods of relative stability.

Can a person die from MS?

Like everyone else, most people with MS die from "natural causes" that include heart attacks, strokes, or cancer. Death caused directly by the plaques of MS is highly unusual. Sometimes a plaque occurs in the part of the brain that regulates breathing and consciousness, in which case death could result if adequate medical care is not provided. In very rare instances, large areas of demyelination could cause swelling of the brain that puts pressure on the life supporting systems, ultimately causing respiratory failure and death.

People sometimes die because of complications of their disease. These complications include choking because of swallowing difficulties, serious kidney or blood infections, or pneumonia. Because most physicians who care for people with MS are aware of these potential complications, they are able to provide the kind of preventive health care that minimizes the risk of their occurrence. The relatively recent availability of a wide range of antibiotic medications has also greatly reduced the numbers of deaths from infection.

Another notable cause of death in MS is suicide. Although the rate of suicide in MS is somewhat higher than the rate in the general population, we still do not have a clear understanding of why this is so. These suicides may be the result of severe depression, the outcome of a person's decision to terminate life in the face of severe and incapacitating disability, or the result of some other factor(s) of which we are still unaware (see Chapter 11 for a more complete discussion of emotional issues in MS).

I know a family in which the mother and son both have MS. No one else in my family has MS. Is it hereditary?

Although MS is not inherited, we pass on to our children the genes that determine all of their characteristics, including the way their immune systems behave. It seems that a certain genetic pattern may make a person more likely to get MS than if those genetic characteristics were not present.

The best way to study how genes influence the likelihood of getting disease is to study twins. Identical twins have the same genetic makeup, whereas nonidentical (fraternal) twins have different genes and are similar to other non-twin siblings. If one identical twin has MS, the chance of the second twin having MS is about 30 percent. For fraternal twins, the chance is 2 percent, the same as for any non-twin siblings. If MS was inherited in the same simple and direct way as eye color, the chance of identical twins both having MS would be 100 percent. The twin studies support the idea that MS is the result of some immune-mediated attack against myelin; is triggered by some factor in the environment; and occurs in those individuals with some genetic predisposition for producing this particular immune response.

What does this mean for a person with MS who is concerned about having children? It means that the probability that one of the children will get MS is fifteen to twenty times greater than it is for people in the general population. While this certainly represents an increased risk, it is important to keep in mind that the risk to these children is still only 3–5 percent. Most MS physicians today will encourage prospective parents with MS to proceed with their family plans based on their feelings about parenting and children, and their personal assessment of their ability to raise their children in a loving and secure environment, rather than on this low risk (see Chapter 13).

Am I susceptible to other autoimmune diseases because I have MS?

There are no generally accepted associations between other autoimmune disorders and MS. There is not, for example, an increased chance of having psoriasis or rheumatoid arthritis because one has MS.

What type of physician should I see for help with my MS? What are the differences between going to an MS center and seeing a private practice neurologist?

You should get treatment from a doctor with whom you feel comfortable and who gives you sound advice. Of course, it is not always possible for someone to know when advice is sound or not. Look for a physician who listens carefully to your complaints and offers suggestions on how to remedy them. A good physician will explain what is known about your symptoms and what options are available to control them. A physician who merely answers all your questions with "That's caused by MS and there's nothing that can be done . . . go home and learn to live with it" may not be giving you the best service. Your physician should be aware of what treatments are available, not only to manage the symptoms of the disease, but also to try to modify the progression of the illness.

Generally, ***neurologists*** are best equipped to answer your questions and give you the guidance you need. Obviously, physicians who see many people with MS and who work at MS centers may be the best choice, not only because they have a broad base of experience but also because they work within a multidisciplinary team of professionals (including, for example, nurses, physical therapists, occupational therapists, psychologists, social workers) who are knowledgeable about specialized aspects of MS care. The variable and complex symptoms of MS have the potential to affect many different aspects of a person's physical, emotional, and social functioning. The members of a multidisciplinary MS team have the expertise to diagnose and treat the varied problems potentially associated with the disease. Additionally, the team approach ensures that a person's care is coordinated rather than spread out among several specialists who are working independently without communicating with one another.

What is a physiatrist?

A *physiatrist* is a physician whose speciality is rehabilitation medicine. Although these physicians prescribe medication, their primary emphasis is on physical treatments (e.g., *orthotics*, mobility aids, and exercise) designed to ease or improve important functions such as walking. While some physiatrists treat MS patients for the full range of symptoms, others see MS patients who are referred to them specifically for rehabilitation purposes.

The neurologist in my managed care program does not specialize in MS. How will I know if I am getting appropriate or up-to-date medical care?

It is not always easy to tell if you are getting the most up-to-date treatment. However, there are several ways that you can educate yourself to find out. The National Multiple Sclerosis Society publishes pamphlets and brochures explaining many symptoms of MS, how these symptoms can be managed, and what can be done to control the disease. Most local chapters sponsor open lecture and discussion meetings throughout the year as well as support groups. Support groups may be particularly helpful because you can listen to what other people with MS have to say about their experiences. If you have a computer and modem, there are several Internet forums that you can access to raise questions and discuss topics of interest with other individuals who have MS.

If you learn about a treatment, medication, or management strategy that you think might be beneficial for you, ask your doctor about it and see what kind of response you get. If you always seem to know more than your doctor, it may be time to consider a change.

How often do I need to get an MRI done?

You may never need an MRI. If your history and physical examination confirm the diagnosis of MS, no additional testing is needed. However, most physicians recommend MRI of the brain at the time of diagnosis to help confirm that the problem is indeed MS rather than some other condition. Since MRI does not reliably predict the course of the disease, there really is no reason why the test should be regularly repeated. However, it might be useful to repeat the test if there is some concern about whether or not the disease is progressing, and if a particular treatment is being considered because of this possibility. The test is best repeated with the same MRI machine used on the first study so that reasonable comparisons can be made.

How do allergies affect MS?

Allergies, such as those to food, animal dander, or pollen, do not cause MS nor do they lead to MS attacks. However, it is possible that an allergic reaction could trigger a pseudo-exacerbation. Unfortunately, some unscrupulous people have deliberately popularized the notion that allergies are the cause of MS so that they can recommend useless and expensive treatment to "desensitize" the person with MS.

Does owning a pet cause MS?

Some years ago, it was suggested that the cause of MS was an infection carried by dogs, possibly canine distemper virus. A report suggested that owning a small dog was associated with a greater risk of getting MS. A national study was undertaken, which showed this was definitely not the case. However, ideas such as this one often seem to linger even though they have been disproved.

What is the EDSS?

Neurologists who see many people with MS need some basis of comparison so that they can communicate findings and conclusions about them in an effective and consistent way. Although the neurologic examination gives a great deal of useful information, it takes a long time to describe the different parts of the examination.

The Expanded Disability Status Scale (EDSS), which is part of the *Minimal Record of Disability*, summarizes the neurologic examination and provides a measure of overall disability—at least as it relates to the ability to walk. It is a 20-point scale, ranging from 0 ("normal examination") to 10 ("death due to MS"). A person with a score of 4.5 can walk three blocks without stopping; a score of 6.0 means that a cane or a leg brace is needed to walk one block; a score over 7.5 indicates that a person cannot take more than a few steps even with crutches or help from another person. The EDSS is used for many reasons, including deciding future medical treatment, establishing rehabilitation goals, and choosing subjects for participation in clinical trials. The major drawback of the scale is that its emphasis on gait impairment ignores disability that results from other impairments such as upper limb problems or memory loss. However, no other scale for MS is as widely used as this one.

Symptom Management

If there is no cure for MS, why do I need to bother seeing a doctor at all?

A close look at medical practice today reveals that relatively few diseases can actually be cured. Most must be treated on an ongoing basis to allow the individuals who have them to function at their best—comfortably and productively. This is particularly true of MS, which can be so varied and unpredictable in its symptoms and associated problems. Periodic medical follow-up will enable you to manage the symptoms you have in order to increase your mobility, enhance day-to-day functioning, improve your comfort and, most importantly, help you to avoid needless complications. Additionally, these visits with your physician will ensure that you have up-to-date, accurate information about available medications and treatments so that you can be an active participant in the management of your MS. You will also be able to learn about upcoming *clinical trials* in which you might be eligible to participate (see Chapter 3 for further discussion of clinical trials).

How often do I need to be seen by the doctor?

How frequently you should be seen and how long a visit should take will be determined by the types of problems you are experiencing. A person with relatively "benign" MS who has very few symptoms can probably do well with just a thorough yearly visit. The person who has more complicated symptoms that require ongoing medical management and a rehabilitative regimen will need more frequent visits. Because the symptoms of MS can come and go over time, you may find that you need to see your physician more frequently at some times than at others. Of greatest importance is that your questions be answered and that a workable treatment and management strategy be understood and agreed upon by you and your physician.

Why do some symptoms come and go while others seem to stay for a long time?

Symptoms of MS occur because of inflammation within the brain and spinal cord. Initially, the inflammation results in swelling (edema), which can cause symptoms. The symptoms start to go away as the swelling gradually subsides. Sometimes this inflammation is severe enough to cause demyelination. Once the myelin has been destroyed, the symptoms tend to remain.

To me, every new symptom feels like an emergency. How do I know when it's important to call the doctor?

A disease such as MS, with its varied symptom picture and unpredictability, tends to make a person very aware of day-to-day changes in the way his or her body feels. Each new symptom or sensation feels strange and perhaps somewhat frightening. In general, if you are experiencing a symptom that is puzzling or bothersome, a telephone call to your doctor is appropriate. As you become more familiar with your MS and the patterns your symptoms tend to follow, you may find that you are comfortable waiting a few days to see if the problem goes away before making the call. Keep track of the changes so that when you do call your physician you are able to describe how and when the problem started. Keep in mind that very few MS-related symptoms are medical emergencies and that most can be handled safely and effectively during normal working hours.

My symptoms are so varied and unpredictable that it's hard for me to know which are caused by MS and which might be due to some other medical problem. How do I know which doctor to call for a new problem or symptom?

The symptoms of MS can be quite varied, appearing in many different parts of your body. It is important for you to be educated about MS and the types of symptoms it tends to cause so that you can make reasonable judgments about what is MS-related and what is not. In general, any symptom that seems to be neurologic and is not otherwise easily explained by some other common illness should be reported to your doctor. Symptoms that are not common in MS, such as chest pain, shortness of breath, stomach pain, and so on, should be discussed with your family physician. Since the neurologist functions as the principal physician for some people with MS, he or she will make an appropriate referral if the problem you are having is unrelated to your MS.

What causes the stiffness in my arms and legs and what is the best treatment for this problem?

Muscle stiffness associated with MS is "spasticity"—an increase in *muscle tone* that can interfere with normal movement of the affected limb even though the strength of that limb might be normal. This increased muscle tone is caused by a dysregulation of nerve impulses in the spinal cord, resulting in too much stimulation in some muscles and too little in others. Spasticity tends to occur most frequently in postural muscles (those that enable us to stand upright), including muscles in the calf, thigh, groin, buttock, and occasionally the back. Spasticity can also occur in the arms. Very mild spasticity can sometimes be managed with appropriate stretching and range of motion exercises (see Chapter 5).

If exercises alone are too uncomfortable or do not provide adequate relief and mobility, antispasticity medications may be used. A variety of medications are available for this purpose, including baclofen (Lioresal®), clonazepam (Klonopin®), diazepam (Valium®), and dantrolene (Dantrium®). Your physician will select the particular medication best suited for your needs; baclofen is the drug most commonly used (see Appendix B). The correct dosage of baclofen will differ from one individual to another. The goal of treatment is to find the dosage level that provides adequate muscle relaxation without producing excessive fatigue or weakness. An additional drug for the treatment of spasticity, tizanidine HCl (Zanaflex®), is expected to be available by prescription in the United States by the end of 1996. The drug has been available in Canada for some time. Tizanidine has been shown to relieve spasticity without causing muscle weakness.

Occasionally, people with MS-related spasticity develop *flexor* or *extensor spasms*. These spasms, which typically last two or three seconds, are disinhibited (hyperactive) spinal reflexes that can occur in response to the slightest of noxious stimuli (e.g., the rubbing of bed sheets against the foot during sleep). Flexor spasms cause both legs to pull upward into a clenched position, while extensor spasms cause the legs to straighten into the stiff, extended position. These uncontrolled spasms can be sufficiently intense and sudden to propel the person out of his or her chair. Baclofen (Lioresal®), diazepam (Valium®), and clonazepam (Klonopin®) are the medications of choice for the management of this problem (see Appendix B).

In the case of severe spasticity that cannot be managed comfortably or effectively with oral baclofen (tablets), a pump can be surgically implanted in the abdomen to automatically administer low doses of liquid baclofen directly into the spinal cord. The pump's usefulness stems from its ability to reduce spasticity with a much lower dose of medication, thus eliminating the side effects that can occur with higher doses of baclofen.

Severe spasticity that does not respond to medications may also be treated with a procedure called a **nerve block** or **motor point block**. An injection of phenol into the affected nerve chemically damages the nerve and interferes with its function for up to three months. This temporary destruction of the nerve prevents the affected muscle from contracting and allows the person to feel more comfortable. The nerve block may also improve gait and mobility. The injections of phenol are usually given by a physiatrist or anesthesiologist using an **EMG** to pinpoint the location of the nerve.

Botox, made from botulinum toxin, may also be used to block a nerve's function, although it accomplishes this via a different mechanism from that of phenol. The botox is injected into the affected muscle at the point where the nerve enters the muscle and prevents the nerve from exciting the muscle to contract. Botox is somewhat easier and safer to use than phenol and can be administered by the neurologist, but may require more repetitive injections to achieve sustained blockage of the nerve.

On rare occasions, surgery is required to cut one particular nerve to the affected muscle without endangering other nerves that are in close proximity. Fortunately, the recent availability of the baclofen pump has greatly reduced the need for nerve blocks or surgery to reduce spasticity.

My doctor has told me that I may be a suitable candidate for a baclofen pump. How does the pump work and how will I know if it is the right treatment for me?

Your physician may recommend the baclofen pump if your spasticity is not adequately controlled by oral baclofen or if you are experiencing intolerable side effects such as drowsiness, dizziness, weakness, or nausea. The pump is a surgically implanted device that is programmed to deliver the correct dose of liquid baclofen (Lioresal® Intrathecal), on a continuous basis, directly into the area surrounding your spinal cord (***intrathecal space***). Because the drug is administered in this way, it is possible to obtain positive results using a lower dose with fewer side effects.

Before implanting the baclofen pump, your doctor will inject a test dose of liquid baclofen into the intrathecal space of your lower back to see how you respond to the medication. The test dose is given in the hospital so that you can be observed for changes in rigidity and spasms and for any side effects you might experience. If the test dose proves to be comfortable and effective, you and your physician will decide whether to proceed with the baclofen pump.

In order to receive liquid baclofen on a regular, long-term basis, it is necessary to implant a pump and catheter into your body. The pump (a round metal disk weighing about six ounces) is placed under the skin of the abdomen during a surgical procedure. A catheter connects the pump to the intrathecal space in your back. The pump is refilled at periodic intervals by injecting the liquid through your skin into the pump's drug reservoir.

The pump has been shown to be a safe and effective treatment for the management of severe spasticity. Its potential to reduce the discomforts and possible complications associated with spasticity makes it a valuable treatment option for you and your physician to consider.

What are contractures and how are they treated?

Contractures are an abnormal, sometimes permanent flexion (bending) of a joint that can occur if significant spasticity goes untreated. When spasticity prevents a limb from moving freely about the joint, some of the muscles and tendons around the joint become shortened. This shortening further constricts movement of the joint. Without treatment, the joint may freeze and become immobilized. Contractures can usually be prevented with a careful regimen of antispasticity medication and physical therapy techniques designed to maintain joint flexibility and mobility.

Severe contractures may require more drastic treatment measures in order to reduce the intractable pain, positioning problems, and possible skin complications that can result. For example, surgery may be performed to sever the affected tendon, thus allowing the contracted limb to be straightened. This irreversible procedure is used only in individuals whose prolonged spasticity has resulted in permanent paralysis of the contracted limbs. By far the best treatment of contractures is to prevent them from occurring in the first place. With the advent of the baclofen pump, this type of unmanageable spasticity should soon become a problem of the past.

At night I experience painful spasms in my legs that make it very hard for me to sleep. Is there anything I can do about this problem?

These painful flexor spasms are involuntary muscle contractions that result from spasticity or increased muscle tone. They seem to occur in response to such stimuli as sheets being rubbed over the skin of the lower limbs. Stretching exercises before bedtime may be helpful, but medication is often necessary. Baclofen (Lioresal®), diazepam (Valium®), and clonazepam (Klonopin®) are the medications most commonly used to treat these spasms. Diazepam and clonazepam are somewhat sedating, making them particularly useful for the management of nighttime spasticity. Both of these drugs can be habit-forming, however, and must therefore be prescribed and used with some caution (see Appendix B). Some people find that the over-the-counter medications threonine and quinine are also helpful with this problem. Be sure to discuss the situation with your physician before beginning any treatment.

My hands and feet often get numb or feel like "pins and needles." Are there any medications for this problem?

"Pins and needles" are one example of sensory symptoms in MS. Sensory symptoms are those that a person can feel but for which the physician cannot see objective evidence during the neurologic exam. Other examples include numbness, tingling, decreased or blurred vision, dizziness, or pain. These symptoms occur because of demyelination in the sensory pathways of the spinal cord or brain. Although they can be quite uncomfortable, sensory symptoms are generally considered relatively benign because they tend to come and go without severely restricting a person's ability to function. Although there is no specific medication for most sensory symptoms, antiseizure medications such as carbamazepine (Tegretol®) and valproic acid (Depakene®) may decrease their intensity. A tricyclic antidepressant medication such as amitriptyline (Elavil®) can provide some relief, particularly if the symptoms are painful (see Appendix B). In the meantime, remember that these symptoms tend to go away on their own and seldom signal significant impairment.

What causes tremor in MS and are there any treatments available for it?

Tremor is an involuntary, relatively rhythmic movement of the arms, legs, or head. While several types of tremor can occur in MS, the most common one results from demyelination in the pathways leading to or from the balance center of the brain (***cerebellum***). Damage in this area of the brain causes an ***intention tremor***, a relatively slow, oscillating (back and forth) movement of a limb engaged in purposeful movement. For example, a person with an intention tremor finds it difficult to perform the finger-to-nose test on the neurologic exam because the intentional movement of the finger toward the nose triggers a tremor in that arm.

Tremor is one of the most difficult symptoms to treat and can be among the most disabling. There are balance and coordination exercises (see Chapter 5) that can help a person to develop compensatory techniques, but the results are far from satisfying. Some people have greater success with relaxation exercises, which seem to lessen the tenseness that sometimes aggravates the tremor. Weights can be placed on the affected limbs to lessen the oscillations somewhat, or weighted utensils can be used for such activities as eating, dressing, and writing (see Chapter 6).

No medication has been developed specifically for tremor. However, some medications designed to treat other conditions have secondary antitremor properties. These include the beta-blocker propranolol (Inderal®), clonazepam (Klonopin®), primidone (Mysoline®), isoniazid (Laniazid®—United States; Isotamine®—Canada), and glutethemide (United States only). While these medications are not usually effective with MS-related tremor, it is impossible to predict who will respond to one or another of the medications and who will not. Therefore, it is worthwhile to try them singly or in combination in an effort to control the tremor.

I take a lot of different medications now—some prescribed by my neurologist and others by my family doctor. Do I need to be concerned about the interactions of all of these drugs?

Everyone needs to be concerned about the actions and interactions of the drugs they take. Each physician involved in your care must know all of the prescription and nonprescription medications that you are taking. Keep a list of all your medications and ask that a copy of that list be included in your medical chart. When the doctor prescribes a new medication for you, feel free to ask about its possible interactions with the others you are taking. Usually there is not an interaction problem, but it makes good sense to ask.

Refer to the Medication Information Sheets in Appendix B for information about the drugs commonly used in MS. You can also ask your pharmacist to give you the "package insert" that comes with each medication, read about your medication(s) in one of the standard drug references, or get information from one of the on-line computer services.

Is there any treatment for my balance problems? People who see me on the street think I'm drunk.

Balance problems in MS, like tremor, are usually caused by damage in the cerebellum. Balance and coordination exercises may offer some compensatory strategies, but there is no effective treatment at this time for damage to the cerebellum. Assistive devices such as a cane, crutches, or a walker will offer you varying degrees of stability and, just as importantly, tell the world that you are not drunk (see Chapter 5). Many people initially take the emotional plunge of using an assistive device for this reason; they would rather be identified as having a physical impairment than as having had too much to drink.

I have always gotten a lot of exercise and been in pretty good shape. Now I feel weakness in my legs in spite of the exercise. What is causing this weakness and is there anything I can do about it?

Weakness in MS is caused by a faulty transmission of impulses from the brain through the spinal cord to the muscle. The problem is not due to a bad or weak muscle. Weakness from poor nerve transmission will not be altered by exercise and, in fact, can be worsened by aggressive exercise that produces fatigue. At the same time, however, inadequate use of the muscle will produce its own kind of weakness, known as "disuse weakness." Therefore, an effective exercise program for weakness must include exercises to strengthen the muscles that have adequate nerve conduction as well as useful movements for the weakened muscles that lack adequate nerve conduction (see Chapter 5). There is currently no medication to treat weakness in MS; researchers are working to identify medications that might improve nerve conduction in demyelinated nerves.

Fatigue has become my most disabling symptom. Sometimes I even feel it right after I wake up in the morning. Is there any treatment for this problem?

Fatigue is one of the most common symptoms in MS. There are four distinct types of fatigue, each with its own management strategy.

◇ Normal fatigue in people with MS is managed with rest just as it is in people without MS.

◇ Exercise-induced fatigue can occur in an arm or leg following repetitive movements. After walking some distance, for example, you might find that one leg begins to drag and feel very weak. This type of fatigue is caused by a temporary blocking in the nerve and is best managed by stopping the walk long enough to allow nerve conduction to restart.

◇ Depression can also cause a feeling of fatigue and is best managed with an accurate diagnosis and a regimen of psychotherapy and, if needed, antidepressant medication.

◇ The most common fatigue seen in MS is also referred to as "lassitude." This fatigue is described as an overwhelming tiredness that seems unrelated to activity level or even time of day. While most people report this type of fatigue in the late afternoon or early evening, it can also occur in the morning. While some people find that a brief rest alleviates this fatigue to some degree, others report that it is unaffected by sleep or relaxation.

Lassitude of this type often responds to neurochemical medications (see Appendix B) such as amantadine (Symmetrel®), pemoline (Cylert®), and fluoxetine (Prozac®).

My MS seems to get worse every summer. I feel so weak and tired when it's that I can hardly move. Why does this happen and is there any solution to this problem?

For many people, heat temporarily worsens MS symptoms. This can occur with as little as a one-degree elevation in core body temperature. There is no evidence that heat actually makes the disease worse. Instead, heat alters nerve conduction (the passage of nerve impulses) and causes a feeling of weakness in the limbs. This same phenomenon often occurs when a person becomes overheated following strenuous exercise or develops an elevated body temperature due to a viral or bacterial infection. In fact, the "hot bath test" for MS was used before current imaging techniques made it unnecessary to capitalize on this heat sensitivity; a person suspected of having the disease was put in a bathtub of hot water to see if MS symptoms could be elicited. Thus, it is not surprising that the heat and humidity of summer make your symptoms feel worse.

Keeping your body cool helps to alleviate this problem and is certainly the best management strategy for the heat of summer and of a fever. Avoid unnecessary heat—hot showers and sunbathing, for example, are not good activities for someone with MS—and make use of air conditioning, cold drinks, or a body cooling system like the ones designed for laborers in heat-intensive occupations (see Appendix D). Body cooling systems come in two basic types and seem to be most helpful for those individuals who are sensitive to the heat rather than the humidity of summer. The simplest cooling system is a vest designed to hold frozen gel packs in front and back compartments (e.g., Steele Vest®). A person can wear this type of vest for driving in a warm car, engaging in outdoor activities, cooking over a hot stove, or just staying cool in a warm house. A somewhat more complex cooling system electronically pumps a cold liquid through a specially designed garment (e.g., the cooling suits made by Life Enhancement Technologies, LLC). Research is currently underway to determine the effectiveness of these types of cooling apparatuses for people with MS.

What types of pain can be caused by MS? What are the best treatments for the different types of pain?

Pain in MS can take different forms. The most common is called *dysesthesia*, referring to a burning sensation caused by abnormalities in the sensory pathways in the brain and spinal cord. Demyelination in the sensory pathways can result in pain, numbness, tingling, itching, or other abnormal sensations. Sometimes the pain is quite severe or sharp, most commonly in the trigeminal nerve of the face. *Trigeminal neuralgia* is often described as a stabbing or shock-like pain along the side of the face. These types of pain do not respond to ordinary pain medications. The preferred treatment is to try to alter the faulty nerve conduction with other types of medications, including antiepileptic drugs such as carbamazepine (Tegretol®), phenytoin (Dilantin®), and valproic acid (Depakene®). Antidepressant medications such as amitriptyline (Elavil®) may also relieve the pain (see Appendix B). Some people find that acupuncture and meditation are effective for dysesthesias.

Unusually severe cases of trigeminal neuralgia that do not respond to any of these interventions can also be treated with an outpatient surgical procedure called a *percutaneous rhizotomy*. Under local anesthesia, the surgeon makes a tiny incision in the side of the face and blocks the function of the trigeminal nerve using one of several possible techniques, including laser surgery, cryosurgery (freezing), and cauterization.

A second, relatively common type of pain or discomfort in MS results from the symptom of spasticity—increased muscle tone and muscle spasms can be quite uncomfortable. Antispasticity medications are the most effective treatment for this type of discomfort.

In addition to these more common types of pain in MS, secondary orthopedic pain can result from changes in a person's posture or gait. If a person begins to walk or stand differently because of weakness or spasticity, for example, these changes can in turn cause pain in the knees, back, or hips. It is important to identify the causes of this type of secondary pain so that an appropriate treatment regimen of physical therapy, gait training, seating assessment (for someone in a wheelchair), exercise, and pain relief can be implemented.

My eye doctor says he can't give me glasses to correct the vision problems caused by MS. What is causing my visual problems and why can't they be corrected?

Visual symptoms are quite common in MS. They can result from damage to the optic nerve or from an incoordination in the eye muscles, neither of which is correctable with eyeglasses. The optic nerve connects the eye to the brain. Inflammation or demyelination in the optic nerve causes *optic neuritis*, which is experienced as a temporary loss or disturbance in vision and possibly pain behind the affected eye. Typically, vision returns partially or fully within a few weeks. While it is quite rare for a person with MS to become totally blind, it is not at all uncommon for an individual to have recurrent episodes of optic neuritis over the course of the disease, usually in one eye at a time. Damage to the optic nerve can result in a blurring of vision, which may or may not totally resolve over time. This blurring of vision is not correctable with eyeglasses because it is the result of nerve damage rather than changes in the shape of the eye. Color vision requires a great many nerve fibers from the eye for accurate transmission and is particularly susceptible to changes from demyelination.

Although episodes of optic neuritis typically resolve spontaneously, acute loss of vision used to be treated fairly routinely with low doses of oral cortisone in order to end the episode more quickly. Recent research has demonstrated that high-dose corticosteroids such as methylprednisolone (Solu-Medrol®) or dexamethasone (Decadron®) are more effective in the treatment of optic neuritis. If visual loss is relatively mild and manageable, the best alternative is probably to wait for the episode to remit on its own. However, a course of high-dose corticosteroids may be prescribed if everyday functioning becomes too impaired.

Optic neuritis can cause a large, noticeable "blind spot" in the center of the visual field, and the person experiences a visual image with a dark, blank area in the middle. This is called a central *scotoma* and is not correctable with either eyeglasses or medication, although steroids may be helpful in the early, acute phase.

Diplopia (double vision), the experience of seeing two of everything, is caused by weakening or incoordination of eye muscles. This symptom is typically treated with a short course of steroids. Patching one eye while trying to drive or read will stop the double image; however, permanent patching of the eye will slow the brain's remarkable ability to accommodate to the weakness and produce a single image in spite of the weakened muscles.

Upon examination, the physician may detect a rhythmic jerkiness or bounce in one or both eyes. This relatively common visual finding in MS is **nystagmus**. Nystagmus does not always cause symptoms of which the person is aware. In the event that it does become troublesome, clonazepam (Klonopin®) is sometimes effective in reducing this annoying but painless problem.

I have developed a lot of problems with my memory and thinking in the last few years. Is there any medication I can take to help with these problems?

Some degree of cognitive change occurs in 50–60 percent of people with MS. Fortunately, the majority of these changes progress quite slowly and are relatively mild. For a complete discussion of cognition in MS, please refer to Chapter 9. The answer to your specific question is that no medication has been found that can treat or manage these changes successfully. You and your doctor should be alert to any signs of depression, which can sometimes mimic changes in cognition and is far more amenable to treatment. Research is currently being done to determine whether the neurostimulant pemoline (Cylert®) is effective in treating cognitive symptoms.

Sometimes the treatment I get for one symptom makes another problem worse (e.g., my bladder medications make my mouth uncomfortably dry, the antidepressant I took interfered with my sex life, the medication I took for pain made me constipated). How can I learn more about these side effects so that I can make reasonable decisions about what is best for me?

Side effects are very common with certain medications and should be discussed with your physician. The MS health care team is quite knowledgeable about frequently used medications and has a great deal of experience with people's reactions to them. Using the information you give them about your symptoms, as well as feedback about the beneficial and not so beneficial responses you are having to the medications, your health care team can help you maximize the positive treatment effects while minimizing side effects. They will usually be able to reduce any unpleasant side effects to a manageable level with minor adjustments in level and timing of dosages. For additional information about medication side effects, you can refer to the Medication Information Sheets in Appendix B, read the "package insert" available at your pharmacy, or consult a drug reference book or on-line computer service for information about a particular medication that has been prescribed for you (see Appendix D).

I've read that people who aren't very mobile are at greater risk for osteoporosis. I am now in a wheelchair most of the time. How can I prevent osteoporosis and what is the treatment for it?

Osteoporosis, defined as a gradual loss of calcium from the bones, which causes them to be fragile and easily broken, is caused by a combination of factors. Hormones, vitamins, genetic predisposition, and level of physical activity all play a role. Anyone who has decreased mobility, particularly a loss of weight-bearing activity (as would be true of a person using a wheelchair most of the time) needs to be concerned about osteoporosis. Additionally, excessive or prolonged use of steroids can lead to osteoporosis. Talk to your physician about your risk for osteoporosis and the advisability of a baseline evaluation to determine the health of your bones. You may be referred to a physical therapist for a regimen of weight-bearing exercises to enhance bone strength. Vitamin D, calcium, and appropriate hormone treatment may also be recommended to you. Do not begin any exercise program or medication regimen without first consulting your physician.

◇ Refer to Chapter 3 for questions and answers about clinical trials, new treatments, and alternative treatments.
◇ Refer to Chapter 5 for questions and answers about exercise.
◇ Refer to Chapter 7 for questions and answers about swallowing.

◇ Refer to Chapter 9 for questions and answers about cognitive symptoms.

◇ Refer to Chapter 11 for questions and answers about emotional changes.

◇ Refer to Chapter 12 for questions and answers about sexual problems.

◇ Refer to Appendix B for a listing of commonly used medications in MS—their indications, instructions for their use, precautions, and side effects.

Recommended Readings

Lechtenberg R. *Multiple Sclerosis Fact Book (2nd edition)*. Philadelphia: F.A. Davis, 1995.

Schapiro R. *Symptom Management in Multiple Sclerosis (2nd edition)*. New York: Demos Vermande, 1994.

Scheinberg LC, Holland NJ (eds.). *Multiple Sclerosis: A Guide for Patients and Their Families (2nd edition)*. New York: Raven Press, 1987.

Selected booklets available from the National Multiple Sclerosis Society (Customer Service: 212-986-3240; Information: 800-344-4867)

◇ *Living with MS*—Debra Frankel, M.S., O.T.R., with Hettie Jones

◇ *What Everyone Should Know About Multiple Sclerosis*

◇ *Things I Wish Someone Had Told Me: Practical Thoughts for People Newly Diagnosed with Multiple Sclerosis*—Suzanne Rogers

◇ *The Rehab Outlook*—Lisa J. Bain and Randall Schapiro, M.D.

Reprint available from the Canadian Multiple Sclerosis Society (416-922-6065)

◇ *Coping with Fatigue in MS Takes Understanding and Planning*—Alexander Burnfield, M.D., M.R.C. Psych.

Facts and Issues (reprints of articles from the National Multiple
  Sclerosis Society magazine, *Inside MS*).

   ◇ *Diagnosis: The Whole Story*
   ◇ *Genes and MS Susceptibility*
   ◇ *Digging for Clues to Fatigue*
   ◇ *Pain: A Certain Four-Letter Word*

3

Treatment Issues

Aaron E. Miller, M.D.
Robert M. Herndon, M.D.

Any discussion of treatments for multiple sclerosis must start with a careful look at what we mean by the word "treatment." To most people, being "treated" for an illness means that they report their symptoms to a physician, are prescribed a medication (an antibiotic, for example), the symptoms go away, and they are cured. In another familiar scenario, the person gets the flu or some other viral infection, goes to the doctor or the pharmacy for some medications to relieve discomfort, and waits patiently for the virus to run its course and go away. In the case of physical injury, the treatment may be even more direct and clear-cut. The person who temporarily cannot walk because of a broken leg is treated for the injury, and walking ability is restored. Of course, the best treatment of all is a vaccination to prevent the disease in the first place.

At the present time, none of these familiar notions of treatment applies in MS. We are unable to prevent the illness from occurring, we do not know how to cure it, we have not found a way to restore damaged *myelin* or lost functions, and the disease is a chronic one that refuses to run its course and go away. While efforts continue in the scientific community to find a cure for MS and restore damaged myelin, the primary

focus of day-to-day medical care in MS is symptom management (see Chapter 2) and efforts to stabilize the disease course.
These efforts to stabilize the disease are the main focus of this
chapter.

In order to understand why efforts to find an effective treatment for MS have been so frustrating, it is important to review
some of the characteristics of the disease. Although we believe
MS to be an *autoimmune disease* that is triggered in genetically susceptible individuals by some viral agent in the environment (see Chapter 2), we do not yet have any definitive answers.
Not knowing the cause of a disease makes looking for its cure
significantly more challenging. Additionally, the disease tends
to progress quite slowly, with a symptom picture that is highly
variable from one person to the next. These characteristics make
it difficult for researchers to know how to evaluate the efficacy
of any particular treatment. If every person with MS looks somewhat different from every other, what symptom or other aspect
of the disease should be looked at to determine if a treatment is
working?

Furthermore, although a review of treatments used in MS over
the fifteen-year period from 1935 to 1950 indicated that 66 percent of the patients improved, none of these interventions has
been shown *over time* to be any more effective than no treatment
at all. Other studies have demonstrated that 70 percent of individuals treated for a recent worsening of their disease will
improve with a *placebo* medication. Thus, treatment of a recent
exacerbation in MS can only be considered effective if it leads
to long-lasting improvement in significantly more than 70 percent of people who are given it.

This brings us back to the question of measuring the outcomes
obtained when evaluating experimental treatments. Recent
research efforts have targeted the number of exacerbations,
length of exacerbations, length of time between exacerbations,
severity of exacerbations, and the total area or volume of lesions
shown on *MRI* as reasonable indicators of treatment impact. In
1981, at the first international conference on therapeutic trials in
MS, it was clear that there had been only one successful treatment trial in MS that would meet current scientific standards. In
that trial of *adrenocorticotropic hormone (ACTH)*, it was
demonstrated that ACTH could shorten attacks even though it
had no effect on the ultimate degree of recovery.

Since that time, there have been several high quality drug trials in MS. There are currently more drug trials in progress than at any time in the history of the disease. These include trials for exacerbating-remitting and secondary progressive MS, and are ongoing in both North America and Europe. Among these are trials of cladribine, *interferon* alpha, roquinimex, oral myelin, mitoxantrone, rolipram, transforming growth factor beta (TGF-beta), and soluble tumor necrosis factor receptor, among others. *As the results from these trials become available, the information will be incorporated into periodic chapter updates available from the publisher.*

This is an exciting time for both individuals with MS and their health care providers. Interferon beta-1b (Betaseron®), the first drug approved by the ***Food and Drug Administration (FDA)*** for treatment of MS, became available in the Fall of 1993. Despite some drawbacks, it has had a noticeable impact on the frequency and severity of attacks in many of those receiving the drug. In 1994, reports were made of the successful trial of methotrexate for progressive MS and successful trials of two new drugs, interferon beta-1a (Avonex®) and copolymer 1 (Copaxone®) for exacerbating-remitting MS. Interferon beta-1a was approved in May 1996, with approval of copolymer 1 expected later in the year. While these offer neither a cure nor any restoration of lost function, they do represent a significant advance in our efforts to stabilize the disease process.

What makes it so difficult for scientists to find a cure for multiple sclerosis?

Physicians and researchers have found it difficult to find a cure for MS because the underlying cause of the illness is not known. Current thinking is that some "environmental" trigger (a viral infection, for example) initiates a process in which the individual's *immune system* inappropriately attacks the myelin in his or her own *central nervous system*. This process probably occurs more readily in people born with a genetic predisposition to the disease. Since we do not know the exact triggers for the initial and ongoing immunological assault, it is difficult to devise specific treatments to prevent it.

The ultimate result of the immunological process is damage to the myelin. Once this damage has proceeded sufficiently, nerve fibers no longer conduct impulses properly and persistent neurologic dysfunction occurs. At present, we do not know how to help the individual repair or restore myelin and therefore we are unable to reverse the neurologic symptoms, i.e., cure the disease. One hopeful sign is that we have recently come to realize that mammals do have some potential capacity for spontaneous repair of central nervous system myelin.

When I have an exacerbation my doctor prescribes intravenous steroids (Solu-Medrol®). Why are steroids prescribed and what is the difference between steroids taken orally and those taken intravenously?

Steroids are a group of chemicals, some of which are naturally occurring hormones. They have many important hormonal functions but they have various additional effects when administered as medications (usually in synthetic preparations). Their utility in MS stems from their ability to close the damaged ***blood-brain barrier*** and decrease inflammation in the central nervous system.

Under normal circumstances, many potentially damaging substances are prevented by the blood-brain barrier from passing out of the blood stream into the brain and spinal cord. During attacks of MS, this barrier can break down and begin to leak, allowing damaging chemicals and cells to pass into the central nervous system. Inflammation then ensues, resulting in both ***acute*** neurologic injury—sometimes with accompanying symptoms—and ***chronic*** damage to myelin. Steroids appear to decrease this inflammation.

Most neurologists caring for MS patients believe that steroids work best when given directly into the veins in high doses. We do not know whether equivalently high doses given orally would be equally effective. In the past, it has been more common to prescribe lower doses of steroids orally. However, recent studies in patients with ***optic neuritis***, a condition that is often the first sign of MS, suggest that this is less effective than high doses given intravenously.

Do steroids have any long-term benefits? I feel much better while I'm taking steroids but my doctor says they should not be used frequently or for very long periods. Why not?

At present, it is unclear whether steroids convey any long-term benefits to people with MS. There is some suggestion that short courses of high-dose intravenous steroids may have a protracted benefit in delaying further disease activity. However, the chronic use of steroids is fraught with many potentially dangerous side effects and is currently thought to be unwise in the treatment of MS. Many people feel better while taking steroids, in part because these drugs have a mood-elevating effect. However, their long-term use can be associated with such side effects as hypertension, diabetes, bone loss (***osteoporosis***), cataracts, ulcers, and hip disease. These potential detrimental effects outweigh the possible benefits when steroids are used on an extended basis.

When I take steroids I get very emotional and have intense mood swings. I also feel very down or depressed toward the end of the treatment. Why does this happen and is there anything to do about it?

Short courses of steroids, even in very high doses, are usually well-tolerated. Many people do have some minor mood changes, both highs and lows. Others may have difficulty sleeping. A much smaller group of individuals may have more severe disturbances in mood or behavior. Lithium, a medication often prescribed for people with bipolar disorder (formerly called manic-depressive disorder), is sometimes used to prevent or manage these mood swings. Carbamazepine (Tegretol®) has also been shown to be very effective. On occasion, antidepressant medications may be prescribed, but they are seldom needed because the "blues" associated with a short course of steroids usually resolve spontaneously before the antidepressants would begin to take effect (usually a few weeks).

Once a promising new treatment has been identified, why does it take such a long time for it to be available for patients?

The process of new drug development is unfortunately very slow, particularly for a chronic disease like MS. The typical sequence initially involves animal studies. This is a crucial first step because an experimental model for MS, ***experimental allergic encephalomyelitis***, exists in laboratory rodents (as well as other species). This allows a quick assessment of the possible benefits of a treatment, as well as the preliminary evaluation of its safety. A promising agent then moves into human clinical trials.

Figure 3-1.   Summary table of steps involved in the development of a new drug).

◇ Phase I   Animal studies
◇ Phase II   Preliminary human clinical trials
       ✚ small, unblinded, open label trials (for safety)
       ✚ double-blind pilot trials (for efficacy)
◇ Phase III Multicenter, randomized, double-blind, placebo-controlled trials
◇ Data Analysis
◇ Application for approval of drug by the FDA
◇ Pharmaceutical company brings drug to market

Human clinical trials begin with very small "open label" (unblinded) trials in which the physicians and subjects both know what drug is being taken. These trials are aimed more at demonstrating the safety of a treatment than its benefit. They are typically of much shorter duration than later studies but still take many months to a year or longer because of the variable nature of MS. The open label trials are then followed by relatively small, ***double-blind***, pilot trials designed to give stronger evidence suggesting that a new treatment may be effective as well as safe. "Double-blind" means that neither the subject nor the investigators know which patients are receiving the real medication and which are getting the placebo (an inactive substance). This procedure is followed in order to prevent hopes and expectations on the part of researchers or subjects from affecting the course or evaluation of the treatment.

If the drug still appears promising, testing will move into Phase III, involving large, multicenter, randomized, placebo-controlled, double-blind trials. In this stage of drug development, typically hundreds of subjects are entered into a study in which some are randomly assigned to receive the medication and others to get placebo. Because MS is a chronic disease in which changes occur relatively slowly in most people, these Phase III trials typically last for several years in order to obtain enough information on which to base fair and statistically valid conclusions.

Following the completion of the trial, another six months may be necessary to analyze the data in a large study and to prepare submission of documents to the Food and Drug Administration (FDA), which is ultimately responsible for the approval of new drugs. The FDA then carefully reviews both the data and the methodology of the trial and must be convinced of both the *effectiveness* and *safety* of the treatment before giving its approval. This process typically takes another six to twelve months. Finally, after approval of a drug, the pharmaceutical company typically needs a few more months to get the drug to market.

Thus, the process is extremely long and arduous, as well as very frustrating for people with MS and their families. However, it is a process designed to assure that everyone receives safe treatments and that no one misses out on the opportunity to take other, potentially useful treatments while taking something that is ineffective. The problem with many of the publicly acclaimed "treatments" that receive so much attention in the press (e.g., snake venom and the removal of tooth amalgams) is that they have not been through this process. In other words, they have not been proven to be effective in a clinical trial and can sometimes be quite harmful.

What is the "placebo effect?"

A placebo is a non-drug substance that is designed to look just like the drug that is being evaluated in a research protocol. One of the main reasons that double-blind trials are routinely employed in MS is the **placebo effect**. Investigators repeatedly find that a substantial proportion of patients with a variety of diseases experience some benefit even when they are treated with a placebo. Although this may occur in part through unconscious psychological mechanisms, some studies have also demonstrated the production of certain chemicals in such patients that may contribute to this improvement. Even though the benefits are not usually sustained, this short-lived effect confounds the study of new drugs. Randomized, placebo-controlled, double-blind trials are used in order to determine the advantage (if any) that the new drug shows over placebo effects. Thus, to demonstrate the value of a new treatment, it must be proved to have a benefit *superior* to that offered by a placebo.

It is important to remember that being treated with a placebo is not the same as receiving *no* treatment. Taking the placebo fosters certain expectations for improvement that are not present when no treatment is given. That is why new drugs are always compared with a placebo rather than with no treatment at all. The drug must demonstrate a specific benefit beyond the placebo effect or the improvement that might occur spontaneously with no treatment.

If alternative treatments like bee stings and cobra venom work well for some people, why aren't they more widely prescribed?

Alternative treatments for MS such as bee stings are often touted as helping people with MS. The problem is that these reports are always "anecdotal"; they consist mostly of individual *claims* of success, without any scientific study. It is well-known that MS often undergoes spontaneous improvement or remission. Furthermore, as discussed previously, virtually every study of MS indicates a significant placebo effect, whereby people taking placebo (non-drug substance) do better than they would with no treatment. Therefore, claims of success with any therapy, including alternative treatments, must be regarded with considerable skepticism unless blinded clinical trials are done. Additionally, some of these treatments, such as bee stings, carry potentially severe risks. Specifically, fatal allergic reactions can occur in some individuals receiving bee stings. These comments are not to suggest that there might not be merit to some alternative treatments, but rather to emphasize the importance of proper scientific investigation under controlled and *safe* conditions.

Who designs clinical trials and decides when and where they will take place and who can participate?

Clinical trials may originate from several different sources. Early trials are often initiated by investigators interested in MS, whereas more definitive trials of promising new treatments are generally initiated by pharmaceutical companies interested in marketing a product. Although these companies have physicians and basic scientists in their direct employment, they usually recruit outside investigators to help plan a clinical trial. Then, depending on the size of the study, additional investigators from other MS centers are invited to participate in the trial in order to enter the required number of patients as quickly as possible.

How can I get into a clinical trial?

Various sources of information about clinical trials are available. The best place to start is with your own physician, who will often be able to direct you to a particular trial. The National Multiple Sclerosis Society can also provide information about the sites participating in particular clinical trials. Some of the local chapters of the National Multiple Sclerosis Society publish newsletters that may announce trials in your area. Many of the member centers of the Consortium of Multiple Sclerosis Centers participate in one or more clinical trials. It is important to remember that each trial has a very specific "protocol" that details the types of patients who are eligible to participate. For some trials, the eligibility criteria are quite restrictive; for others, the criteria are more liberal. Your willingness to participate in a clinical trial is greatly appreciated by investigators because successful completion of such studies is the only way that we will definitively identify effective new treatments. Do not be discouraged if you do not meet the entrance criteria for a particular trial. Keep informed—the next one might be right for you.

Why should I participate in a clinical trial if I have a fifty percent chance of getting the placebo instead of the real drug?

There are several reasons to participate in clinical trials.

◇ It has been demonstrated repeatedly in MS trials that even those subjects who receive the placebo usually do better than they would have done without any intervention.

◇ Clinical trials are the best mechanism currently available to identify effective treatments; therefore, your participation ultimately helps investigators answer important questions.

◇ Standard, accepted treatments continue to be allowed under the research protocols of most placebo-controlled trials. For example, acute exacerbations could be treated with steroids in the interferon beta-1b (Betaseron®) and interferon beta-1a (Avonex®) trials.

◇ With Betaseron® and Avonex® currently available, and Copaxone® expected to be available in late 1996, it is likely that we will shift away from placebo-controlled trials to drug comparison trials in which a proposed new drug will be compared with the most effective available drug. Thus, any proposed new drug would have to demonstrate its superiority over those that have already been approved for use. Participants in this type of drug comparison trial would therefore be randomly assigned to either the proposed drug or one that has already been shown to be effective in treating MS.

Why do I have to be able to walk in order to be in a clinical trial?

The entrance criteria for particular trials are very specific. Many of the trials require that subjects be able to walk, sometimes without the use of aids. This requirement is made because it is often more difficult to detect changes in disease activity in individuals whose illness is more advanced, and the inclusion of people with more advanced disease might cause investigators to discard potentially useful treatments because they erroneously failed to detect a benefit. This situation might arise, for example, when neither the group receiving the drug nor the placebo group seemed to progress very much during the course of a trial.

Why were Betaseron® and Avonex® originally tested only on people with relapsing-remitting MS?

Betaseron® and Avonex® were originally tested on people with relapsing-remitting MS because investigators thought those with milder disease would be more likely to show a benefit from the treatment. Also, previous studies had shown that it might be easier to demonstrate an effect by measuring a reduction in attack rate than by showing a reduction in disease progression.

My MS used to be relapsing-remitting. Now that it seems to be secondary progressive, would Betaseron® or Avonex® still be appropriate treatment for me?

Betaseron® and Avonex® have both been approved by the FDA for treatment in individuals with relapsing-remitting MS. We simply do not know if these medications are effective in people with secondary progressive MS because studies have not yet been done. A large clinical trial of Betaseron® has recently begun to try to answer this question. We do not know any specific biological factor to suggest that such individuals would behave differently than those with relapsing-remitting disease, but we will not know for sure until the trial is completed several years from now.

Once I start taking Betaseron® or Avonex® how long will I need to take the medication?

No one knows how long a person "needs" to take these medications. Since neither medication completely prevents disease activity, the occurrence of an occasional attack in someone taking one of these medications does not necessarily mean drug failure. Follow-up data from the original group of 372 individuals with ambulatory, relapsing-remitting MS in the interferon beta-1b trial indicate the continued benefit and safety of Betaseron® for at least four to five years. Compared with those treated with a placebo, the group treated with high-dose Betaseron® (the same dose that is currently prescribed for patients) had about a 30 percent reduction in annual exacerbation rate and showed no increase in total amount of lesion area in the CNS as detected with MRI.

After a year or longer, however, there is some evidence that approximately 38 percent of individuals develop substances in the blood that have been found to neutralize the effect of Betaseron® in certain test tube analyses. These substances are probably *antibodies*—proteins of the immune system that protect the body from foreign substances such as viruses and bacteria. The development of this neutralizing effect appears to be associated with a reduction in treatment benefits. Follow-up data from the Betaseron® trial indicate that the exacerbation rate of the subgroup of treated individuals who developed the antibodies was significantly higher than the exacerbation rate for those who did not develop antibodies; in fact, it did not differ from the exacerbation rate for the group receiving a placebo. Unfortunately, there is no FDA-approved, commercially available test for these antibodies at the present time. This means that there is no simple way for a person to determine his or her likelihood of developing antibodies to Betaseron®. Although similar neutralizing antibodies were reported in some of the patients in the Avonex® trial, no data are currently available on the relationship between these antibodies and disease activity in people taking Avonex®.

In general, people taking Betaseron® should remain on the medication unless they are clearly showing frequent attacks, significant disease progression, or severe side effects. Of course, the availability of newer effective treatments will require continual reassessment of an individual's situation.

I have been taking Betaseron® for more than two years and I still don't feel better. Does this mean that the drug isn't working for me?

In the clinical trial of interferon beta-1b (Betaseron®), there was no evidence that the drug made the treatment group "feel better." The treatment was found simply to reduce the number and severity of exacerbations in relapsing-remitting MS. Although a significant effort has been made to inform people about the possible benefits and limitations of this treatment, it is clear that many people harbor a hope that it will make them feel better. This is not particularly surprising since most people's life experiences with medical treatment in general, and medication in particular, is that it is designed to make a person feel better.

In a recent study of one hundred individuals eligible for Betaseron® (funded by the National Multiple Sclerosis Society at the University of California, San Francisco), a significant proportion of those surveyed had misconceptions about the drug's potential effects. More than 80 percent expected that the drug would reduce their level of physical discomfort and improve their overall quality of life. Unfortunately, these misconceptions may cause people to become disappointed or dissatisfied with the drug's effects and stop taking it prematurely, even if it may be working for them in ways they cannot readily see or feel.

Since it is not possible to evaluate the extent to which Betaseron® is working successfully for any one individual at any particular point in time, it is advisable for you to remain on the drug unless you are having frequent attacks, rapid disease progression, or severe side effects.

Why do Betaseron® and Avonex® have to be taken by injection?

Injection is the only route of administration that has been shown to be effective at the present time. Betaseron® and Avonex® are proteins, and proteins are degraded in the stomach and intestinal tract. The degradation products may not have the same effects in modulating the immune system that the intact molecule has.

What will happen if I lose track of the date and forget to give myself a shot of Betaseron® or Avonex®?

Missing an *occasional* Betaseron® injection is not thought to be harmful. If that should happen, just give yourself the injection at the next most appropriate opportunity and continue the every-other-day routine from that point. If you miss a dose of Avonex®, take it as soon as you remember and continue on a weekly schedule. Do not, however, take two doses within two days of each other.

Why are Betaseron® and Avonex® so expensive and will the cost of these drugs ever come down?

Betaseron® is very expensive for several reasons. First, the technology to develop and produce this genetically engineered drug, which is grown in and harvested from bacteria, is complex and costly. When a new drug is marketed, the very expensive costs of developing the product are passed along to the consumer. It is important to realize that for every drug that does reach the marketplace, dozens of others have failed to achieve that goal. The costs of testing those unsuccessful drugs must also be recouped through sales of the drugs that are approved.

Unfortunately for the public, pharmaceutical companies, like all other businesses, have a fiduciary obligation to their stockholders to try to maximize profits. Therefore, new drugs are generally quite expensive, especially those without similar competitive medications. With the approval of additional treatments, many people expect that competition may bring down the cost of these drugs.

I have recently been diagnosed with MS and have no apparent symptoms at this time. Should I start taking Betaseron® or Avonex® right away?

The decision to begin one of these medications should be made jointly by the individual and physician. In general, the person whose disease shows signs of relatively recent activity is the likeliest candidate to benefit from the treatment. People who have had very rare attacks or have very "benign" MS may not do better with treatment.

What are the long-term side effects of taking Betaseron® or Avonex®? Will I get cancer because of these drugs?

No severe, long-term side effects have as yet been recognized with the use of these treatments. However, it is important to realize that only very small numbers of people have taken the drug for more than a few years. There is nothing at present to suggest an increased risk of cancer in people taking Betaseron® or Avonex®. Follow-up data from the original group of 372 individuals with ambulatory relapsing-remitting MS in the interferon beta-1b trial showed a significant drop in the numbers of people experiencing flu-like symptoms and injection-site reactions. While 76 percent of the high-dose treatment group experienced flu-like symptoms during the initial months of the clinical trial, only 3–8 percent of this group reported these symptoms through the next five years. Similarly, the injection-site reactions experienced by 80 percent of the high-dose group in the early months of the trial were reported by 44–50 percent of this group in years four and five. Thus, most people taking Betaseron® over an extended period of time seem to be doing so with relatively little problem or discomfort. In the Avonex® trial, 4 percent of patients discontinued the drug due to adverse effects; modest side effects, including flu-like symptoms, muscle aches, fever, chills, and weakness, diminished with continued treatment. Four percent of patients experienced mild injection-site reactions.

If I have an exacerbation while I'm taking Betaseron® or Avonex® can I still be given intravenous steroids?

Individuals taking Betaseron® or Avonex® may still be treated with intravenous steroids in the same manner as those not on the medication.

What new drugs are currently being tested for MS and how do they differ?

Many new drugs are currently being evaluated for the treatment of MS and are at various stages of development. Among the agents in more advanced testing are oral myelin (Myloral®), roquinimex (Linomide®), and cladribine (Leustatin®). Oral myelin is being tested because of an immunologic phenomenon known as "oral tolerance." When foreign proteins are injected into the body, the organism mounts an immune response against that substance (known as an **antigen**). However, when that same antigen is administered orally, the organism becomes tolerant to it. This is the same mechanism that allows us to consume foods without interference from the immune system. We believe that people with MS, for reasons that are not known, have an **autoimmune disease**, which causes their immune system to attack the body's own myelin, mistaking it for a foreign substance. The hope of this trial is that by orally administering myelin, the person will become tolerant of the antigens within it and the autoimmune attacks will decrease or be eliminated. A large multicenter trial of oral myelin is well along and will be completed in March 1997. No additional subjects are being enrolled.

A large trial of roquinimex began in the Fall of 1995. Roquinimex is a drug that has a variety of effects that modulate the immune system (as does Betaseron®, for example). It has been found to be very effective in preventing an animal model of MS known as experimental autoimmune encephalomyelitis (EAE) and had promising results in two small trials in people with MS. The medication is administered orally. The current trial will involve over seven hundred patients whose neurologic condition has been worsening. It is anticipated that enrollment will be completed in late 1996 and subjects will continue on treatment for three years.

Cladribine is a potent immunosuppressive drug that has previously been used to treat an unusual form of leukemia known as hairy cell leukemia. It has powerful toxic effects on lymphocytes and may be beneficial in MS through this action. The drug was reported to be very successful in slowing progression of the disease in a relatively small pilot trial. A multicenter trial is currently underway. The drug is administered by injection. Blood cell counts, including platelets (which are important elements to prevent bleeding), must be monitored closely.

I have read that there will soon be new treatments available for MS. How will I know whether to continue with Betaseron® or try one of the new treatments? Will any of these treatments be used in conjunction with Betaseron®?

Interferon beta-1a (Avonex®) was approved by the FDA in 1996. Although closely related to interferon beta-1b (Betaseron®), Avonex® is administered by intramuscular injection once a week, rather than by subcutaneous injection every other day, as Betaseron® is given. Since intramuscular injections are more difficult to self-administer, some people may need to be given their injections by a health care professional or other caregiver. Like Betaseron®, Avonex® was found to reduce the frequency of clinical exacerbations as well as the number and volume of active brain lesions in people with relapsing-remitting MS. Additionally, Avonex® was found to reduce the risk of disability progression (as measured by the *Expanded Disability Status Scale (EDSS)* in these individuals. However, since the Avonex® trial included only those individuals with little or no disability, no conclusions can as yet be drawn concerning the impact of Avonex® on the disability progression of individuals with more severe symptoms. People who are doing well on Betaseron® with minimal side effects will probably have little reason to switch to Avonex®. Since Avonex® generally has fewer side effects, it may be preferred by individuals who are not tolerating Betaseron® well.

The third drug, copolymer 1 (Copaxone®), is completely unrelated to the interferons. It is believed to "fool" the immune system in some way and thereby prevent further damage to myelin. Copaxone® is administered by daily subcutaneous injection. Both Copaxone® and Avonex® were tested in relatively mildly affected individuals with relapsing-remitting disease. Copaxone® may be particularly effective in *very* mildly affected individuals. Again, people doing well on Betaseron® should probably not switch to Copaxone®. When a person who has never been treated is deciding which agent to start, the pros and cons of each drug should be discussed with the physician.

We do not have any information concerning the relative effectiveness of these agents. No agent has yet been adequately tested in people with progressive MS, although a large trial of Betaseron® is underway in this group of patients. Many MS investigators would like to see a trial combining one of the interferons with copolymer 1. However, such a trial will be very expensive and it is not clear who would pay for it if it were undertaken.

My family is worried about my using Betaseron® because of the reported suicides. What is the risk of depression and/or suicide with this drug?

Depression is very common in people with MS. Fortunately, however, it is usually not severe and generally responds well to combinations of psychotherapy and medication. Nevertheless, suicide occurs more frequently among people with MS than among comparable groups of people without the disease. In the Betaseron® definitive trial, four suicide attempts and one completed suicide occurred. Because of the frequency of depression and suicide in the MS population (see Chapter 11) and the small number of events in the trial, one cannot conclude that these episodes of depression were caused by the drug. It is known, however, that very high doses of interferon, such as those used in cancer treatment, do cause depression. As a result of concerns about interferons and depression, the emotional state of patients receiving Betaseron® has been followed carefully since marketing of the drug began. Severe depression and suicide appear to be rare among individuals taking Betaseron®.

The best recommendation is that people with a previous history of severe affective disorder [depression or bipolar (manic-depressive) illness] or previous suicide attempts should probably not take either interferon beta-1b (Betaseron®) or interferon beta-1a (Avonex®). Individuals with milder forms of depression can probably safely take Betaseron® or Avonex® under close supervision. Family members, other loved ones, and caregivers should be advised to be alert to any changes in mood and report them promptly to the physician. Sometimes the physician will wish to consult with a psychiatrist before starting a person on interferon beta-1b or interferon beta-1a, even though no suicide attempts or serious depression occurred in individuals in the Avonex® trial.

I have been reading about Betaseron® on the Internet and most of what I've read has been about the problems people have with it. I'm concerned about the side effects of Betaseron® and I'm reluctant to try it because I don't want to feel worse than I already do.

The Internet has been a useful forum for people to exchange views and information about MS. It is probably a fact of life, however, that people tend to report negative effects and side effects more commonly than they "go on record" with positive feelings. Certainly, side effects do occur with Betaseron®. Most common are flu-like symptoms that occur primarily in the first few months of treatment. For the majority of people, these are relatively mild and can be managed by taking injections at night and using minor analgesics (pain relievers), such as ibuprofen or acetaminophen. Also annoying are local injection-site reactions. Most typically these are confined to the appearance of red blotches and, perhaps, minor pain. Only infrequently do more severe reactions occur that may necessitate stopping the medication. We now have experience with over 35,000 individuals taking Betaseron®. In general, with proper education and support from physicians and nurses, the medication is well tolerated and people can readily continue taking it. Overall, perhaps about 15 percent of people need to discontinue treatment for one reason or another and, certainly, not all of these are because of side effects.

What is immunosuppressive therapy and will it make my MS better?

Immunosuppressive therapy utilizes treatment agents that dampen the body's natural immune response, which is designed to protect it from foreign substances. In MS, we believe the immune system mistakenly attacks the person's own myelin as if it were foreign. By suppressing the immune system, such therapy may reduce the severity of this attack and thus reduce further damage to the myelin in the nervous system. Immunosuppressive drugs such as cyclosporine and methotrexate have been shown to slow the progression of MS. Cyclosporine, however, proved too toxic for widespread acceptance by physicians or their patients. Methotrexate has been used in cancer treatment, for immunosuppression in organ transplantation, and for the treatment of rheumatoid arthritis. In relatively low doses, it has been shown to slow the rate of progression in MS. However, methotrexate is potentially toxic to the liver, and treatment with this drug must be carefully monitored. It is not compatible with nonsteroidal anti-inflammatory drugs (e.g., aspirin or ibuprofen) or with alcohol, so that the use of methotrexate involves a number of restrictions. It is currently being used in some individuals with progressive MS. There is some evidence that azathioprine may slow progression in MS, but the effect, if it exists, is small and somewhat controversial. All treatments currently available or in advanced stages of testing are aimed to reduce further damage. Of course, individuals with MS often improve spontaneously. The longer symptoms of MS have been present, the lower the likelihood that this spontaneous improvement will occur.

Is it possible to replace or repair the myelin that has been destroyed by MS?

It is not currently possible to enhance or improve myelin repair in MS. However, recent animal and laboratory investigations have shown that myelin repair occurs spontaneously in mammals and that this repair can be enhanced in animals. Some myelin repair occurs naturally in MS, particularly early in the disease, and this may be an important aspect of recovery from attacks. Further study is underway to try to find ways to enhance myelin repair in humans.

I have a friend who is taking 4-AP for his MS. What is 4-AP and is it likely to help me?

4-AP, which stands for 4-aminopyridine, is a chemical that affects channels in nerve fibers that control the passage of potassium. In so doing, it appears able to improve temporarily the transmission of impulses through these fibers. Some individuals with MS experience improvement in neurologic symptoms when they take this substance orally. It seems particularly likely to help people whose MS is heat-sensitive. 4-AP is not approved by the FDA and therefore is not routinely available at pharmacies. However, a physician can legally write a prescription for the chemical to be made up for a patient by a *compounding* pharmacy, which will put the substance into a medicinal form.

The problem is that 4-AP has a number of potentially serious side effects, most noteworthy of which is seizures. Furthermore, it has a low *toxic-therapeutic index*, meaning that the dose that may cause problems is not very much higher than that which may be beneficial. Because compounding pharmacies do not have the same high level of standardization controls that exist for prescription drugs marketed by regulated pharmaceutical companies, a lack of precision about dosage may pose significant risks to people who obtain the substance from compounding pharmacies. At the present time, investigation of this drug in a commercially prepared, controlled-release formulation is continuing. We hope that such trials will demonstrate a benefit for individuals with MS and that the drug can then be made available safely.

Oral myelin is sold at my local health food store. Will this product help my MS symptoms?

Oral myelin is currently being tested as a treatment to reduce or prevent further relapses of MS. As indicated previously, a specific preparation of the drug is in large scale clinical trial. Unfortunately, preparations touted as containing oral myelin are presently being sold at many health food stores. Such products are essentially unregulated. The amounts of oral myelin that they contain are unknown, but usually much smaller than what is being tested. Furthermore, the source of the product is generally not indicated. Certain herds of cattle, though *not those in the United States*, have harbored a fatal, transmissible disease

that *may* pose risks to humans. Extreme precautions have been
taken to eliminate any risk to subjects in the FDA approved trial
of Myloral®, *but the same cannot be said for these uncontrolled
products distributed through health food stores.* Furthermore,
until the completion of the large trial underway, we do not know
whether people taking oral myelin fare better, the same, or even
worse than individuals taking a placebo. It must further be
emphasized that there is no reason to believe that oral myelin
will improve MS symptoms. Rather, if it works, it will reduce
the chances of further damage.

**One of my friends recommended that I try marijuana to relieve
my MS symptoms. Is marijuana an effective treatment for MS?**

Smoking marijuana has been reported by some individuals to
benefit some of their symptoms, particularly spasticity. Small
clinical trials of orally administered tetrahydrocannabinol, the
active chemical in marijuana, have failed to demonstrate this
benefit. The use of marijuana has not been legalized for the
treatment of MS.

**My friends and relatives are always pushing me to try different
diets and vitamins. Does diet have any effect on this disease?**

Many diets have been touted as being useful for MS, but none
has ever been proven so in a controlled trial. While some of
these, (e.g., the popular Swank diet) are generally healthful, others are extremely demanding, inconvenient, and possibly harmful. The same is true for vitamins and other supplements, *none*
of which has been shown to help MS. It is clear, however, that
maintenance of good health and physical condition is valuable
and may help a person with MS cope better with the physical
and emotional challenges of the neurologic disease. Thus, a diet
such as the American Heart Association diet—which strikingly
resembles the Swank diet—may be worthwhile if a person with
MS wants to follow a nutritional regimen.

Recommended Resources

AVONEX Support Line (800-456-2255)
BETASERON Customer Service (800-788-1467)
National Multiple Sclerosis Society (800-FIGHT MS)

Recommended Readings

Giffels JJ. *Clinical Trials: What You Should Know Before Volunteering to Be a Research Subject.* New York: Demos Vermande, 1996.

Sibley WA. *Therapeutic Claims in Multiple Sclerosis (4th edition).* New York: Demos Vermande, 1996.

Selected booklets available from the National Multiple Sclerosis Society (Customer Service: 212-986-3240; Information: 800-344-4867)

◇ *Research Directions in Multiple Sclerosis*—Stephen C. Reingold, Ph.D.

References in this area become outdated very quickly. The most accurate, up-to-date information about treatments and drug trials is available through the National Multiple Sclerosis Society Society (800-344-4867).

4

Nursing Care

June Halper, MSN, RN.CS., ANP

Multiple sclerosis can affect many aspects of a person's functioning over its long and unpredictable course. Some of the problems caused by the illness, such as weakness, imbalance, optic neuritis, or bladder and bowel symptoms, are a direct result of *plaque* formation in the *central nervous system*. Others, including skin breakdown, can result from the lack of mobility caused by the illness. Much has been learned in recent years about successful management of these primary and secondary problems in MS. With education and support provided by the health care team, people can learn to manage their symptoms and avoid unnecessary problems and complications.

The nurse can be a helpful ally in these management efforts, whether as a member of an MS center's health care team, in the community's Visiting Nurse Service, on a hospital inpatient service, in a rehabilitation facility, or in the home. A primary goal of nursing care in MS is to help people learn effective, preventive self-care in order to manage smaller problems before they become major ones. This chapter has as its focus three areas in which nursing plays a key role—bladder function, bowel management, and skin care.

Bladder Function

The neurologic changes in MS sometimes interfere with bladder function. These changes can be distressing and occasionally disabling, but they are manageable with effective interventions including education, thorough diagnostic testing, medications, and self-care activities.

The urinary system includes the kidneys, which filter impurities from the bloodstream and excrete them in the urine; ureters, the small tubes that transport urine from the kidneys to the bladder; the urinary bladder, which stores urine until it is time to void (urinate); and the **urethra**, which transports the urine out of the body. In order for normal urination to occur, the detrusor or bladder muscle must contract to expel urine at the same time that the internal and external sphincters are relaxed to allow the urine to pass freely out of the body. In normal function, the urine is collected slowly, causing the bladder to expand. When approximately six to eight ounces (180–240 ml) of urine have accumulated, nerve endings in the bladder send a message to the

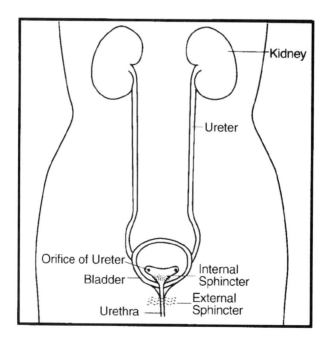

Figure 4-1.   Diagram of the urinary system.

voiding reflex area of the spinal cord which, in turn, sends a message to the brain signaling the need to urinate. The brain then sends a message back to the spinal cord that signals the voiding reflex to contract the **detrusor muscle** and relax the urethral sphincter. Thus, a functional urinary system depends on an intact nervous system.

In multiple sclerosis, the excretion or elimination of urine can be altered in the following ways:

Failure to store urine, usually seen in a small, spastic bladder, results from **demyelination** of the pathways between the spinal cord and the brain. The bladder fills quickly and sends messages to the spinal cord, which, because of demyelination, is unable to forward the message to the brain. As a result, voluntary control of urination is interrupted and voiding becomes a reflex response to repeated signals from the spinal cord. Failure to store can result in symptoms of **urinary urgency** (having to get to the bathroom quickly), **urinary frequency** (feeling the urge to urinate even when urination has occurred very recently), dribbling, **incontinence** (wetting oneself), and **nocturia** (being awakened at night by the need to urinate).

Failure to empty urine occurs when there is demyelination in the voiding reflex area of the spinal cord. Even though the bladder fills with large amounts of urine, the spinal cord is unable to send the necessary messages—either to the brain that the bladder is full or to the bladder and sphincter. The resulting absence of either voluntary or reflexive voiding causes the bladder to overfill. Failure to empty results in a large, **flaccid** (atonic) bladder and symptoms of urgency, dribbling, hesitancy, and incontinence.

Combined dysfunction can result from a failure to store/failure to empty combination called **detrusor-external sphincter dyssynergia (DESD)**. Combined dysfunction involves a lack of coordination between muscle groups, whereby the detrusor and external sphincter contract simultaneously, trapping urine within the bladder. Both urgency and hesitancy may occur, as well as dribbling or incontinence.

It is important to remember that a particular symptom does not point to a particular type of bladder failure. In fact, each of the primary urinary symptoms—urgency, frequency, hesitancy, incontinence, and nocturia—can be caused by any of the functional abnormalities that have been described. Careful evaluation is needed in order to identify the cause of the problem and select appropriate treatment measures.

I have just been diagnosed with MS. What are the chances that I will develop problems controlling my bladder or bowel?

Multiple sclerosis can affect the motor and sensory pathways from the brain and spinal cord that control both bladder and bowel function. Over the course of the disease, as many as 80–90 percent of people develop transient or persistent urinary symptoms. Bladder symptoms can occur at the onset of the illness or at any time thereafter. They can usually be controlled with medications, self-care activities, and some possible modifications in lifestyle. Bowel problems occur somewhat less frequently but are still common enough that everyone with MS needs to be aware of their relationship to the disease and familiar with effective prevention and management strategies.

The most important thing to remember about bladder and bowel symptoms in MS is that they can be helped. The MS health care team is familiar with these problems and their management. Although you may initially find it difficult or uncomfortable to discuss bladder and bowel questions with your doctor or nurse, the more open you are about any problems you are having, the more quickly and easily you can learn effective management techniques and avoid unnecessary complications and discomfort.

I have recently begun having trouble controlling my urine. All of a sudden, without any warning, I have to get to the bathroom immediately or risk wetting myself. What is the treatment for this problem?

The sudden sensation of having to urinate quickly is called urinary urgency. It usually results from the bladder's failure to store urine properly or from a failure to store/failure to empty combination (bladder detrusor-external sphincter dyssynergia— DESD). A careful evaluation is needed in order to determine the cause of the urgency. Urgency resulting from a failure to store can be managed with an **anticholinergic** medication, such as oxybutynin chloride (Ditropan®), which controls spasms in the bladder and other smooth muscles of the body by inhibiting transmission of parasympathetic nerve impulses. Certain tricyclic antidepressants, most notably imipramine (Tofranil®), share these anticholinergic properties and have been found to be useful in controlling urinary muscle contractions (see Appendix B). Feelings of urgency resulting from the bladder's failure to empty or from DESD are best managed with a treatment regimen that includes anticholinergic medication and ***intermittent self-catheterization (ISC)***.

What is intermittent self-catheterization?

If the bladder fails to empty properly or the bladder and sphincters do not work together in the proper rhythm, your physician may suggest that you do intermittent self-catheterization (ISC) on a scheduled basis—from one to five times a day. ISC can be thought of as physical therapy for your bladder because it promotes regular filling and emptying (expanding and contracting) of the bladder muscle and may help restore normal function. You begin by emptying your bladder as thoroughly as you can. Then you drain the residual or remaining urine by passing a ***catheter*** (a very thin, hollow, plastic tube that resembles a straw) into your bladder through the urethra. The catheter stays in your bladder until the urine stops draining—no more than a minute or two—and is then removed. With a little practice, the procedure is easy, quick, and painless. ISC can be done while sitting on the toilet, lying on the bed, or even in the public restroom of your favorite restaurant. Your doctor or nurse can instruct you in the appropriate use, care, and cleaning of the urinary catheter.

What kinds of tests will the doctor do to find out why I am having problems urinating?

A number of tests are used to diagnose urinary problems. Your physician will first determine whether a urinary tract infection (UTI) is causing your urinary symptoms. Infections in one or more of the structures of the urinary tract are caused by bacteria and can be detected by microscopic examination of a urine specimen. A test called a ***urine culture and sensitivity (C&S)*** will be used to identify the particular bacteria that is present and the antibiotic to which it is sensitive. The bacteria from a midstream urine sample is allowed to grow for three days in a special laboratory medium and then tested for sensitivity to a variety of antibiotics. This allows your physician to prescribe the antibiotic most likely to kill that bacteria. An antibiotic that commonly cures UTI may be prescribed until the results of the C&S are known.

In order to determine whether your urinary symptoms are caused by the bladder's failure to empty, failure to store, or combined dysfunction, the doctor can evaluate your ***post-void residual (PVR)***. You will be asked to drink ample fluids for a day or two before the test and two glasses just prior to the PVR. As soon as you feel the need to urinate, you will do so and the amount of urine will be measured. After you have urinated, the nurse will pass a catheter into the bladder to drain and measure the urine remaining in the bladder. It is important to determine if urine is being retained in the bladder because urine that is not voided can cause a urinary tract infection. Depending on the results of this test, your doctor may suggest a program of self-catheterization and/or an anticholinergic medication to manage your symptoms.

In most instances, the results from this simple test, in combination with your body's response to this treatment regimen, will provide ample information about the source of your urinary symptoms. Further testing may be required if the physician is still unable to diagnose the problem. In an intravenous pyelogram (IVP), dye is injected into your vein so that sequential X-ray pictures can be taken of the kidneys, ureters, and bladder. Ultrasound technology (utilizing sound waves) can also be used to determine the presence of stones or other abnormalities in your bladder. A somewhat more invasive test, a urinary ***cystoscopy***, which can be done in a urologist's office or in the hospital, allows the physician to examine the inside of the bladder.

Sometimes when I feel that I have to urinate I find that I have trouble getting started. I feel the pressure to empty my bladder but nothing comes out. Is there anything I can do about this?

The inability to initiate urination in spite of the sensation of a full bladder is called urinary hesitancy and usually results from the bladder's failure to empty properly. Patience almost always pays off; people find that the urinary stream usually starts within a minute or two. You can try running water in the sink to help relax the urinary sphincter. "Tickling" the opening to the urethra (the opening behind a woman's vagina or the tip of a man's penis) with a moist tissue may also promote relaxation. If these techniques do not produce results, you may tap lightly on the lower part of your abdomen. Do not press or hit yourself too forcefully as this might worsen the problem.

Speak to your physician if you are unable to manage the hesitancy. A medication such as baclofen will relax the sphincter to allow the bladder to empty more effectively.

After I finish urinating I sometimes feel that my bladder is still full. Nothing more comes out but I'm afraid to leave the bathroom in case of an accident. How can I tell if there is more urine left in my bladder?

The sensation of a full bladder after voiding can be caused by the bladder's failure either to empty or store properly. A "post-void residual" can be done to determine if you are retaining urine in your bladder and what treatment would be most beneficial. As indicated, it is important that you be able to empty your bladder fully, using whatever combination of medication and/or ISC is appropriate, both to maintain your personal comfort and to reduce your risk of bladder infections.

I'm so worried I'll have a bladder accident that I hardly drink anything any more. My doctor says that I need to drink fluids so that I won't get bladder infections. What can I do to handle this problem?

Urine, which consists of solid and liquid waste substances that are not needed by your body, is manufactured continuously by the kidneys. It is important for urine to be diluted with water because urine that contains more solid particles than liquid will increase your risk of infection. Many people who experience urinary urgency or frequency restrict their intake of fluids in the hope of relieving their symptoms and freeing themselves from the bathroom. As a result, their urine becomes too highly concentrated with solid particles (resulting in a dark brownish appearance) and therefore more susceptible to infection. You should drink between six and eight glasses of fluid per day, early in the day if you prefer in order to avoid having to go to the bathroom at night. You can also get fluids in such foods as soup, Jell-O®, fruits, puddings, and compotes. In addition to reducing your risk of bladder infections, adequate fluid intake will help you to maintain satisfactory bowel function.

Identifying the cause of your bladder accidents will make it possible for your physician to design a bladder management program, possibly including medication and scheduled voiding, in an effort to "train" your bladder and help reduce the risk of accidents.

Sometimes I wet myself without even knowing that it is happening—I can't feel either the urge to urinate or the urine itself. Why is this happening and is there anything I can do about it?

Spontaneous voiding (urinary incontinence) can occur in MS for a number of reasons. Because uninhibited bladder spasms and a weakened bladder muscle can both cause urine to pass out of the bladder before the urge to urinate is felt, post-void residual testing is required to determine the cause of the problem. Diminished sensations in the genital area will reduce a person's awareness of the urge to void and perhaps even of the sensation of being wet. Usually a treatment regimen consisting of ISC and/or a trial of anticholinergic medication will be sufficient to control the incontinence. If the bladder dysfunction that is causing the incontinence does not respond to this type of treatment regimen, your neurologist will probably refer you to a **urologist** for more extensive bladder studies to determine if some other problem is contributing to your symptoms.

I seem to be getting up three or four times during the night to urinate. This is very unusual for me. Is there anything I can do about this problem?

The first step in dealing with nocturia, as this problem is called, is to make sure that you do not have a urinary tract infection. Then your physician or nurse will do a PVR to determine the probable cause of the problem. Nocturia is most commonly caused by spasms in the bladder muscles that result in the bladder's failure to store urine properly. It can usually be treated very effectively with a bedtime dose of either imipramine (Tofranil®) or desmopressin (DDAVP Nasal Spray®) (see Appendix B).

I think I have memorized the location of every bathroom in the city. Is there anything I can do when I'm going out so that I don't constantly have to be near a toilet?

The urinary symptoms of urgency and frequency, which sometimes make people feel as though their lives are controlled by the location of the nearest bathroom, can usually be treated and managed once they are properly diagnosed. Your health care team can diagnose the source of these symptoms and prescribe a course of medication and/or ISC that will allow you to regain control of your bladder.

Once this sense of control is regained, you will feel more confident about venturing farther from the bathroom. Most people still find that they feel more comfortable if, upon arriving at their destination, they check out the location of the bathroom so that they can get there without having to search for it. Some people choose to wear some protective pad (e.g., Serenity® or Depends®) so that they do not have to panic about possible leakage. If you know that you have trouble controlling your bladder for long periods of time and that you are going to be in a situation in which getting to a bathroom quickly is impossible (a football game, a wedding, or a long bus ride, for example), you can discuss with your doctor the occasional use of a drug such as desmopressin or imipramine.

What are the symptoms of a urinary tract infection and what are the treatments for it?

Urinary tract infections can sometimes occur without any apparent symptoms or discomfort. More often, however, an infection causes symptoms such as urinary urgency and frequency, a burning sensation, abdominal pain, an elevated body temperature, increased spasticity, and possibly foul-smelling, dark-colored urine. Urinary tract infections most commonly occur in the bladder and are usually treatable with oral antibiotics. An infection in the upper portion of the urinary tract, including the kidneys and ureters, is more serious and potentially more debilitating. Kidney infections are usually accompanied by a high fever and may require intravenous treatment with antibiotics. Both types of infection are treated by increased fluid intake and rest, as well as close medical monitoring.

Individuals who are particularly prone to urinary tract infections may be prescribed an antiseptic, such as methenamine (Hiprex® or Mandelamine®), to use on a routine basis to "cleanse" the urine and reduce the number of bacteria (see Appendix B). Additionally, maintaining an acid urine will help in the prevention of urinary tract infections because the organisms that cause infections do not grow as easily in an acidic environment. You can make your urine more acid by following certain dietary guidelines. Increase your daily intake of: (1) protein, such as that found in meat, fish, fowl, eggs, and gelatin; and (2) cranberries (and their juice), plums, and prunes. The cranberry juice, which provides a replacement for the vitamin C found in citrus fruits, should be taken at frequent intervals throughout the day because vitamin C is processed and excreted very rapidly by the body. Decrease your intake of citrus fruits and juices (grapefruit, oranges, lemons, and tomatoes); milk and milk products; beverages or antacids containing sodium carbonate or sodium bicarbonate (use Gelusil® or any other aluminum-type antacid in their place); non-citrus fruits and vegetables; potatoes, lima beans, soy beans, greens, spinach, and dried vegetables.

To treat chronic, recurrent UTIs, your physician may prescribe long-term, low-dose antibiotics such as sulfamethoxazole (Septra® or Bactrim®) in an effort to suppress bacterial activity and reduce the risk of infection (see Appendix B).

I feel very weak when I have a bladder (urinary tract) infection even though I never seem to run a very high fever. Does this mean that the infection is making my MS worse?

Any type of infection is likely to cause a feeling of weakness and an apparent exacerbation of symptoms, especially one that causes an elevation in body temperature. This is referred to as a *pseudo-exacerbation* because it is caused by the underlying infection and not by an actual progression of the disease. The important strategy when this occurs is to treat the infection promptly, thus removing the trigger for this temporary worsening of the symptoms. A pseudo-exacerbation and accompanying weakness typically remit or disappear once the infection is brought under control.

Is a urinary tract infection ever life-threatening?

A urinary tract infection can be life-threatening if left untreated and allowed to spread into the kidneys. Since all blood is filtered through the kidneys, the infection can pass into the bloodstream and cause serious problems.

Are there different types of urinary catheters? How do I know what type of catheter is best for me?

The type of catheter used for intermittent self-catheterization resembles a straw and is called a straight catheter. One end is tapered and has a small hole called a port. This end is inserted into the bladder for urinary drainage. The other end has a larger opening that allows the urine to flow into the toilet or a collecting device.

A **Foley catheter** is an **indwelling catheter** that remains in the bladder for longer periods of time, allowing continuous drainage into a collection bag. The tapered end has a balloon that is inflated when the catheter is placed into the bladder. The balloon is filled with sterile water while in the bladder and emptied when the catheter is withdrawn, but cannot be felt by the person at any time. A Foley catheter is used for continuous drainage of urine when bladder function cannot be improved by the other means discussed in this chapter or if a person is experiencing skin breakdown (**decubitus** ulcer) because of chronic wetness that cannot be otherwise managed.

My doctor wants me to do intermittent self-catheterization. Why can't I just use a Foley catheter all the time so I don't have to be bothered?

ISC is a strategy to maintain and sometimes improve bladder tone and bladder function. It prevents infections, reduces symptoms, and prevents the long-term complications of chronic urinary tract infections. People may find that their bladder symptoms are more problematic some times than others; they may need to do ISC for a period of time and then find it unnecessary for a while. A Foley catheter is used by people who are unable to manage their bladder function with medications or self-care, either because their symptoms cannot be controlled or their other symptoms interfere with their ability to do ISC.

The urinary system is normally closed to the outside environment even when a person self-catheterizes. Once an indwelling catheter is inserted into the bladder, this closed system remains open at all times, making the person susceptible to ongoing infections, the development of bladder stones, and other complications of the urinary system. Foley catheters are now thought of as the last resort when other treatments are not viable.

Is it possible to use a Foley catheter for some situations and catheterize myself the rest of the time?

Some people who self-catheterize regularly can insert Foley catheters for situations when ISC is not possible. Airline flights or long car trips, for example, make ISC somewhat problematic. The Foley catheter is inserted prior to the journey and then removed. Because of the increased risk of infection with an indwelling catheter, it is very important to discuss the advisability of this strategy with your physician; it may be reasonable for some individuals but not others. Anyone using a Foley catheter needs to increase fluid intake to minimize the risk of infection. You can resume your normal ISC bladder routine once the Foley catheter is removed.

Will my bladder symptoms ever get better or go away?

This is not an easy question to answer. Many people report that their bladder symptoms improve or disappear, at least temporarily, with the appropriate use of medications and ISC. Others report that their bladder dysfunction waxes and wanes but never fully disappears. As with other symptoms of MS, bladder symptoms vary from person to person and from one period of time to another. The key to bladder management is accurate knowledge about what is causing the problem followed by appropriate action to minimize complaints and control symptoms.

Are there any surgical procedures that would take care of my bladder symptoms?

No surgical procedures can resolve bladder problems caused by neurologic changes. In certain rare instances, when none of the medications or self-care techniques have successfully relieved urinary symptoms, surgery (e.g., suprapubic *cystostomy*, *sphincterotomy*, *transurethral resection*) is performed to help bladder management.

Bowel Function

The gastrointestinal tract, which is responsible for the digestion and absorption of food and the elimination of waste, is composed of the following parts:

◇ the mouth, in which digestion is initiated by the chewing process and the addition of saliva;

◇ the esophagus, which connects the mouth to the stomach;

◇ the stomach, which stores food and advances the digestive process;

◇ the small intestine, where the digestive process is continued;

◇ the large intestine, where stool is formed;

◇ the rectum, in which the stool is stored just prior to defecation; and

◇ the anal canal, which contains the internal and external sphincters that normally remain closed to prevent leakage.

Stool normally passes into the rectum just prior to a bowel movement. When the rectum becomes full, it sends nerve impulses to a critical area of the spinal cord. The stool then passes through the anal canal, where it encounters first the internal sphincter, which opens reflexively in response to signals from the spinal cord, and then the external sphincter, which responds to signals from both the spinal cord and brain. The external sphincter is under "voluntary control," which means that a person can consciously tighten it to prevent defecation until the time and place are convenient. As with the urinary system, a

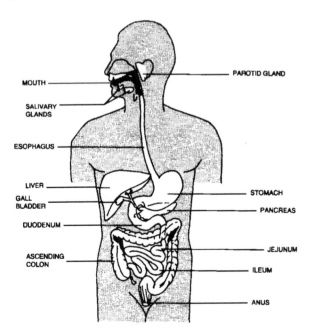

Figure 4-2. The gastrointestinal tract.

functional gastrointestinal system is dependent on a functional nervous system.

Changes in bowel function can be manifested as **constipation**, bowel urgency, or loss of bowel control (incontinence). People rarely complain about loose stools or diarrhea unless they have taken excessive amounts of laxatives or stool softeners. Constipation, by far the most frequent bowel complaint in MS, refers to infrequent, incomplete, or difficult bowel movements. The management of constipation in MS is important not only because of the abdominal discomfort it can cause, but also because of its potential for exacerbating other symptoms such as spasticity and urinary urgency and frequency.

Several factors conspire to produce MS-related constipation:

◇ Demyelination in the brain or spinal cord and reduced physical movement can each slow the passage of stool through the bowel. Because the body continuously draws moisture from the stool as it makes its way through the body, stool that remains in the intestine for extended periods of time becomes overly dry, hard, and difficult to pass.

◇ Dry, hardened stool can also result from decreased sensation in the rectal area. A person with decreased sensation may not experience the need to have a bowel movement, with the result that the stool remains in the rectum for an overly extended period of time.

◇ The same problem sometimes occurs because weakened abdominal muscles make it difficult to push the stool out of the rectum.

◇ A reduced fluid intake (usually in response to anxiety over bladder problems) will also cause the body to absorb more water from the stool.

◇ Certain medications slow bowel function and therefore contribute to the stool's loss of moisture.

Bowel changes in MS can be successfully managed with a self-care program that starts with a thorough evaluation of your dietary habits, medications, past and present bowel habits, and physical requirements for safe and comfortable toileting. If needed, an individualized bowel management program can be initiated with the help of the physician and nurse; successful bowel management then depends on the patience required to find the right combination of dietary changes, medications, and a consistent regimen. In general, a healthy bowel program consists of adequate fluid intake, a high fiber diet, adequate exercise, and a consistent, relaxed time for bowel evacuation, preferably thirty minutes after a meal when the *gastrocolic reflex* is at its strongest.

Are the bowel and bladder symptoms I have related? Some of my friends with MS have one or the other symptom but not both.

Bowel and bladder symptoms in MS may be related to one another, but they do not necessarily have to be. Spasms resulting from impaired neurologic function can cause symptoms of urgency and frequency in both the bladder and bowel systems. Weakened musculature can also interfere with the emptying process in either system. A full bowel can press on the bladder, causing symptoms of urinary urgency and frequency. Individual factors, such as diet, amount of exercise, and pre-illness patterns are more likely to affect a person's bowel regimen independently of what is occurring with the bladder.

My doctor says that drinking more fluids will help with my constipation, but when I drink I have difficulty controlling my urine. I can't decide which problem is worse!

Increasing your fluid intake is certainly one important method for improving bowel function. It is generally recommended that you drink two quarts of fluid every day. Be sure to discuss any problems you are having with urinary control with your physician or nurse so that they can recommend appropriate management techniques. The dilemma, of course, is that both problems are annoying and uncomfortable. Bladder problems need to be addressed first so that you can manage the high fluid intake needed for satisfactory bowel function. It may take some time and patience on your part to balance your bladder and bowel management, but it can be accomplished in ways that will reduce your symptoms, make you more comfortable, and avoid future complications.

Are there special diets that can help me with my bowel problems?

In addition to increased fluid intake, it is equally important to add fiber to your diet, usually in the form of bran, grains, fresh fruits and vegetables, prunes and prune juice. Fiber increases the moisture-retaining bulk of the stool, allowing it to pass more quickly and easily through the intestinal tract. Also be sure that you engage in some form of physical exercise each day to help promote regular bowel function.

What should I do if increasing my intake of fluids and fiber doesn't relieve the constipation?

In addition to the high fiber diet and increased intake of fluids, you can take a natural bulk supplement (made from the psyllium seed) such as Metamucil® on a daily basis, as well as a stool softener such as Colace®. These over-the-counter products will help to keep the stool soft enough to pass easily through your system. Regular adherence to this type of high fiber regimen will be sufficient for most people to control constipation. If the problem continues, your physician will probably recommend that you use a *mild* laxative such as Milk of Magnesia® every other night or so, and perhaps a glycerin suppository thirty minutes before you plan to move your bowels. Bisacodyl (Dulcolax®) suppositories can also be tried if the glycerin suppository is ineffective. Those who are unable to move their bowels even with these additional measures may require a Therevac Plus® or Fleet® enema to move the bowels. The Therevac Plus® is generally preferred because it is the size of a suppository and therefore much easier to use. As you can see, there are a variety of steps that can be taken to control constipation and create a comfortable bowel regimen. The goal is to maintain a consistent schedule of bowel evacuation using the mildest form of intervention that will encourage your body to function on a regular and comfortable basis.

Why can't I just use a laxative or enema whenever I need to move my bowels?

Laxatives and enemas should ideally be used only to help evacuate impacted stool that has remained in your bowel for a prolonged period. You might need a laxative or suppository to empty the bowel if you have not moved your bowels in more than four or five days and the stool has become too dry and difficult to pass. These products should be used only on an intermittent, as-needed basis because their chronic use can actually slow the bowel and increase constipation. As noted, the more effective technique for treating constipation is with a management regimen that prevents it in the first place.

If I'm so constipated most of the time, why do I sometimes seem to have diarrhea at the same time?

Occasionally, people who become severely constipated will find that looser stool from higher in the intestinal tract leaks around the impacted (dry and hard) stool. The solution to this problem is to remove the impacted stool with either a laxative or enema, and then begin a structured bowel program to retrain the bowel.

Sometimes I have bowel accidents even though my stomach is not upset and I don't have diarrhea. I lose control of my bowels without even realizing that it is going to happen. What is causing this and is there anything I can do about it?

Neurologic impairment in MS can cause spasms in the involuntary muscles of the bladder and bowel just as it does in the voluntary muscles of the legs and arms. These spasms can lead to involuntary loss of bowel control. Additionally, full or partial loss of sensation in the rectum allows it to fill with stool without your being aware of this fullness. The rectum stretches beyond normal capacity and then empties unexpectedly in response to an involuntary relaxation of the anal sphincter.

The most effective management of this infrequent but distressing problem is to retrain your bowel by establishing a bowel regimen. This regimen should include the dietary changes already discussed, as well as having a *consistent* time for moving your bowels. The frequency of evacuation matters less than the regularity of the interval and particular time of day that you choose. After breakfast every other day would be appropriate for one person; every day after lunch might be more comfortable for someone else—it does not matter as long as you stick with a consistent schedule. Whichever time you choose, make sure to allow yourself a quiet, relaxed period of time in the bathroom. Some people find that hot liquids such as coffee or tea help to stimulate the urge to defecate. If necessary, your physician may supplement this bowel regimen with an anticholinergic medication to relieve the spasms. Bowel retraining can take several weeks or even months, but it will help you to avoid bowel accidents and feel more in control of your body.

It has become increasingly difficult for me to move my bowels even with the use of laxatives and suppositories. I have not had a bowel movement in more than a week and don't know what to do.

A week is too long for most people to go without a bowel movement. In general, a person should take measures to have a bowel movement once three or four days have passed. You should notify your physician or nurse so that you can receive assistance emptying your bowel. In all likelihood, your bowel has become impacted with hardened stool that you will not be able to pass without help. Once your bowel has been emptied, the doctor or nurse will help you to establish a regimen to retrain your bowel and thus avoid the prolonged use of laxatives and/or laxative suppositories. Chronic use of these products results in "tolerance" to them so that the bowel will no longer respond to the medications in them.

Skin Care

The skin is the largest organ of the body. An intact skin protects the organs by maintaining body structure and preventing infections.

The risk of skin changes and skin breakdown is increased when people who are severely disabled with MS become less active, sitting or lying for longer periods. Continuous pressure on any area of skin decreases the flow of blood to that area. Without the flow of blood to bring oxygen and other nutrients, the skin can become damaged or die in a process referred to as ulceration. Pressure sores (also known as *decubitus* ulcers) occur most frequently in areas where the skin is thin and lies over protruding bones that cause pressure (the base of the spine and around the elbows, heels, and ankles). Additionally, a person who has increased muscle tone and spasticity is at greater risk of skin breakdown because the skin has a tendency to rub against supporting surfaces and become irritated. Bowel and bladder incontinence can also increase the risk of skin breakdown because the accumulation of moisture can cause ulcers around the genital region.

Good skin care requires an adequate intake of nutritious foods and fluids as well as frequent changes of position, comfortable

MULTIPLE SCLEROSIS: THE QUESTIONS, THE ANSWERS

seating with even weight distribution, skin cleanliness and moisturizing, and frequent skin checks to identify current and potential problems. Once skin breakdown occurs, it requires prompt medical and nursing attention. Pressure sores are very slow to heal and the most effective treatment is prevention.

Now that I use a wheelchair much of the time, my doctor has ordered a special seat cushion. How is this cushion going to help my skin?

A good cushion for your wheelchair helps to distribute your weight evenly and prevent any single area of skin from being put under constant pressure. In addition to using this specially designed cushion, it is important for you to shift your weight regularly, either by yourself or with someone else's assistance. This will periodically relieve pressure on the skin of your lower back, buttocks, and thighs, and allow the blood to circulate freely. A physical therapist can teach you wheelchair activities that are specially designed to relieve pressure on the skin and prevent decubitus ulcers.

How can I tell if I am developing a problem with my skin?

The best way to determine if you are developing skin problems is to be on the lookout for changes in skin coloring. Since it is difficult for you to get a clear view of the areas that are most prone to irritation, you may want to use a mirror for self-examination of at-risk areas. It is also advisable for you to be given a fairly regular "once over" by a nurse or family member. This is particularly important if you have experienced any loss of sensation, since this loss would probably prevent you from becoming aware of the sore. The earliest sign of a pressure sore is usually a reddening of the skin, which gradually becomes blistered and then opens. Sometimes the first sign is a soft, blackened area under the skin. If the sore is allowed to progress, fluid will begin to ooze from the opening, which gradually becomes wider and deeper.

Since my most recent MS exacerbation I have spent many hours of the day in bed. Should I be using a special type of bed or mattress?

Anyone who spends many hours of the day in bed should be evaluated by a nurse familiar with skin care. The nurse will

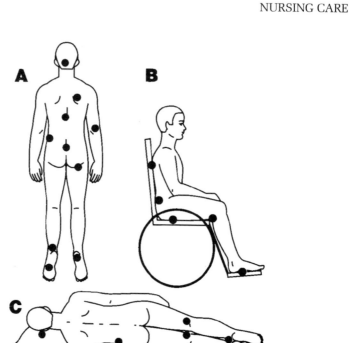

Figure 4-3. Dots show pressure points
when lying on back (**A**), when sitting (**B**),
and when lying on side (**C**).

examine your skin, paying particular attention to the areas over
bony projections (e.g., base of the spine, hips, heels), and evaluate your body alignment in bed. This type of examination will
enable the nurse to identify current and potential skin problems
and make any necessary recommendations about the use of special bedding, including a special air mattress, mattress overlay,
or other products designed to prevent skin breakdown. In addition to appropriate bedding, it is important for you to turn and
reposition yourself at least every two hours throughout the day
and night.

Why is skin breakdown a serious problem for someone with MS?

Skin breakdown is a serious problem for anyone. A pressure sore
can develop in a few hours but take several months to heal. Once
a sore has formed, long periods of immobility are required to
relieve pressure and provide adequate air to the affected area.
Such periods of immobility can easily cause troublesome sec-

ondary problems. Untreated sores can lead to an infection of the underlying bone (osteomyelitis), which is difficult to treat. Since the skin protects the body from outside infections, its breakdown can allow the tissues underneath to become infected. This type of infection might ultimately lead to septicemia (blood poisoning), which can be life-threatening.

I recently developed a pressure sore on my buttocks. What is the treatment for this type of sore?

Any area of the skin that has become reddened should be massaged regularly with a skin lotion. You should change your position frequently so that the area has plenty of exposure to the air. Be sure to notify your doctor or nurse immediately if you have already developed a small opening in the skin. Your physician will start you on a treatment regimen that involves keeping the area clean (with a providone iodine solution such as Betadine®), dry, and pressure-free. If the sore has gone below the surface of the skin, the wound will be kept dry and open until the deeper area has healed. The nurse will monitor the status of the sore on a regular and frequent basis and keep your physician informed. Since the sore is on your buttocks, you will need to remain in bed and on your side or stomach for fairly long periods each day in order for it to heal. If the decubitus continues to grow deeper or wider, you will probably need to go into the hospital for further treatment involving antibiotics to prevent infection and immersion in a whirlpool-type bath for deep cleansing of the area. While in the hospital, you may also be given a special Clinitron® bed that promotes healing of the skin. A flotation effect, created by tiny, constantly moving, silicone balls, relieves pressure on your skin without your having to move or turn.

My doctor has said that I may need surgery for a pressure sore. Why would surgery be needed and how is the procedure done?

Occasionally, pressure sores do not respond to the measures already described. The blood circulation in the area of the sore may simply be too impaired for the healing process to proceed. If your decubitus has continued to worsen in spite of all treatment efforts, surgery may be required to close it. During surgery, any dead (necrotic) tissue in the area will be removed. A piece (flap) of skin from another area of your body that has better circulation may then be grafted onto the area of the sore. In the rare instances in which this type of surgery is required, healing of both the grafted skin and the area from which it was taken is generally quite successful.

Does my diet have anything to do with the condition of my skin? Are there any foods that will protect me from skin breakdown?

Skin integrity depends on activity and exercise, your general state of health, and adequate nutrition. While one factor alone is unlikely to cause skin breakdown, a combination of deficits in any of these areas can certainly lead to problems. No specific food or diet will protect your skin from breaking down. Your best strategy for avoiding skin breakdown is to keep your skin clean, free of urine and other irritants, and moisturized; learn the exercises you need to know in order to enhance circulation and relieve areas of pressure on your body; and maintain a healthy diet.

I know that lying constantly in one position can be harmful to my skin, but it is very difficult for me turn myself over. Is there anything I can do to make the turning easier so that I don't have to ask my husband (or aide) to help me turn?

Your physician can refer you to a physical or occupational therapist for a home evaluation of this problem. Depending on your physical abilities and the type of bed you have, these professionals can help you learn ways to maneuver yourself independently. Some people can make use of bars on the side of the bed to pull themselves over. There is also a bedsheet available that has fabric strips to allow people to turn and position themselves in bed.

Recommended Readings

Carroll D, Dorman J. *Living Well with MS*. New York: HarperCollins, 1993.

Lechtenberg R. *Multiple Sclerosis Fact Book*. Philadelphia: F.A. Davis, 1995.

Maloney F, Burks J, Ringel S. *Interdisciplinary Rehabilitation of Multiple Sclerosis and Neuromuscular Disorders*. New York: J.B. Lippincott, 1985.

Rosner L, Ross S. *Multiple Sclerosis. New Hope and Practical Advice for People with MS and their Families*. New York: Simon and Schuster, 1992.

Schapiro R. *Multiple Sclerosis: A Rehabilitation Approach to Management.* New York: Demos Vermande, 1991.

Schapiro R. *Symptom Management in Multiple Sclerosis (2nd edition).* New York: Demos Vermande, 1994.

Scheinberg L, Holland N. (eds). *Multiple Sclerosis: A Guide for Patients and Their Families (2nd edition).* New York: Raven Press, 1987.

Selected booklets available from the National Multiple Sclerosis Society (Customer Service: 212-986–3240; Information: 800-344-4867)

◇ *Understanding Bladder Problems in MS*—Nancy J. Holland, Ed.D., and Michele G. Madonna, R.N., M.A.

◇ *Facts and Issues* (reprints of articles from the National Multiple Sclerosis Society magazine, *Inside MS*).

◇ "Me? Use a Catheter?"

◇ *Understanding Bowel Problems in MS*—Nancy J. Holland, Ed.D., with Robin Frames.

5

Physical Therapy

Angela Chan, B.P.T.

The *physical therapist* is a health care professional trained to evaluate and improve movement and function of the body, with particular emphasis on physical mobility, balance, posture, fatigue, and pain. Many factors affect the abilities of people with MS to be as physically active as they would like to be. Physical therapy (PT) has as its goal to help people meet the mobility challenges and physical demands in their family, work, and social lives while accommodating the physical changes brought about by the disease.

In PT, the therapist and person with MS work as a team to minimize limitations imposed by MS, maximize functional ability and overall quality of life, and prevent debilitating complications. The therapist recommends various treatment strategies following a thorough physical and functional evaluation. The individual provides the determination and commitment to follow through with the treatment regimen as well as valuable feedback to the therapist. It is only with this feedback that the therapist can accurately determine if the treatment is working effectively and make any necessary revisions in the treatment plan. There are three important components to a successful PT program:

◇ education for people with MS and their family members about the physical problems caused by the disease, and what can and cannot be done to alleviate current problems and prevent future ones;

◇ an individualized exercise program designed to deal with these problems; and

◇ mobility enhancement through the use of a variety of mobility aids, adaptive equipment for the home, office, and automobile, and education about community resources.

Evaluation

How will I know if I need to be seen by a physical therapist?

Your first contact with a physical therapist is likely to be initiated by your physician. A person with MS is most commonly referred to PT by the physician for an exercise regimen designed to help one or more symptoms. If your physician has not yet mentioned PT to you, you can ask whether it would be beneficial to you and if it is available in your area. Many people maintain intermittent contact with the physical therapist over the course of their MS, consulting the therapist for treatment recommendations as specific physical problems become bothersome and affect their ability to engage in normal activity. Periodic evaluation by a physical therapist is helpful not only in managing current problems but also in identifying and preventing potential ones.

How do I get in touch with a physical therapist?

When referring you for physical therapy, your physician will probably select a therapist in your area and tell you how to make contact. Many physical therapists work in health care facilities such as hospitals, community health centers, and rehabilitation centers. Others have a private practice, seeing patients in their office or in the patients' homes. Depending on where the therapist works, most PT services are funded by Medicare, Medicaid, or a private insurance plan. In Canada, PT is covered by the provincial health care plan or private insurance plans. Some private practitioners who work in an outpatient center or in the home are available only on a fee-for-service basis.

How will the physical therapist evaluate my problems?

The physical therapist will perform a thorough physical and functional assessment that includes evaluating your posture and body movements; measuring muscle strength; assessing flexibility of the muscles, tendons and joints; assessing your ability to discriminate sensations such as heat and cold, pain, pressure, touch, and movement; and evaluating your mobility at work, at home, and in the community.

Mobility is an area of specialty for most physical therapists—improving your ability to get around is the therapist's primary objective. The therapist performs a gait analysis to assess your capabilities in walking and mobility; this involves observing how you walk and identifying causes of change in your normal walking pattern. In gait analysis, as in posture assessment, actions and interactions of various body parts are studied. The actions of each leg individually and both legs in sequence are observed, together with such factors as speed, rhythm, stride length, step length, and distance. The "what" and "when" of any walking device will also be noted.

The assessment also includes taking a comprehensive history that focuses on the impact of the illness on role performance and satisfaction at home and at work, as well as overall quality of life. Family members, friends, and caregivers can provide useful background information and share their perspectives of the impact of MS on a person's life. However, each individual with MS is unique in being able to describe his or her own frustrations and limitations and in setting personal goals for physical therapy.

Both the therapist's assessment and your personal history are essential when determining the factors that contribute to your problems. Together they form the basis of the physical therapist's plan of action, the strategies that the therapist will work with you to implement in order to maximize your mobility and enhance your physical and functional capabilities.

The Role of Exercise

Are there different types of exercise?

There is wide variation in the types of exercise that a physical therapist may recommend.

◇ *Strengthening exercises* are designed to make the body stronger. Weights, exercise elastic, or machines may be used to provide resistance so that your muscles have to work harder. Regular workouts build up muscle size and increase your ability to perform exercise. The physical therapist will design an exercise program to strengthen specific weakened muscles. Depending on the strength of these muscles, weights or other forms of resistance may be recommended.

◇ *Range of motion exercises* are performed to ensure that each joint is moved throughout the full range of available movement, with the objective being to maintain joint flexibility. Joint mobility is dependent on many factors; tightness of the joint capsule, ligaments, and tendons may individually or in combination restrict joint movements. Joint stiffness may occur when swelling is present or after an injury. If movement of the joint does not occur on a regular basis, the joint will become stiff and interfere with normal movement.

◇ *Stretching exercises* are recommended for muscles and tendons that have lost their elasticity. When muscles and tendons around a joint lose this elasticity, the person feels stiff and finds it difficult to move. These exercises help to maintain the elasticity or stretchability of tissues and to prevent **contractures.**

◇ *Resisted exercises* are performed against some form of resistance, e.g., weights or exercise elastic, and help promote and maintain strength.

◇ *Fitness exercises* are designed to maintain general health and well-being rather than for a specific problem or symptom.

◇ *Exercises for cardiovascular fitness* are designed to increase heart rate and thus improve blood circulation and aerobic function.

The exercises prescribed by the physical therapist can also be divided according to the degree of assistance required by the person performing them: *active exercises* are performed completely independently; *active assisted exercises* require some assistance by another person; *passive exercises* are performed by a helper (therapist or caregiver) if a person is unable to perform them independently. Thus, a person performing *active range of motion* exercises might do leg extensions at a variety of angles; the person engaged in *passive range of motion exercises* would need the therapist or caregiver to move the leg into the appropriate positions.

In what ways will exercise help my MS?

Exercises can help your MS by developing and strengthening those muscles that continue to have adequate nerve conduction and by helping to maintain the tone of those with inadequate nerve conduction. Exercise will train your muscles to work better individually or together and may thereby improve coordination in your arms and legs. Thus, an exercise program can help you learn ways of walking and moving that compensate somewhat for the neurologic changes caused by MS. Exercises are also used to improve range of motion and to help relieve mild **spasticity**, balance problems, and some types of pain. It is important to remember, however, that exercise cannot reverse the disease process or undo damage that has been done to the nervous system.

How can I find out what type of exercise is best for me?

Exercises designed to address your particular needs are best prescribed by your neurologist or physical therapist. Trainers in a fitness or health club can develop a general fitness program for you, but keep in mind that they probably do not understand MS and the ways in which neurologic changes affect your body. Be sure to check with your physician before beginning any type of exercise program.

Are there any types of exercise that are harmful to me now that I have MS?

No specific exercises are harmful to individuals with MS. Common sense will be your best ally here. In general, your body will tell you how it is responding to exercise and will certainly let you know if it cannot tolerate the exercise program you have chosen. Be careful not to exert yourself to the point of exhaustion or raise your body temperature so much that you activate your MS symptoms. Although these momentary symptoms are indicative of being overheated rather than of any kind of disease activity or progression, they can be uncomfortable and unnerving. Regular, moderate exercise with periodic rest breaks will enable you to get maximum benefit from your exercise program and avoid unnecessary discomfort.

Is weight training helpful for the weakness that I feel in my arms and legs?

The weakness you are experiencing in your arms and legs is probably the result of impaired nerve conduction to the muscles involved, and the feelings of weakness are probably caused by neurologic changes rather than by weakness in the muscles themselves. Weight training cannot improve nerve conduction and thus will not improve neurologically-based weakness. Weight training is good for developing and strengthening muscles that *do* have adequate nerve conduction. Your neurologist can evaluate the weakness in various parts of your body and advise you as to its causes. A physical therapist can then design for you a fitness program that specifically addresses the types of weakness you are experiencing.

How can I exercise effectively now that I have lost so much strength in my arms and legs?

If you are unable to perform active exercise because of problems with weakness, spasticity, or imbalance, the physical therapist can work with you on assisted and passive exercises that are more appropriate for your needs. It is important to remember that exercise programs are not all designed for strength or endurance; exercise is equally important for maintaining flexibility, range of motion, posture, and muscle tone.

I feel so fatigued most of the time that my regular daily activities use up all the energy I have. How can I possibly exercise when I feel so tired?

Reduced energy level and reduced endurance are common problems for people with MS. Fatigue is recognized as a real and valid symptom that may have a variety of causes. The physical therapist can help you understand the various causes of your fatigue and explore with you ways of optimizing your energy and reducing fatigue. You may be able to conserve energy and minimize tiredness by doing various activities in a slightly different way, making more effective use of tools or strategies to save time and reduce unnecessary effort, or creating small rest periods in your day. Walking or mobility aids are sometimes prescribed to increase a person's ability to cover greater distances with less fatigue. Additionally, the physical therapist can teach you types of exercise that are less physically strenuous and demanding than ones you might have done in the past. Exercise does not have to be fast or vigorous in order to provide you with substantial benefit. In fact, an important benefit of some exercises is increased relaxation.

Should I join a health club or an exercise class to get my exercise?

Some general fitness exercises can be performed in a health club or in an exercise class setting. Added benefits of exercising outside the home are socialization, encouragement and feedback from the instructor and fellow participants, and the benefits of a structured program. Going out to participate is also evidence of commitment. Keep in mind, however, that the staff members in a health club are generally not trained to understand or treat neurologic symptoms. Consult with your physician before beginning any exercise program. If you require an exercise program that is more appropriate to your physical symptoms, your physician will refer you to a physical therapist.

Is swimming a good exercise for me?

Water is an excellent medium for exercise. It allows weakened muscles to move more easily while providing sufficient resistance to help strengthen other muscles. Water also helps to stabilize a person who has balance problems. Because swimming is a highly coordinated physical activity involving the whole body, it helps to regulate breathing and build endurance. Your physical therapist can develop a personalized exercise program for you to do in the water.

It is advisable to gather some information before you go to a swimming pool. How far is it from the changing room and the toilet to the pool? Is someone available to provide assistance in and out of the pool if necessary? What is the temperature of the water? Although people react differently to water temperature, many with MS cannot tolerate heat. A water temperature of 86° F seems to be the most comfortable for individuals with MS. The temperature of a "therapeutic pool" is frequently too hot.

If you are experiencing any MS-related bladder symptoms that might interfere with your comfort in the swimming pool, talk them over with your neurologist or nurse before beginning a swimming program.

Is there any reason for me to stop playing the recreational sports that I enjoy?

The answer to this question depends on the symptoms of MS that you are experiencing and their impact on your enjoyment of any particular sport. If you can physically play the sport, even if not as well as before, then you should probably continue to do so. Too many people stop playing sports as soon as they are diagnosed or because they can't play as well as they did in the past. There is no reason to stop playing your sport unless you feel that you are putting yourself at risk of injury. Stopping prematurely will deny you recreation and enjoyment, as well as the benefits of exercise and the continued challenge to your body. The point is to adapt to change, not to stop living because of it.

Because of MS I'm not getting as much exercise as I used to and I'm putting on weight. What should I do?

Weight control is an issue of concern for almost everyone, and becomes more challenging when symptoms of MS make a person less mobile and more fatigued. Some form of aerobic exercise on a regular basis promotes general health and well-being. Numerous exercise programs are offered by community Parks and Recreation Programs, the local YMCA, or health clubs. With the help of your physician or physical therapist, choose the type of exercise that meets your needs and interests. If your endurance and ability are limited, you might consider a senior's fitness program as another option. Additionally, it may be necessary to reduce your food intake somewhat in order to compensate for your decreased activity level. Ask your physician to recommend a balanced, low-fat diet that can help you control the weight gain.

My posture seems to have changed since I've had MS. Are there exercises that will improve my posture?

Posture is a key area in the PT assessment. The therapist will observe the position of your head, neck, shoulders, body, pelvis, hips, knees, ankles, and feet. Standing posture as well as posture during movement are noted. The physical therapist is able to identify areas of muscle weakness and/or stiffness and develop corrective movements targeting these areas. Maintaining good posture is important not only for the sake of your appearance, but also to prevent uncomfortable muscle and joint strain and secondary back problems that can arise from standing, sitting, and moving improperly.

Is yoga helpful to a person who has MS?

Yoga is an excellent form of exercise for people with MS because it involves a lot of stretching exercises for the whole body. The controlled breathing exercises promote relaxation of the mind and the body and help people to be more in tune with their bodies. As with any other form of exercise, it is important that the yoga exercises be tailored to your particular physical needs and limitations.

Is Tai-Chi a good form of exercise for someone with MS?

Tai-Chi is another excellent form of exercise for individuals with MS. Tai-Chi movements are slow and controlled with periodic quick changes in position. Many of the movements in Tai-Chi require good balance; try to perform your exercise routine close to a grab bar or railing in case you need to steady yourself. Once learned, performing Tai-Chi can also be relaxing. This form of exercise requires mental discipline and controlled breathing.

My neurologist has referred me to a physical therapist for treatment of pain I have developed in my shoulders, back, and legs. How can exercises help without causing me more pain than I'm already feeling?

Physical therapists contribute to pain reduction through non-medication means, including the use of heat or ice treatments, exercise, and teaching proper positioning or support for the body. Problems with balance and ambulation often cause changes in posture, and these postural changes can gradually result in secondary pain in the lower back, hips, and knees. The use of *ambulation aids* such as crutches or walkers can also contribute to secondary pain in the shoulders and upper back. In evaluating your pain symptoms, the initial task for the physical therapist will be to determine the source of the problem. If the pain is a result of changes in your posture, balance, or gait, the

therapist may design a treatment regimen that involves education about the mechanism of your problem as well as exercises
designed to improve the impaired functions that are contributing to the pain. Rather than giving you additional pain, the exercises involved will actually reduce pain by alleviating its causes. Additionally, the therapist may recommend the use of a new
or different mechanical aid, such as a cane, walker, or wheelchair, if any of these would contribute to a reduction in the pain
you are experiencing.

Can exercise help me with my balance problems?

Balance and safety are areas of primary concern for the physical
therapist and common problems for many with MS. Impaired
balance in MS results primarily from **plaques** in the **cerebellum** and **brainstem**, but can also be caused by impaired sensation in the soles of the feet and weakness and/or stiffness of any
part of the leg. Even vision impairment may contribute to poor
equilibrium. The physical therapist will assess your balance in
the standing, sitting, and kneeling positions, as well as while
you are walking. Balance problems that are caused by damage
in the cerebellum and brainstem cannot be corrected by exercise. However, the therapist can recommend particular exercises designed to maximize your ability to maintain your balance
or help you to compensate for changes in your ability to balance. The therapist may also prescribe a walking aid such as a
cane or a walker. Safety is a primary concern since impaired
balance can lead to falls resulting in bruising, swelling, pain,
and even fractures.

**Since my last exacerbation I have been unable to walk. Will
exercising my legs help me to walk again?**

Walking is a complex motor activity that is dependent on many
functions working in a coordinated fashion. Exercising your
legs will maintain flexibility of the joints and muscles, encourage the muscles to work to their best potential, and prevent further muscle deterioration. Therefore, depending on the degree
and location of demyelination that occurred during your last
exacerbation and the amount of spontaneous recovery you
experience, leg exercises might facilitate your efforts to walk
again. However, there is no guarantee since exercise cannot correct neurologic damage done by the disease. Even if walking is

not possible, exercising your legs will help you to sit properly and thereby prevent the pain and stiffness that can result from prolonged sitting.

Can exercise help a person who is unable to walk and spends most of the time in a wheelchair?

Exercise is extremely important for the person who is no longer able to walk. In its various forms, exercise enhances flexibility, posture, strength, and endurance, each of which contributes to comfort and physical well-being. Stiffness in the legs affects a person's ability to sit upright with proper foot positioning. Passive range of motion and stretching exercises can help to relieve this type of stiffness. Exercises for the arms, upper body, and trunk are very important for maintaining good posture, which, in turn, reduces the risk of back and hip strain. Maintaining upper body strength also facilitates transfers in and out of the wheelchair or bed. Additionally, upper body exercises can strengthen the neck or torso and thereby increase a person's ability to sit comfortably for longer periods of time. Any exercise regimen that enhances the mobility of the person in a wheelchair also reduces the risk of skin breakdown (see Chapter 4). People who spend long periods of time in a wheelchair are taught specific exercises designed to shift their weight and thus relieve pressure on areas of the body that are particularly prone to skin breakdown.

My foot is turning in. Are there exercises that can make this better?

When a foot "turns in," the muscles and tendons on the inside of the foot become shortened and the muscles turning the foot out are weakened due to disuse. Without exercise, the ankle joint becomes stiff. Passive and active exercises for the muscles controlling the ankle are vitally important in this situation. The physician or physical therapist may also suggest a special type of leg brace to help with this problem. The key is to begin the treatment regimen before changes to the muscles and joints become permanent.

What exercises can I do to relieve the stiffness I feel in my body?

Stiffness in MS is most often related to the common symptom of *spasticity*, which is caused by a dysregulation of nerve impulses in the spinal cord (see Chapter 2). Very mild spasticity in MS can often be managed effectively with a regimen of stretching and range of motion exercises. These exercises are very important for maintaining flexibility of the muscles and tendons and thereby reducing further stiffness and other complications. The physical therapist will design a specific stretching program for you. Keep in mind, however, that exercises alone may not be sufficient to treat your spasticity. If the stiffness continues or worsens, or if the exercises become too difficult or uncomfortable for you to do, your physician will probably recommend that you use medication in combination with exercise to manage the spasticity.

Walking and Mobility Aids

I've begun to stagger so much when I walk that people think I'm drunk. What can I do about this problem?

Staggering is a symptom of poor balance that is usually caused by disease activity in the cerebellum or brainstem. At this time, no medication or other treatment is very effective for this problem. There are two major consequences of impaired balance; the first is the risk of potentially dangerous falls; the second, unfortunately, is that others often perceive the person who staggers to have a drinking problem. Depending on the cause and extent of your balance problems, your physician or physical therapist will probably recommend a mobility aid such as a cane, forearm (**Lofstrand**) crutch, or walker. The use of a mobility aid will provide you with extra stability and will also send a clear signal to any observer that there is a medical cause for your staggering.

The physical therapist will determine which type of aid is most beneficial for you by evaluating how much additional stability you need. A single cane, for example, adds a point of stability only on one side of your body. A **quad cane**, which has four short legs attached to a small platform at its end, provides greater stability by giving you a broader base on which to lean. The therapist may recommend that you use two canes or crutches if you would benefit from a stabilizing point on each side of your body. If these do not provide sufficient stability, the thera-

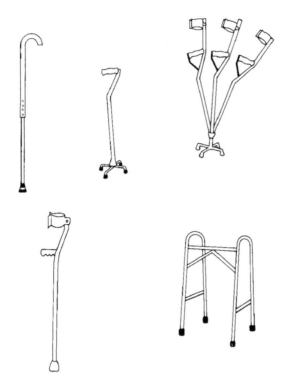

Figure 5-1.   Walking aids. Left to right: straight cane, quad cane, quad cane with swivel-action base, forearm crutch, and walker.

pist may recommend a walker. Because a walker moves directly in front of you, it provides greater stability and also reduces fatigue. Bear in mind that as your needs change, the type of aid that is recommended for you will change as well.

I seem to trip a lot and I've even had a few falls. Why is this happening?

Weakness of your foot or hip muscles, stiffness in your legs, fatigue, and poor balance could, individually or in combination, contribute to tripping and falling. Since falls can have major consequences, the first step in the management of this problem is to identify its source. Having diagnosed the problem, your physician will provide the necessary treatment and/or make the appropriate referral. If, for example, your falls are primarily the result of *foot drop*, you will probably be referred to an *orthotist* or physical therapist for an *ankle-foot orthosis (AFO)*.

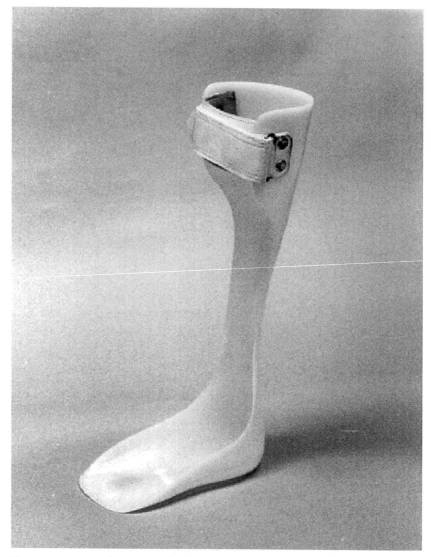

Figure 5-2. A plastic ankle-foot orthosis.

The AFO is a plastic brace that supports a weakened ankle so that you can walk with a heel-to-toe motion and avoid catching your toe on the ground. If tripping is primarily the result of leg weakness, you will probably be referred to a physical therapist for a treatment regimen of exercises and evaluation for a mobility aid such as a cane or walker. If the tripping and falling occur primarily when you are already tired from overexertion, the physical therapist may recommend that you use a mobility aid such as a motorized scooter when you need to cover longer distances.

How will I know if I need to use a walker?

Most people seem to feel that a walker makes them look more disabled, and would therefore prefer to try various types of unilateral supports, e.g., a cane, forearm crutch, or quad cane, before having to switch to a walker. The physician or physical therapist will recommend that you use a walker if you need more stability in order to maintain balance and avoid hazardous falls. A walker also requires less energy. Some walkers have (two or four) wheels, hand brakes, a seat, and a basket for carrying things. The specific walker should be selected with special attention to your individual needs. You may find that a particular type of equipment works best for you in one situation while another type of aid is more useful in a different situation; the major objectives are to maintain stability and safety, conserve energy, and get the job done.

If I use a leg splint or brace, will my leg muscles become weak or useless?

A foot or leg splint is generally prescribed because of muscle weakness. In other words, the splint does not cause weakness; rather it substitutes for muscles that are already weakened due to lack of adequate nerve innervation. Since it is true that certain muscles in the foot are not required to work as much when a splint is used, the physical therapist always prescribes stretching and active exercise to be done during the hours the splint is off. This will ensure the preservation of normal movement, which will, in turn, promote normal muscle action in both legs as well as the rest of the body.

Although I can walk around the house, I can't walk more than a block without getting weak. What should I do? I don't want to be stuck at home all the time.

Weakness and fatigue are limiting your ability to walk distances. Depending on your physical needs, the type of neighborhood in which you live, and your regular mode of transportation, a mobility aid such as a wheelchair or motorized scooter could greatly enhance your mobility and ability to enjoy life outside your home. People often believe that as long as they can walk at all, they have no use for this type of equipment. As a result, they use all of their available energy just getting from point A to point B and then have no energy left to enjoy themselves or get back again! A scooter is actually designed to be used by a person who is independent, ambulatory, and on the go. By using a scooter to get from place to place, you conserve your energy and also get more things accomplished.

You will probably find that your family and friends are very supportive of your decision to use a mobility aid. You will once again be able to participate with them in a variety of activities that previously felt too difficult, too tiring, and too slow, including trips to restaurants, the shopping mall, the zoo, a museum—and even Disney World.

Do not buy any piece of equipment without first consulting with a health care professional. Your physician can help you to identify the exact nature of your walking problem and energy shortage. If your needs can be met with a mobility aid, a physical therapist can help you choose the type that would be most useful. Too much money is involved to make any decisions based solely on the advice of a salesperson, no matter how well-intentioned he or she may be. Equipment should meet your current needs as well as your future needs. A salesperson does not understand your medical condition and the potential changes you may experience in the future, and therefore cannot and should not advise you on what is the best equipment for you.

What is the difference between a manual wheelchair, a motorized scooter, and an electric wheelchair? How do I know which is best for me? Does insurance pay for any of them?

A manual wheelchair is a non-motorized mobility device. A person who wants to use this type of wheelchair without assistance from another person needs to have sufficient upper body strength to propel the chair. If you have significant upper body weakness or fatigue, another person will need to assist you. The advantage of this type of mobility aid is that it is collapsible and hence easy to transport. Some people who are quite ambulatory most of the time keep a lightweight, portable wheelchair in the trunk of the car for use in places like shopping malls that have great distances to cover.

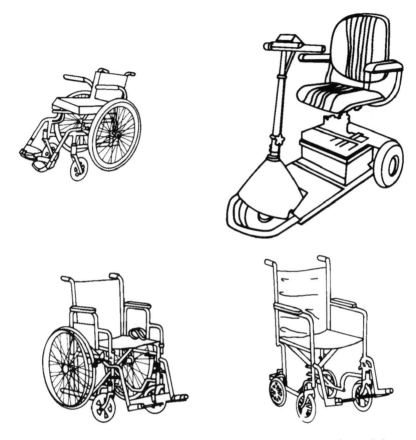

Figure 5-3.   Different types of wheelchairs. (**A**) sports chair, (**B**) scooter, (**C**) standard wheelchair, and (**D**) chair with small wheels, which must be pushed.

A motorized scooter is a vehicle that resembles a golf cart. It typically has three or four wheels, runs on rechargeable batteries, and is driven by a thumb push mechanism. To use a scooter effectively, you need to be able to stand and transfer into the seat. This requires standing ability, a fairly high degree of mobility, and adequate balance. Electric scooters can be disassembled and put into your car. Depending on the size and style of your car, it is possible to install an electric lift that will raise the heaviest parts of the scooter into the trunk. Scooters now come in a bewildering variety of styles, sizes, and weights. Some are designed primarily for indoor use while others can travel very well over outdoor terrain. All can be taken on an airplane as checked baggage.

A motorized wheelchair has a battery and is driven with a stick control by the person sitting in the wheelchair. This type of chair is useful for the person who cannot stand and transfer independently, and needs more seating support than is provided by the seat of an electric scooter. Its major limitation is that it is not collapsible or easily transportable. The person who wants to use an electric wheelchair independently within the community will probably need a wheelchair-equipped van for transportation. Both the scooter and the motorized wheelchair are good alternatives for someone who does not like the feeling of being pushed from behind. It is quite easy to "wheel" alongside a companion, carrying on a conversation and feeling completely independent.

Many factors must be considered before deciding what equipment is best for you. Your physician and physical therapist can evaluate your physical requirements and tell you which option(s) would be best for you. Once you know which types of equipment would meet your needs safely, the physical therapist will assist you to think through the following questions: Where do I want to be able to use this equipment? Where will I store the equipment when I am not using it? How will I transport it from one place to another? Will I be able to get the equipment in and out of my home? Will I be able to use this equipment independently or will I need someone else's help? Answering these questions will help you to select the particular equipment that meets your needs most effectively.

Some government agencies and insurance plans pay the entire cost or a portion of the cost of mobility equipment. Since physical therapists are aware of the different funding sources and their requirements, they may be able to help you to apply for funding.

If I start to use a wheelchair to go long distances, will I lose the ability to walk?

No. Inability to walk is caused by demyelination, not by using a wheelchair. Due to increased fatigue or diminishing endurance, you may wish to use a wheelchair or scooter to increase your mobility at work or in the community. Or you may begin to use a mobility aid for high energy outings such as trips to malls, museums, or the zoo. Using the mobility equipment to enhance your life and broaden your scope of activities will not cause your symptoms to worsen. A mobility aid is not the cause of weakness or fatigue—it is the solution to these two common problems.

Should I purchase a secondhand wheelchair?

Like eyeglasses, mobility equipment is prescribed specifically to fit you. Each person has a different physical build as well as different MS symptoms that must be accommodated. A tall, heavy person with balance problems and a weak right side would need a very different size and style of equipment than a small person whose primary symptom is severe fatigue. Since your prescription for mobility equipment takes into account all of your specific physical characteristics and symptoms, your mobility aid is not interchangeable with that of another person.

It is difficult for me to get around town to do my errands and take care of household business without having someone to help me. Can a physical therapist be of help with this problem?

In addition to recommending the appropriate mobility equipment, the physical therapist is one of several possible sources of information about transportation in your community (including MS Care Centers, your local chapter of the National Multiple Sclerosis Society, and other members of your health care team). The therapist may help you to obtain a disabled license plate from the local motor vehicle department, which will enable you to make use of handicapped parking spaces. The therapist can also show you how to apply for access to any available public transit programs for the disabled, or for a designated disabled parking spot near your home, school, or work place.

This is only a sample of the questions commonly asked of physical therapists. Questions more specific to your own situation should be directed to your own therapist. Although two individuals with MS may seem to have the same symptoms, the underlying causes of these symptoms may be quite different. It is best to get an individual assessment of your particular situation.

Acknowledgment

Appreciation is extended to D.J. Chrysler and C. Lee of the Physiotherapy Department of St. Michael's Hospital, Toronto, for their valuable contribution to this chapter.

Recommended Readings

Blonsky R. *The Exercise Program (2nd edition)*. New York: Demos Vermande, 1988.

Kraft GH, Catanzaro M. *Living with Multiple Sclerosis: A Wellness Approach*. New York: Demos Vermande, 1996.

Schapiro R. *Symptom Management in Multiple Sclerosis (2nd edition)*. New York: Demos Vermande, 1991

Selected booklets available from the National Multiple Sclerosis Society (Customer Service: 212-986-3240; Information: 800-344-4867)

◇ *Moving with Multiple Sclerosis*—Iris Kimberg, M.S., O.T.R., R.P.T.

◇ *The Rehab Outlook*—Lisa J. Bain and Randall T. Schapiro, M.D.

Facts and Issues (reprints of articles from the National Multiple Sclerosis Society magazine, *Inside MS*).

◇ *Digging for Clues to Fatigue*

◇ *Getting a Grip on Gait*

Reprint available from the Canadian Multiple Sclerosis Society (416-922-6065)

◇ *Coping with Fatigue in MS Takes Understanding and Planning*—Alexander Burnfield, M.B., M.R.C. Psych.

6

Occupational Therapy

Jean Hietpas, O.T.R., L.C.S.W.

Due to the nature of the disease process, the symptoms of multiple sclerosis can vary greatly from one individual to another. For some, the symptoms may be slight, such as tingling in the hands or mild weakness. For others, the symptoms may be more severe, possibly including problems such as **paresis** (weakness), balance problems, alterations in sensation, fatigue, difficulty with coordination, vision loss, speech disturbances, and **cognitive impairment**.

In addition to the variety of symptoms, a person with MS can also experience variation in the progression of symptoms. Some people experience fluctuations between periods of **remission** (recovery) and episodes of **exacerbation** (worsening). Others experience increasingly severe symptoms over the course of time with little or no remission (see Chapter 2).

Occupational therapy assists individuals to manage both the variety of symptoms and the variations in symptom progression. The therapy focuses on maintaining everyday living skills that are essential for independent living, such as dressing, bathing, grooming, meal preparation, writing, and driving. The **occupational therapist** (OT) tailors treatment to specific individual needs and deficits based on the variation in MS symptoms and disease progression. The goal of treatment is to develop and support individual abilities and adaptations that promote functional independence in everyday living and maintain quality of life.

The OT addresses four major areas that are essential to maintaining independence:

◇ upper body strength, movement, and coordination;

◇ aids to independent living (including practice with ***activities of daily living*** *(ADL)* skills, ADL equipment, wheelchairs, and environmental access);

◇ compensatory strategies for impairment in thinking, sensation problems, or vision loss;

◇ fatigue management through education about energy conservation, work simplification, and stress management.

The OT uses both assessment and treatment tools to manage MS-related problems. Assessment, which is often an ongoing process, involves both the expertise of the OT and the active participation of the person with MS. As part of the assessment process, you will be asked about your home and work environment, including your ability to maneuver around your kitchen, bathroom, and living area, as well as access in and out of your home or work situation. The OT will also evaluate your sitting and standing abilities, as well as the strength and ease of upper body movement. Once problem areas have been identified, the OT will work with you to develop a treatment plan to correct or manage these problems.

I'm experiencing increasing weakness in my hands and fingers. Will exercise make my hands strong again? What exercises are best for this problem?

Our hands are the "doing" centers for many of our everyday tasks. Many of the jobs we need to do become frustrating and difficult when hand strength and coordination decrease. The weakness that you experience as the result of MS is due to reduced nerve conduction rather than weakened muscles. Therefore, the primary goal is not necessarily to increase hand strength (although for some people the hands do become stronger), but to maintain existing dexterity and muscle strength as much as possible. Your OT will prescribe active range of motion exercises such as opening and closing the hands, and mild resistance exercises such as a thera-putty exercise program. Exercise programs need to be individualized so that the appropriate muscles are involved, especially if stiffness or spasticity is present.

It seems to take so much effort just to get up in the morning and deal with bathing, dressing, and breakfast. Is there something I can do to make those tasks easier and less tiring?

The principles to keep in mind with all of your activities of daily living (ADLs) are to simplify your life and conserve energy. When MS fatigue interferes with your ability to perform the basic physical tasks, take time to think about your routine. Contemplate how you can simplify, plan, and reorganize your routine to conserve your energy. Examples of energy conservation might include such simple changes as taking a shower in the evening so that you have less to do in the morning. If you are heat-sensitive, consider taking a cool or lukewarm shower rather than a fatigue-producing hot shower. Build two- to three-minute rests into your schedule so that you do not get overly exhausted. Consider selecting your clothes for the next day and putting them on a bedside chair before you go to bed in the evening. As you purchase clothes now and in the future, try to select items that are easy to take on and off and require a minimum of energy to maintain. Similarly, plan your breakfast the night before, and leave the nonperishable items and dishes on the counter or table so that they are ready to use in the morning.

My hands feel weak and clumsy most of the time. Is there anything to help tie my shoes and button my shirt?

A variety of products are now available (see ADL equipment on p. 123) to help with frustrating tasks such as tying shoes and buttoning shirts. Various options are available if you are able to bend over and reach your shoes, including "no-bows," a spring-loaded lace tightener; velcro shoe closures; and even one-hand shoe-tying techniques. If you are not able to reach your feet, you can replace your cotton shoelaces with elastic ones that will turn your tie shoes into slip-ons. With the elastic laces tied in place, have a shoemaker stitch the shoe tongue in place and use a long-handled shoehorn to put on your shoes. Another simple solution is a well-fitting pair of slip-on shoes. Some people find it tiring and difficult to pull on their socks. A gadget is available that will help you to pull a sock over your toes and up the calf more easily.

Buttoning is made simpler with a buttonhook, which is used to pull the button through the buttonhole with a minimum of strength and dexterity. Some people prefer to wear shirts with large, easy to grasp buttons, pullovers, or polo-type shirts, which have very few buttons. Catalogues containing these and other products are available for consumers. You will discover numerous ways to streamline many aspects of your daily routines as you begin to look for ways to conserve time and energy.

Dressing is becoming a tiring and time-consuming task. What kinds of clothing are simple to put on, simple to take care of, and still look good enough for me to wear to work?

Energy conservation is important to consider in the dressing process. Generally, over-sized clothes or shirts and blouses with large buttons down the front are easier to get on and off. Likewise, loose-fitting slacks with an elastic waist are comfortable and easy to pull on and off (see reference list under clothing). Adaptive aids such as dressing sticks, sock aids, and long-handled shoehorns can be helpful when you are trained by an OT to be proficient in their use (see references under ADL equipment).

Women can add a scarf or jewelry to almost any kind of pullover shirt or sweater to enhance it. Men may find it useful to wear clip-on ties or to leave their neckties tied so that they need only be slipped over the head and tightened. Dress shirts can remain permanently buttoned except for the top buttons. Another strategy is to remove the buttons, close the buttonholes, and reattach the buttons on top of the buttonholes. Velcro pieces can then be sewn behind the buttonholes and on the original button sites for easy closure.

What underwear can a man get on and off without standing up that is also convenient for bathroom functions?

Several companies specialize in adaptive clothing for health care needs. A man's velcro closure underpant can be taken on and off from a seated position (see "Avenues Unlimited" catalogue). The President's Committee on Employment of People with Disabilities created a resource list of clothing for people with disabilities (see reference list under clothing). Many companies have free or minimal charge catalogs for mail-order shopping.

Getting on and (especially) off the toilet has become difficult. Are there any modifications I can make that will ease this problem?

Several modifications can be made to facilitate toileting, some having to do with your body mechanics, others with adaptive equipment. It is important to pay attention to the placement of both your arms and feet when changing from the seated to standing position. With your feet placed firmly in front of you, use your hands and arms to push off from the toilet seat. To go from a standing to a sitting position, place yourself squarely in front of the toilet seat, bend your knees until you can touch each side of the toilet seat with your hands, and then lower yourself slowly to the seat.

The simplest mechanical aid to help you get on and off the toilet is a secure grab bar on the wall next to the toilet. Obviously, this is only effective if the toilet is adjacent to a wall.

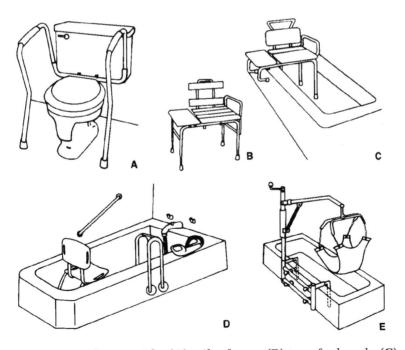

Figure 6-1 Bathroom aids. (**A**) toilet frame, (**B**) transfer bench, (**C**) bathing bench, (**D**) shower chair, lifeguard rail, diagonal grab bar, and hand-held shower hose, and (**E**) patient lifter and bath attachment.

An over-the-toilet commode frame allows for adjustability in the height of the seat and provides bilateral armrests to assist you in lowering and raising your body. A number of other medical equipment items such as an elevated toilet seat and side rails can be helpful. These items are available through a local medical supplier or through the ADL equipment companies referenced at the end of this chapter. An OT can be helpful in determining which piece of equipment best suits your needs.

I'm concerned that I'm not adequately cleaning myself after toileting. Are there ways to do this more effectively?

Independence in toileting is a very personal matter, yet one that can be problematic because of poor sitting balance or limited use of the hands. Try using a wet washcloth to wipe yourself or have a squeeze bottle with warm water to rinse yourself after toileting. Several toileting aids, such as a toilet paper holder, are available through ADL equipment suppliers (see reference list). Also available are portable or permanently installed bidets that rinse and, in some models, dry the posterior portion of the body.

Getting in and out of the shower-tub combination has become difficult for me. Do you have any suggestions for making this job easier and safer?

It is important to make sure that the transition or transfer in and out of the shower stall or tub-shower is safe. Both balance and a certain amount of strength are necessary for safe transfers. If your balance is in question, the easiest solution is to install a grab bar to hold onto during the transfer. Grab bars should be permanently mounted to the wall (your local hardware store can recommend a handyman to install them). Your physician or an OT can assess your upper body strength to determine if you are able to use a grab bar to assist with the transfer safely and independently. If your upper body strength is not sufficient or if your lower body is too weak, the OT may recommend a tub transfer bench for a seated transfer in and out of the tub-shower.

A shower chair or bench is the answer if your standing balance and tolerance are not sufficient to allow you to stand confidently during your shower. They are available through your local medical supply company and can be found in the Yellow Pages under medical equipment. A shower chair should be adjustable in height so you can set it to your comfort. A hand-held shower hose will make a seated shower more enjoyable, and a non-slip mat in the tub or shower stall will help prevent a fall.

Getting up and out of a chair is becoming harder for me. What is the best type of chair for me to sit in and are there any recommended techniques or gadgets that will make it easier for me to get up again?

The best type of chair is one that is relatively high off the ground and has solid arms. Height is critical—it is always more difficult to get out of low, soft, easy chairs. Chairs are generally 17" or 18" from the floor to the top of the seat. You can add a 2"–3" foam cushion to raise the height of your chair or add leg extenders (rubber cups that fit on the legs of the chair) to raise the seat height. It will be easier to get up from a chair if you scoot forward first and then push up from the chair with your hands on the arms of the chair. If these adaptations are not sufficient, there are portable lifter cushions that you can place on your own chair, or chairs with built-in lifter seats, that will gently propel you out of a seated position. Many of the companies that offer these products are referenced at the end of the chapter under chair lifts or ADL equipment suppliers.

My bed is so low that I have a hard time getting out of it. Are there ways to modify my bed that will solve this problem?

Getting up from low surfaces can be difficult. First, pay attention to your body mechanics: try rolling onto your side, facing the edge of the bed, and pushing yourself up with your bottom arm while swinging your legs over the side of the bed. If you have trouble rolling over onto your side, you can purchase sheets with fabric pull strips sewn onto them or grab bars that can be attached to the sides of your mattress. Once in a sitting position on the edge of the bed, try to push yourself up with your hands. If the bed is too low or too soft for you to be able to push yourself upright, you can raise the height of the bed by placing it on wood blocks. Strategically placing a grab bar on the wall next to your bed, or a floor-to-ceiling pole next to the bed, can allow you to pull yourself from a sitting position to a standing position. Floor-to-ceiling poles are available through your local medical equipment suppliers listed in local Yellow Pages of your telephone directory.

I'm looking for a new car. Is there anything in particular I should take into consideration when selecting one?

Take your time when selecting a new car. Try to anticipate what your needs might be in the future as well as thinking carefully about your present needs. For example, a stick shift or standard transmission car might seem more appealing to you now, but can cause future difficulties if you develop weakness or incoordination in your left foot. Compare the ease with which you can get in and out of different models. Operate the door handles, gear shift, turn signal, windshield wipers, horn, cruise control, radio, air conditioning, and seat adjustments to see how easy to manipulate and accessible they are. Always purchase air conditioning in the automobile to prevent fatigue on a hot day. Consider a tilt steering wheel and power seats to give you maximum adjustability and comfort.

Try lifting packages in and out of the back seat and the trunk of the car. Large parcels, grocery bags, a small child, and possibly a wheelchair or other piece of adaptive equipment are examples of the "cargo" that people often need to be able to maneuver in their cars. Vehicles with a lower trunk opening allow you to take items in and out without having to lift them as high off the ground. You may find that a four-door sedan allows easier access to back-seat storage space for crutches or a wheelchair, or that a station wagon or hatch-back vehicle better fits your needs. A minivan or van is also an option to consider if you currently use a power mobility device such as an electric scooter, or anticipate using one in the future. Refer to the list of recommended resources at the end of the chapter for further information about vehicles and vehicle modifications.

Being able to drive my car is very important to me, but my right leg doesn't move as quickly and reliably between pedals as it used to. I've heard about hand controls and I'm wondering whether they could work for me.

Thousands of people operate vehicles with the use of hand controls. They work well for someone who has good upper body control but limited lower body function. Since safe driving depends on a variety of functions, including eye–hand coordination, head and neck flexibility, adequate vision, and reasonable reaction time, it would be well worth your while to seek a driving evaluation before investing in equipment for your car. Ask your physician, OT, or the local chapter of the MS Society for the name of the nearest driver evaluation program. The major car companies also offer listings of driver evaluation programs as well as the names of companies that will perform adaptive modifications on your car (see Vehicle Modifications under Recommended Resources).

Hand controls come in a variety of styles and configurations. They most often are attached to the steering column and look like additional sticks protruding from it. Acceleration and braking are accomplished by pulling the control toward you or pushing it away from you. If turning the steering wheel has become more difficult because of hand or arm weakness, a round knob can be attached to the steering wheel.

When I do the laundry, I have to carry it up and down fourteen stairs. Is there anything I can do to make this process easier and safer?

Carrying items can be dangerous if your standing balance is unstable. Break the task into small, light loads rather than carrying one large load. Or put the laundry in a bag with a drawstring and pull it up and down the stairs behind you. Depending on your staircase, you may be able to create a simple pulley system that allows you to pull the laundry bag up and down the stairs with a minimum amount of strength and exertion. Another solution might be for a family member or neighbor to carry the laundry up and down the stairs. Do not hesitate to recruit assistance for tasks that become too difficult or too dangerous for you to do alone.

Some people find that the sorting and folding of laundry is time-consuming and tiring. Ask family members to presort their own clothes into dark and light piles before bringing them to the washing machine, and to make sure that each item is turned right side out. You can also tell them that anything that is given to you turned inside out will be given back to them clean but still inside out. Depending on the ages of your family members, you might even ask each person to take care of his or her own laundry!

We are planning to redo the bathroom and kitchen in our home. What kinds of modifications would you recommend?

Accessibility and ease of use are the main factors to consider in making home modifications. Several good references to home modifications are available (see reference list).

When designing for accessibility in the bathroom, important features to consider include door width; adequacy of space in which to maneuver; the height and shape of the sink and toilet; the accessibility of the medicine cabinet and other storage areas; access to the shower stall; and the shape and style of faucets and shower heads.

Likewise, a well-designed kitchen can make meal preparation more pleasurable and less exhausting. Carefully placed appliances, counters, sinks, cabinets, and work areas should be considered and discussed when remodeling your kitchen. You will want to be able to reach the items you need without having to do a great deal of walking back and forth or reaching. As with any other long-term, expensive decisions and purchases, try to think not only about your present needs but also your potential needs in the future. You might plan for your countertops to be lower than usual in case you want or need to do more of your cooking from a seated position. Similarly, you might want to consider overhanging countertops that would allow space for your legs if you were working from a seated position. You are well-advised to consult with an OT as well as a general contractor who is knowledgeable about accessibility before proceeding (see Appendix D for resources related to architectural adaptations).

I enjoy cooking but find that I get worn-out from the effort and weakened by the heat. Do you have any suggestions for solving these problems?

Many nutritious, simple, and easy-to-prepare foods are now available that shorten the amount of time required for preparation. For example, instant oatmeal provides a nutritious and tasty breakfast, and items such as instant rice, instant potatoes, instant soups, frozen vegetables, and frozen meals are easy to prepare.

A microwave, convection oven, or toaster oven create little or no heat and quicken meal preparation time. If you are now using a standard oven or doing a lot of stove-top cooking that makes the kitchen overly warm, you might want to consider the use of a "cool vest." This handy garment looks like an outdoor vest designed to hold frozen gel packs. Wearing this vest during cooking or any other uncomfortably warm activity can keep you cool and reduce that uncomfortable, heat-induced fatigue that is so common in MS.

Make sure that the kitchen is organized, clean, and neat so you have an open work area. Having a stool in the kitchen to sit on during meal preparation and clean-up assists in conserving your energy. Use a dishwasher or recruit family assistance for tasks that are difficult for you.

We eat a lot of fresh vegetables and make salads for our meals, but peeling, chopping, and cutting have become difficult. Are there any techniques or gadgets that will make this task less difficult?

Many types of blenders and food processors are available at your local hardware or department store. These devices save on the effort and time needed to prepare vegetables. Select kitchen knives that have a good solid grip and are easy to maneuver. Good Grips®, for example, has a built-up handle with a non-slip surface and a serrated edge on the blade. Dycem® is a non-slip material designed to anchor bowls and cutting boards while you work. Some cutting boards are designed to hold or stabilize the item you are cutting (see ADL equipment under Recommended Resources). You might also ask a family member to help you wash and cut a two- or three-day supply of vegetables at one time and store them in plastic containers or bags in the refrigerator. Another solution might be to take advantage of the convenience packs of ready-to-eat salad vegetables now carried by many grocery stores.

In addition to using proper utensils and convenience foods, try to conserve your energy by gathering all the items you need for the job in one place before starting to do your food preparation.

I enjoy talking on the phone, but holding the phone is tiring and awkward. Is there anything I can do so that I don't have to give up talking to my family and friends?

Several good telecommunication products and services are available that will make talking on the phone easy and enjoyable. Speaker phones permit hands-free operation so that you can speak and listen without having to hold the receiver. If you wish to have a private conversation, try a hands-free telephone headset, (available at Radio Shack). The telephone company also offers an operator-assisted service for disabled individuals who are unable to dial a telephone number.

If you are experiencing problems with your hearing or vision that interfere with independent phone use, your phone company has various no-charge services. Contact your local phone service to find out if you would benefit from any of these programs, or see the reference list under telecommunications at the end of this chapter.

Going to the grocery store is a major ordeal. The aisles are crowded, I can't reach many of the items I need, and getting the grocery bags into my house is exhausting. There must be an easier way!

Grocery shopping can be a major ordeal for many people, and it is compounded for those with physical problems. Plan what you need and make a list prior to going to the store. Try to shop during off-peak times when the store is less crowded. Know your grocery store (some stores have printed maps indicating which products are stocked in each aisle) and bypass the aisles you do not need. Request shopping assistance at customer service for items that are out of your reach. Often an employee will accompany you while you shop, or the requested items will be waiting for you at customer service. Although you may initially feel reluctant to ask for this kind of help, most people find that store employees and other shoppers are more than happy to provide assistance.

A few grocery stores have electric scooters available for public use and some stores provide a delivery service. In most supermarkets, a store employee is available to carry the groceries to your car. When you return home, ask a family member to carry the groceries from the car, or carry the perishable items in a separate bag or backpack and leave the other items for later, when you have more energy.

If getting to the grocery store becomes impossible, call your local stores and ask if they will take a telephone order for delivery. While it can be very frustrating to have to rely on someone at the store to pick out your items (particularly fresh fruits and vegetables), you will probably find that the process works fairly well once you and the store's employees have gone through it a few times.

I've belonged to a bridge group for years. Lately I haven't gone to the group because I'm afraid of dropping the cards. Do I have to give up card playing?

It is important not to give up the things that you love to do. Card holders come in a variety of shapes and sizes for different kinds of card games. The card holder called the Four Suiter® is popular and attractive, (see ADL Equipment under Recommended Resources). Playing cards with large numbers and symbols are also readily available.

Numbness and tingling in one of my hands causes me to drop things. Is there anything I can do about this problem?

Sensory symptoms that include numbness and tingling have a tendency to come and go intermittently in MS (see Chapter 2). At the present time, no available treatment is likely to have any lasting impact on the numbness and tingling that you are experiencing. The best approach is to learn how to accommodate these symptoms in order to protect yourself from burns or other injuries, and your possessions from unnecessary breakage.

The decreased sensation and dexterity that often accompany numbness and tingling are the likely cause of your tendency to drop things. You drop something because you are less able to feel it in your hand. Visual contact with the object in or near your hands is very important to compensate for this decreased sensation and dexterity, so try to keep an eye on what you are doing. Use cups with large handles that accommodate your whole hand rather than one or two fingers. Also, using a coffee mug with a lid, such as the kind used for travel, will help avoid painful burns. Try using a pen that has a thicker body and perhaps a rougher surface. Slow down enough to make sure that you have a good grip on dishes and other breakable items, and consider purchasing a set of unbreakable dinnerware. You may find that you need to carry each item with two hands in order to ensure its safety and yours. Isotoner® gloves or rubber gloves are useful for some tasks to improve your grip and compensate for sensation loss.

I feel tightness in my neck and arm muscles. Are there stretches or other exercises that might help me with this?

Maintaining flexibility and range of motion in the neck and arms is very important to prevent tightness. Stretching is the best way to accomplish this. A good exercise program must be individualized. An OT or PT can assist you in creating the right program for your particular needs.

Exercise can also be fun and can include activities such as swimming, yoga, Tai-Chi, and exercise groups. It is very important to create a program that you enjoy and can commit to do on a regular basis (see Chapter 5).

Shortly after my baby was born I began experiencing a great deal of fatigue and weakness in my arms and legs. I don't have much help available and need to learn how to handle my daughter safely, particularly as she becomes more active. Do you have any suggestions?

Principles of energy conservation and good body mechanics will be important as you analyze the various tasks you must perform to take care of your daughter safely. Instead of carrying the baby in your arms, experiment with a sling or infant carrier that you can strap to your torso. If carrying your baby in this manner is too tiring, explore what options you have for child equipment with wheels, such as a bassinet, stroller, or portable crib. Wash, change, and dress your baby at counter height, and use a safety belt on the changing table. Kneel while washing her in the bathtub and use an infant-size, lightweight tub with a non-slip surface inside the big tub when the child is young. Consider using disposable diapers as well as easy-on and easy-off clothing with few fasteners.

Learn to rest when your child rests. Prioritize tasks and spread the more difficult jobs throughout the week. Remember to relax and take care of yourself as well as your new baby.

I've heard that a home computer can be very useful for someone who is disabled. How could a computer help me and where should I go to find out which computer would best meet my needs?

The most important question to ask yourself is, "how could a computer be useful for me?" You might, for example, come up with a list of tasks that includes the following: letter writing; filing information and creating mailing lists; bookkeeping and finances; electronic mail and online communication; drawing graphics; sending and receiving information via fax; playing computer games. The next step is to try using a computer. Take a computer literacy course, and talk to friends about ways in which they use their computers. In other words, try to find out whether you are likely to be able to enjoy and make effective use of a computer before you go to the expense of purchasing one.

Now you are ready to go to a computer store and spend time with a salesperson who can explain the jargon and describe the various types of equipment and accessories that are available. It is very helpful to have a friend along, preferably someone who knows more about computers than you do. When talking with the salesperson, it is important that you be quite specific about your disability. A computer system can be adapted for many kinds of visual, sensory, and motor problems. If you find that the salesperson is simply trying to sell you a computer without taking time to understand your needs, try a different salesperson or a different store. References and resources listed at the end of the chapter can also direct you to materials describing various adaptations such as screen magnification to help with decreased vision, keyboard adaptations, and voice recognition to compensate for upper extremity incoordination.

I have a significant tremor in both of my hands, which makes it difficult for me to write legibly or eat without making a mess. It's very important to me to be able to continue doing these things independently. Are there any gadgets that would help with this problem?

Tremor is one of the most difficult and frustrating of MS symptoms (see Chapter 2). Fortunately, a number of well-designed writing and eating aids can alleviate some of the problems it can cause in your daily life. The first step is to try dampening the tremor with weights. A weighted pen with a good grip might help improve your handwriting. A weighted mug and weighted spoon or fork can help you get food to your mouth more smoothly and with less spillage. Wearing a one- or two-pound velcro closure wrist weight during such activities as writing and eating might also be helpful. However, weighted utensils and wrist weights will not be particularly useful if you tire easily or if your arms are extremely weak. Some people find that a pen holder compensates for the tremor and improves legibility. One such holder resembles a rounded paperweight with a hole for your pen and grooves for your fingers. You write by grasping the molded holder with your entire hand and moving it along the page. Plastic writing "guides" are also available to help you write in straighter, more legible lines. Similarly, dinner plates with a curved edge will contain the food and prevent it from scattering onto the table. Drinking glasses are available with lids to prevent spillage.

Recommended Readings

Alliance for Technology Access. *Computer Resources for People with Disabilities: A Guide to Exploring Today's Assistive Technology.* Alameda, CA: Hunter House, 1994.

Bell L, Seyfer E. *Gentle Yoga: A Guide to Gentle Exercise.* Berkeley, CA: Celestial Arts, 1987.

Enders A, Hall M. *Assistive Technology Sourcebook.* Washington, D.C.: Resna Press, 1990.

Garee B (ed.). *Parenting: Tips from Parents (Who Happen to Have a Disability) on Raising Children.* Bloomington, IL: Accent Press, 1989.

Rogers J, Matsumura M. *Mother to Be: A Guide to Pregnancy and Birth for Women with Disabilities.* New York: Demos, 1990.

Robbins K, Rosenthal B. Making everyday activities easier. In: Scheinberg LC, Holland N (eds.). *Multiple Sclerosis: A Guide for Patients and Their Families (2nd edition).* New York: Raven Press, 1987.

Schapiro R. *Symptom Management in Multiple Sclerosis (2nd edition).* New York: Demos, 1994.

Webster B. *All of a Piece: A Life With Multiple Sclerosis.* Baltimore: Johns Hopkins, 1989.

Wolf J. *Fall Down Seven Get Up Eight.* Rutland, VT: Academy Books, 1991.

Wolf J. *Mastering Multiple Sclerosis: A Guide to Management (2nd edition).* Rutland, VT: Academy Books, 1987.

National Multiple Sclerosis Society (800-624-8236)

Independent Living Series

I. Managing Home Environment

General Information
Domestic Appliances
Housecleaning Aids
Reaching Aids
Storage
Lifting Aids
Walking Aids

II. Grooming / Dressing

Clothing and Footwear
Dressing Aids
Grooming Aids

III. Food Preparation

Cooking Utensils
Dishwashing Aids
Food Preparation Aids
Tableware and Cutlery

IV. Bathroom Adaptations

Bath Lifts
Bathing Aids
Bath, Shower and Transfer Seats
Grab Bars
Plumbing Fixtures
Showers
Toilets and Toilet Seats

Booklet avalable from the National Multiple Sclerosis Society

◇ *At Home with MS: Adapting Your Environment*—Jane E. Harmon, O.T.R.

Activities of Daily Living (ADL) Equipment

Access with Ease, Inc. Catalog (800-531-9479)
Maddak, Inc. Aids For Daily Living Catalog (201-628-7600)
Northcoast Medical ADL Catalog (800-235-7054)
Sammons Orthopedic and ADL Products (800-323-5547)
Smith & Nephew Rolyan, Inc. ADL Catalog (800-558-8633)

Chair Lifts

Pride Health Care (800-800-8586)
71 S. Main Street
Pittston, PA 18640
Sears Home Health Care Catalog (800-326-1750)
20 Presidential Drive
Roselle, IL 60172

Clothing

"The Clothes Line" in *Paraplegic News*, September 1987, pp. 15–20.

"Clothing For Handicapped People: An Annotated Bibliography and Resource List" available from The President's Committee on Employment of People with Disabilities, Washington, DC. 20210.

Avenues Unlimited Catalog (800-848-2837)

Fashion Ease Catalog, 1541 60th Street, Brooklyn, NY 11219

J.C. Penney's "Easy Dressing" Catalog (800-222-6161)

Sears Home Health Care Catalog (800-326-1750)

Support Plus / Fashionable Catalog (508-359-2910)

Wardrobe Wagon Catalog (800-WW CARES)

Computers

Lazzaro, Joseph. Adaptive Technologies For Learning and Work Environments, 1993. American Library Assoc., Chicago, IL.

Assistive Device Center, Sacramento State University, School of Engineering and Computer Science, Sacramento, CA. 95819. 916-278-6422

IBM National Support Center For Persons With Disabilities. P.O. Box 2150, Atlanta, GA. 30055

Trace Center Information Center, 1500 Highland Avenue, University of Wisconsin, Madison, WI. 53705. 608-262-6966.

Home Modifications

Eastern Paralyzed Veterans of America, 75-20 Astoria Boulevard, Jackson Heights, NY 11370. 800-444-0120.

Accessible Building Design (In English and Spanish)

Planning for Access: A Guide to Planning and Modifying Your Home

Parenting

Adaptive Parenting: Idea Book I (Through the Looking Glass, 2198 Sixth Street, Suite 100, Berkeley, CA 94710; tel: 510-848-1112; 800-644-2666).

Parenting with a Disability (Through the Looking Glass, 2198 Sixth Street, Suite 100, Berkeley, CA 94710; tel: 510-848-1112; 800-644-2666).

Telecommunications

AT&T Special Needs Center (800-233-1222)
GTE Special Needs Center (800-821-2585)

Vehicles/Vehicle Modifications

Ford Mobility Motoring Program (800-952-2248)
P.O. Box 529
Bloomfield Hills, MI 48303

GM Mobility Assistance Center (800-323-9935)
P.O. Box 9011
Detroit, MI 48202

Mobility Products & Designs, Inc. (Hand Control Information)
(800-488-7688)
14800 28th Avenue North
Minneapolis, MN 55447

7

Speech and Voice Disorders

Pam Sorensen, M.A., C.C.C.-SLP

MS lesions in the brain can interfere with muscle control in the lips, tongue, soft palate (the soft muscle tissue extending back from the roof of the mouth), vocal cords, and diaphragm (the dome-like muscle under the lungs that plays an important role in breathing). These muscles control speech production and voice quality as well as the process of swallowing. A person who develops problems with speech or swallowing is usually referred by his or her physician to a **speech/language pathologist**, who specializes in the diagnosis and treatment of speech and swallowing disorders. Problems with speech production and voice quality are discussed in this chapter while MS-related swallowing difficulties are the subject of Chapter 8.

Normal speech and voice production is complex, requiring the following five systems to work smoothly together:

◇ *Respiration*—using the diaphragm to fill the lungs fully, followed by slow, controlled exhalation for speech.

◇ *Phonation*—using the vocal cords and airflow to produce voice of different pitch (highness or lowness of tone), loudness, and quality.

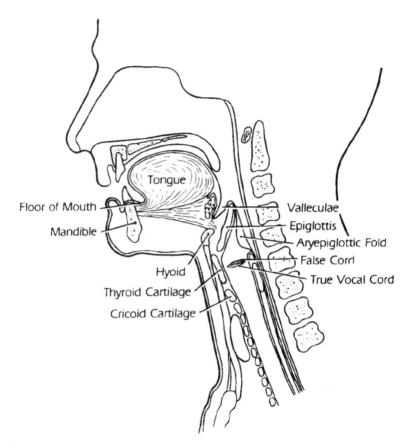

Figure 7-1 Side view of mouth and throat.

- ◇ *Resonance*—raising and lowering the soft palate to direct the voice to vibrate in either the mouth or nose and further affect quality.
- ◇ *Articulation*—making quick, precise movements of the lips, tongue, and soft palate for clarity of speech.
- ◇ *Prosody*—combining all of the above elements for a natural flow of speech, with adequate speaking rate, appropriate pauses, and variations in loudness and emphasis to enhance meaning.

Approximately 25–40 percent of people with MS experience speech and voice disorders during the course of the disease. The disorders are caused by spasticity, weakness, slowness, and incoordination of the muscles in the tongue, lips, soft palate, vocal cords, and diaphragm.

Dysarthria is the term used to describe motor speech disorders that result in the slurred or unclear articulation of words. Impairments in volume control, articulation, and emphasis have been reported as the three most common features of dysarthria.

◇ Impaired volume control refers to a voice that is too quiet, too loud, or tends to fluctuate because of poor breath support and control.

◇ Poor articulation results in speech that is slurred and sometimes difficult to understand in conversation.

◇ Problems with emphasis result in speech that is slowed or unnatural because of inappropriate pauses, placement of excess and equal stress on each word, or difficulty varying pitch and loudness to emphasize important words.

The term **dysphonia** refers to disorders of voice quality. Dysphonia commonly involves the following features:

◇ Harsh voice quality resulting from spasticity or too much muscle tone in the vocal cords that gives the voice a strained, brassy sound.

◇ Impaired pitch control due to tremor or spasticity in the vocal cords, which results either in pitch breaks (similar to the "cracking" that is heard in an adolescent whose voice is changing), or in a monotone voice (lacking the pitch variation that produces a natural line of melody while speaking).

◇ Hypernasality is a nasal speech quality caused by weakness, slowness, or incoordination of the soft palate that allows too much air to resonate in the nasal cavity.

◇ A pitch level that is higher or lower than usual (caused by changes in muscle tone) or an uneven, gravelly voice quality (caused by trying to speak when there is very little air left in the lungs).

◇ Breathiness (caused by vocal cords that allow too much air to escape).

◇ Hoarseness (resulting from vocal cords that fluctuate between coming together too tightly and too loosely) that sounds similar to laryngitis.

Problems with speech and voice can come and go. They sometimes worsen temporarily with MS exacerbations or during
bouts of severe fatigue, and then gradually improve. Depending
on the course that the disease is following, these symptoms may
also progressively worsen. Anyone who experiences problems
with speech or voice that interfere with everyday communication should request a physician's referral to a speech/language
pathologist, who is trained to evaluate symptoms and design an
individualized treatment program. Therapy can alleviate many
types of speech and voice problems; the sooner that therapy is
begun, the greater the improvement is likely to be.

What will the speech/language pathologist do to evaluate my voice and speech?

A speech/language pathologist first completes an *oral peripheral examination*. This includes examining the oral muscles that
are necessary for speech—the lips, tongue, and soft palate—and
assessing their functioning in terms of strength, speed, range,
accuracy, timing, and coordination. The teeth and hard palate
are also examined. You may be asked to stick out your tongue;
wag your tongue from side to side as quickly as you can; lick
your lips around in a circle and then change directions; puff up
your cheeks and resist pressure on your cheeks to release the
air; show your teeth; pucker your lips; alternate between a
pucker and a smile; say "pataka" as quickly and evenly as you
can.

A *voice evaluation* assesses the function of the vocal cords,
respiratory muscles, and soft palate as they relate to pitch, loudness, and voice quality. You may be asked to fill your lungs
deeply, say "ahhh" for as long as you can; repeat "ah" many
times quickly; count as high as you can in one breath; sing up
the scale ("do, re, mi . . ."); and count from one to ten while gradually increasing your volume from a whisper to a shout.
Referrals to an ear, nose, and throat (ENT) specialist for examination of the vocal cords or to a pulmonologist for a baseline
pulmonary (lung) function test may also be indicated.

A *motor speech evaluation* assesses how well all systems
work together: breath support and control, voice production, resonance, articulation, and flow of speech. The precision of your
pronunciation (articulation) and the ease with which you are
understood by others (intelligibility) are measured at the sound,

word, sentence, and conversational levels. A baseline sample of
your speech may be tape-recorded. Conversational speech may
be analyzed for its natural flow (prosody): Are there appropriate
pauses or do they occur too often or at illogical places? Are
important words emphasized with more loudness and higher
pitch to enhance meaning, or are all words spoken with the same
or no emphasis? The rate at which you speak may also be measured in order to determine if your speech is too fast or too slow
when compared with the norm.

What is involved in the treatment of speech and voice problems?

Therapy is recommended with a speech/language pathologist
if speech or voice problems interfere with everyday communication needs. The type and amount of treatment vary with each
individual. A treatment plan can be devised based on your specific problem areas and communication needs. Therapy usually begins with learning about normal speech and voice production. Daily home exercises for the lips, tongue, soft palate,
vocal cords, and diaphragm are taught to strengthen and
improve coordination in these muscles. Active self-monitoring
is essential and can be enhanced with the use of a tape
recorder, Voice Lite® (an instrument that becomes brighter as
loudness increases), spirometer (an instrument that measures
how deeply you fill your lungs), and speech analysis computer software.

You may be taught new strategies and compensatory techniques for improving the clarity of your speech, including slowing down, overarticulation (exaggerated enunciation), phrasing,
strategic pauses, and syllable tapping (tapping as you say each
syllable). Practicing these techniques in increasingly more difficult and less structured speaking situations, during individual
and then group therapy sessions, can help to stabilize these new
skills. Training family members in ways to provide you with
useful cues can help promote treatment carryover outside the
therapy sessions.

If necessary, training can be offered in the use of appropriate
equipment, such as a voice amplifier (with headset microphone
and loudness control) or an electronic communication aid.
Home programs to enhance progress can be developed that
incorporate use of a mirror during oral exercises and the use of
a tape recorder while reading aloud. A referral may also be made

to a neurologist, ENT specialist, pulmonologist, respiratory therapist, or occupational therapist.

My thoughts still flow as well as they used to, but I can't speak as quickly and clearly now. It sounds as though I have a mouthful of marbles. What is causing my speech to sound so slurred?

Feeling "out of sync," as if your mouth is unable to keep up with your thoughts, is a common complaint. Clear speech requires precise, rapid, coordinated movements of your lips, tongue, and soft palate. MS can cause the mouth and throat muscles to become weaker and less coordinated, resulting in the neuromuscular speech disorder called dysarthria. Slurred speech or imprecise articulation is a common feature of dysarthria. It can occasionally become severe enough to interfere with the efforts of others to understand what you are saying.

A speech/language pathologist can help you improve the clarity of your speech. First, it is important to become consistent in identifying when your speech sounds slurred. This may require you to improve your self-monitoring skills by evaluating your own tape-recorded speech samples. Hearing the problem is the necessary first step to being able to make adjustments. The following techniques are helpful in improving speech clarity:

◇ Slow down. Do not try to speak as quickly as you did before. Your oral muscles and breathing probably cannot keep up with your thought process and the rate at which you want to say words. Concentrate on a slower speaking rate.

◇ Overarticulate. Open your mouth a little more while talking, and exaggerate the movements of your tongue, lips, and jaw.

◇ Pause strategically. Instead of trying to quickly say too many words at once, it is better to break it down and learn to pause at logical places in long sentences. This takes extra time and planning, but can promote clear speech.

Talking seems to take much more effort than it used to. I can get very tired and not have enough breath to say complete sentences loudly enough for others to understand me. Why is this happening? What can I do about it?

Talking is a complex activity that we take for granted until something like MS interferes. Clear, audible speech requires physical effort and precise timing by many muscle groups. Speaking for extended periods can thus be quite tiring, particularly for those individuals who also experience MS-related fatigue. A speech/language pathologist can help you become efficient at speaking loudly while simultaneously learning to pace yourself.

Adequate breath support and control are needed for loud speech. Air is the "gasoline" needed to drive the necessary muscles. You start by completely filling your lungs, using your diaphragm to inhale quickly and deeply. Then slowly extend your exhalation to produce words. It is important to identify how many words are loud enough before you run out of air and lose necessary volume. Then you can begin to modify your speech and breathing patterns to raise your volume and improve audibility. Plan pauses for breathing rather than saying too many words in one breath—a technique called "phrasing." For example, you may find that breaking sentences into five-word breath units helps you to maintain adequate loudness.

Besides teaching diaphragmatic breathing exercises and phrasing techniques, the speech/language pathologist can provide other options, as needed. For example, the "push technique" requires you to push down with your elbows on the armrests of your chair while talking. This can help your vocal cords come together more strongly and therefore help create a louder voice. Using a spirometer can assist you in observing and measuring how fully you are filling your lungs. A tape recorder, Voice Lite®, and computer programs that analyze speech volume can give feedback on how loud you sound and if you are reaching the goals set in therapy. Voice amplifiers with headset or collar microphones are sometimes recommended when loudness cannot be improved to a functionally adequate level. However, a speech/language pathologist should first evaluate the problem, recommend the most appropriate equipment, and then train you in its use.

Sometimes I avoid talking to others because it feels bad not to be understood. People seem to lose interest because it takes more time to listen to me. Sometimes they even nod when I know they aren't understanding what I'm saying. What should I do?

You are not alone in your frustration. People with MS and moderate to severe dysarthria often experience similar feelings.

Some also express resentment that their impaired speech causes others to "talk down" to them in the mistaken belief that they are not capable or intelligent. A useful strategy is to let people know about your speech difficulty and explain what assistance you need from them. It takes time and practice to feel comfortable asserting yourself in these ways. You might try out the following explanation: "The reason my speech is slow and hard to understand is because of my MS. My brain works fine, but my lips and tongue don't always cooperate." You can then give your listener guidance in how to respond to you by saying, "I am trying to speak clearly, but please tell me when you don't understand." These simple statements will help you and your listeners to feel more comfortable because they give your listeners permission to talk about any difficulty they might have in understanding what you are saying.

We live in a fast-paced world. Assess the situation and watch the body language of your listeners. This will enable you to judge which people and situations can allow the extra time that you need. Estimate the time needed and ask first: "Do you have . . . minutes to talk about . . .?" It is important that you do not avoid talking to others. It can be a challenge, but you have a right as a speaker to be understood and a responsibility to let listeners know what you need from them. A speech/language pathologist can help you become comfortable and proficient in this process. It is best to build your comfort level gradually with this new approach, first with a therapist and then family and close friends, before trying it with strangers.

If my speech gets any worse, even my family will not understand what I am saying. Are there other ways of communicating that I can learn?

The speech problems typical of MS can usually be improved with therapy. Although your speech may not be as loud, precise, fast, or flowing as it was, learning the appropriate techniques will usually allow you to be adequately understood by others. However, alternative modes of communication are necessary in certain situations. Many options are available, ranging from the simple to the "high tech." Selection depends on your specific needs, abilities, and financial resources. Some of the simpler communication aids include light and buzzer switches to get the attention of others; yes/no signals, eye blink systems, alphabet charts to spell out messages with finger or eye movements, and picture/word communication charts.

Many electronic and computer-assisted forms of communication also are available. They vary in size, portability, complexity, function, input, output, and cost. Some are laptop size for you to type in the message and have it printed out. Others can be programmed so that one key stroke produces a frequently used complete sentence. Some computers actually speak the messages you program in or type. Because of the variety and complexity of the available technology, you should be evaluated by a speech/language pathology and occupational therapy team that has expertise in this area. This specialty team can help you identify the type of equipment best suited to your needs by taking into account whatever physical limitations you may have, as well as your visual-motor, cognitive, and communication skills. You can then purchase or construct the appropriate communication aid and be properly trained in its use.

Do speech and voice problems caused by MS ever remit like other MS symptoms?

If you experience slurred speech only during times of fatigue, you may also notice that these symptoms remit when you are rested. If speech and voice problems result from MS exacerbations, they may improve or resolve following treatment with high-dose steroids. Thus, managing fatigue and treating MS exacerbations can at times help speech and voice symptoms to remit. However, referral to a speech/language pathologist is recommended if symptoms persist even when you are rested, or one month after medical treatment is received for an MS exacerbation.

Why doesn't my voice sound the way it used to? Sometimes it seems hoarse, as if I have laryngitis. Other times it sounds strained or harsh.

Your voice quality is largely determined by how your vocal cords function. MS can cause spasticity, weakness, slowness, and incoordination of any muscle group. Your vocal cords are muscles, too, and can therefore undergo these changes. This can occur temporarily during MS exacerbations and continuously during MS disease progression. The types of voice problems or "dysphonia" that are characteristic of MS include harshness, hoarseness, breathiness, and hypernasality.

A harsh, strained voice quality occurs when there is too much muscle tone or tightness in the vocal cords due to MS spasticity. Baclofen (Lioresal®), a medication to relieve spasticity (see Chapter 2 and Appendix B), may be helpful. Voice therapy may help to reduce harshness by emphasizing relaxation techniques for your throat and vocal cords, improving breath support, promoting "easy onset" of your voicing, and speaking with a breathy quality. The "yawn-sigh" approach, in which the vocal cords are automatically relaxed during a yawn to promote a softer voice quality during the exhaled sigh, may also help with this problem.

A hoarse voice quality results when something interferes with the way your vocal cords come together during speaking. Hoarseness is a combination of harsh and breathy voice qualities. Your vocal cords may fluctuate between coming together too tightly (harsh) and too loosely (breathy), resulting in hoarseness. When hoarseness lasts more than seven to ten days, it is important to have an ENT specialist evaluate medical causes that can be treated, such as colds, allergies, abnormal growths, and paralysis. After these are ruled out, voice therapy that emphasizes increasing breath support and loudness, lowering your usual pitch, and self-monitoring for a "clear" target voice quality may reduce the problem.

What causes my voice to fluctuate so much? It doesn't seem to be within my control. Sometimes I have bursts of loudness. Other times my pitch changes or my voice turns off mid-sentence.

Such wide variations in pitch, loudness, and voice control are probably due to MS lesions in the cerebellum, the part of the brain responsible for regulating and coordinating complex voluntary movements. Cerebellar lesions can interfere with the vocal cord action required to produce vocalizations. You may experience sudden changes in pitch because of uncontrolled fluctuations between vocal cord elongation (high pitch) and contraction (low pitch). Bursts of loudness may result from abrupt vocal cord tension and diaphragm contraction. Intermittent aphonia (the loss of voice in mid-sentence) may occur because of unexpected parting of the vocal folds, when they should be vibrating together to produce voice. Continuous vocal cord tremors may interrupt the smoothness of your voice quality.

These problems are difficult to treat in voice therapy. Medications that reduce spasticity are sometimes helpful. Voice therapy that emphasizes active self-monitoring using a tape recorder, speech analysis by computer software, and reduction of physical effort during voicing may also be beneficial.

How often and for how long will I need to see the therapist?

The frequency and duration of your therapy depends on the type and severity of your problems and your communication needs. However, there is typically much that can be accomplished in two months of twice weekly, hour-long outpatient visits.

Recommended Readings

Colton R, Casper J. *Understanding Voice Problems—A Physiological Perspective for Diagnosis and Treatment.* Baltimore: Williams & Wilkins, 1990.

Darley F, Brown J, Goldstein N. Dysarthria in multiple sclerosis. *J Speech Hearing Research* 1972;15:229–45.

Farmakides M, Boone D. Speech problems of patients with multiple sclerosis. *J Speech Hearing Disorders* 1960;25:385–89.

Sorensen P, Brown S, Logemann J, Wilson K, Herndon R. Communication disorders and dysphagia. *J Neuro Rehab* 1994;8:137-43.

8

Swallowing

Jeri A. Logemann, Ph.D.

In addition to the problems with speech and language discussed in the previous chapter, the *speech/language pathologist* is also trained to diagnose and treat symptoms related to the swallowing mechanism.

Normal swallowing is a rapid, safe, and efficient process that occurs in four stages:

◆ *Stage One—Oral Preparation*

When food is placed in the mouth, chewing reduces it to a consistency appropriate for swallowing. Chewing requires the coordinated action of lip, tongue, and jaw muscles to move the food onto the teeth, pick up the food as it falls from the teeth, mix it with saliva, and replace it onto the teeth. The saliva that is mixed into the food during chewing helps with the digestion process and acts as a natural acid neutralizer. Chewing takes a variable amount of time depending on the amount and thickness of food put in the mouth. When chewing has reduced the food to a consistency appropriate for swallowing, the tongue subdivides it and forms a ball or bolus of the right size to be swallowed. The thicker or more viscous the food, the less a person can swallow at one time. Trying to swallow too much food at one time is uncomfortable and may result in gagging.

◆ Stage Two—Oral Stage

The tongue pushes the bolus of food up and backward through the mouth, applying pressure to the tail end of the bolus. As the tongue pressure pushes the food backward, the movements of the tongue and bolus stimulate sensory nerve endings; these, in turn, signal the brain to trigger a series of muscle contractions in the pharynx (throat), called the "pharyngeal swallow."

◆ Stage Three—Pharyngeal Stage

The triggering of the pharyngeal swallow sets in motion a series of neuromuscular actions. The soft palate (the soft portion at the back of the roof of the mouth) lifts and closes the back entrance to the nose, preventing food or liquid from entering the nasal passages. The larynx (voice box) lifts up, and the epiglottis (the thin strip of cartilage that hangs down at the back of the throat) closes down to help prevent food or liquid from entering the trachea (windpipe). The base of the tongue and the walls of the throat move toward each other until they touch. This movement generates the pressure needed to push the food through the throat. The airway (to the lungs) automatically closes to prevent accidental **aspiration** of food or liquid into the lungs. The valve at the bottom of the throat relaxes and opens to allow the bolus to pass easily into the esophagus (food canal leading down to the stomach).

◆ Stage Four—Esophageal Stage

Muscle contractions propel the bolus through the esophagus, and the valve at the bottom of the esophagus opens to let the food enter the stomach.

In normal swallowing, it takes approximately two seconds for the food to move through the mouth and throat before entering the esophagus. Once in the esophagus, it takes anywhere from eight to twenty seconds for the food to travel to the stomach. When the swallowing mechanism is working normally and efficiently, food particles and liquids seldom make their way into the airway or windpipe. This usually happens only when someone is doing two things at once, such as talking or laughing while trying to swallow. A person who tries to talk while eating may begin to cough or choke because a particle of food has slipped into the airway. Once a normal swallow is completed, very little food is left in the mouth, throat, or esophagus.

What is dysphagia?

Dysphagia means difficulty swallowing. Approximately thirty muscles in the mouth and throat and eight *cranial nerves* are involved in the swallowing mechanism. *Lesions* in the *brainstem* and/or the cranial nerves can cause problems at any point in the swallowing process, from the time the food enters the mouth until it reaches the stomach. A slowing of the nerve impulses that control the mechanisms of swallowing can interfere with the voluntary movements involved in chewing, with the initiation of the pharyngeal swallow, or with the strength or range of movements that are required to push the food through the mouth, throat, or esophagus. Reduced muscle strength or coordination can allow particles to remain in the mouth, throat, or esophagus after the swallow is completed. Food particles remaining in the mouth and throat may be accidentally aspirated into the lungs any time that a delay in the pharyngeal swallow allows the airway to the lungs to remain open. Food or liquid can also escape into the nose or windpipe if there is a malfunction in the valves in the throat. The type of dysphagia a person develops will depend on the particular neuromuscular actions that are impaired. The problems most commonly seen in MS are a delay in the initiation of the pharyngeal swallow and a slowing of the passage of food through the pharynx.

What are the chances that I will develop a swallowing problem?

Most people with MS never experience this type of symptom over the course of the illness. Whether or not you develop a swallowing problem will depend entirely on the location of demyelinating lesions. Dysphagia can result if muscles of the mouth, throat, or esophagus are affected by the neurologic disease process. We do not know the exact percentage of people with MS who develop a swallowing problem, nor do we know if there are any specific characteristics that will predict whether someone will develop a swallowing problem. You should talk with your doctor about seeing a speech/language pathologist for a swallowing evaluation if you are finding it more difficult to chew or swallow your food, or seem to be coughing or choking during or after meals.

I have been referred for a swallowing evaluation. How is the evaluation done and what will the test be able to tell me about my swallowing problem?

The speech/language pathologist will take a complete clinical history and evaluate your ability to control the muscles of your mouth and throat. During this examination, you will be asked to move your lips, tongue, and soft palate in various ways and to produce speech samples that require different types of muscle control. You will also be asked questions about your diet, the kinds of foods that are difficult for you to eat, and the difficulties that you have noticed in eating or swallowing. You may be asked, for example, about episodes of coughing or choking during or after a meal, how long it usually takes you to eat a meal, whether your voice becomes hoarse or gurgly during or after eating, the frequency with which you get respiratory infections, and whether you experience frequent heartburn or indigestion.

The swallowing assessment usually also involves a radiographic study called *videofluoroscopy* (modified barium swallow). The barium you are given to swallow makes the structures of your mouth, throat, and esophagus visible on X-ray. The movements of these structures as you swallow different types of foods are recorded on videotape. During this examination you will be asked to swallow varying amounts of liquids and solid foods with different consistencies. You may also be asked to chew and swallow a cookie with a small amount of barium on top.

This radiographic test is designed to help you, your physician, and the speech/language pathologist understand the specific nature of your swallowing problem. Depending on the results of the test, the speech/language pathologist may ask you to do various swallowing exercises in an attempt to improve or strengthen your swallow. You also may be given instructions on the safest ways to eat (e.g., optimal positioning of your head and neck, the size and frequency of meals, the correct way to chew) as well as the safest kinds of foods to eat (e.g., blenderized food, thickened liquids). The goal of this intervention is to identify ways to make it easier for you to continue to eat safely and comfortably.

If the speech/language pathologist recommends swallowing therapy, what does this treatment involve and for how long am I likely to need it?

Swallowing therapy usually involves exercises to strengthen the muscles used in swallowing and to improve the coordination of muscles during swallowing. Therapy often involves practicing muscle movements and learning safe swallowing strategies. Each person is different, so the exercises and techniques you are given may differ from those prescribed for someone else. The length of time swallowing therapy needs to be continued will also vary from one individual to another. Generally, however, a month or so of twice weekly therapy sessions will provide you with enough training to proceed independently with your swallowing practice. Some people need to continue to exercise daily to keep their muscles operating at maximum strength and efficiency.

Now that I have started having trouble swallowing, how often will the doctor want a swallowing evaluation?

There is no set schedule for swallowing evaluations. Generally, the evaluation should be repeated if you have had a change in your symptoms. For example, you will need a reevaluation if you begin to cough more frequently or have a gurgly voice during or after eating. Sometimes your doctor will want regular reevaluations of swallowing to see if a particular medication has a positive effect on your swallowing ability. *You* may also ask for a reevaluation if *you* notice changes in your swallowing ability. You may not cough or have a gurgly voice, but you may notice that swallowing is more difficult or that it requires more energy and effort to swallow or more time to eat a meal. If you feel your swallowing has changed, it is a good idea to ask your physician for a swallowing reevaluation.

Why do I sometimes have trouble swallowing liquids but have no trouble at all with solid foods?

Some people have more difficulty swallowing liquids, particularly if there is a delay between the end of the oral stage of swallowing (the movement of food through the mouth) and the beginning of the pharyngeal stage of swallowing (the movement of the food through the throat or pharynx). Since the airway remains open until the pharyngeal stage of swallowing has actually begun, the longer the delay, the greater the chance that liquid can slip into the airway and lungs. Because liquids have a thinner consistency than solids, they generally move faster and with less muscle effort than solids. Liquids are therefore likely to find their way into the open airway before solid foods do. People with multiple sclerosis sometimes develop a problem in triggering the pharyngeal stage of swallowing. When this occurs, they may have a tendency to cough or choke when trying to swallow liquids. Adding a thickening agent to the liquids you drink can often help to alleviate this problem.

Why are some solid foods more difficult than others for me to swallow?

Because solid foods are thicker in texture than liquids, they require a great deal more pressure to push backward through the mouth and throat. Some solid foods are naturally thicker than others (peanut butter is the worst, of course). Generating more pressure requires greater muscle strength. If neurologic changes are impeding the muscle action in your mouth, the resulting weakness may affect your ability to swallow solid foods. You will probably have more trouble swallowing the thickest foods and less trouble with thinner ones.

Weakness in the muscles used for chewing can also affect your ability to swallow. If chewing is difficult or tiring, you may be trying to swallow foods that are only half chewed. These half-chewed foods are much more difficult to swallow than foods that have been broken down to a softer consistency. If you are having trouble chewing, you may benefit from chewing exercises or from chopping or blenderizing the food before putting it on your plate. If you notice that your chewing gets weaker throughout a meal, you may want to eat five smaller meals rather than three larger ones.

I seem to have a mouthful of saliva much more often than I used to, and I sometimes start to choke on it. Is there anything I can do about this problem?

A mouthful of saliva that is not easily swallowed may result from a delay in triggering the pharyngeal swallow. You may benefit from swallowing therapy designed to improve the triggering mechanism and reduce the delay. You should talk with your speech/language pathologist about exercises for this problem. Excess saliva may also occur when you are not feeling or paying attention to the need to swallow. It may be helpful to become aware of the need to swallow more often and to receive cues from others. You may also want to keep a lozenge in your mouth to stimulate more saliva, which will, in turn, stimulate more swallows. A sour candy may naturally stimulate more swallows than a more mild or less tasty lozenge.

I used to swallow automatically, without even having to think about it. Now I'm having a problem starting and finishing the swallow. Sometimes I even feel as though I haven't swallowed everything that needs to go down. Why is this happening and can I do anything about it?

This problem probably indicates both a delay in the pharyngeal stage of swallowing and muscle weakness that allows food particles to remain in your mouth or throat following each swallow. These problems can sometimes be alleviated with swallowing therapy: certain icing techniques can help trigger the pharyngeal stage of swallowing; exercises may strengthen muscles used during swallowing. Sucking on a sour candy or taking a very small sip of sour lemonade between every few bites of food may help you to trigger these swallows more efficiently. A safe swallow strategy such as "hold your breath, swallow, clear your throat, and swallow again for each bite or sip" can help to clear out leftover food or liquid from the throat.

I have been told to cut my food into very small pieces (or put it through a blender) and thicken all the liquids I drink because I am coughing or choking more often. The problem still seems to be getting worse. What will happen if I can't solve the choking problem?

If you cannot solve the choking problem with therapy, modified swallowing techniques, or changes in the consistency of your food, your doctor may recommend that you begin nonoral (not by mouth) feedings. Frequent coughing or choking is an indication that you may be aspirating food or liquids into your lungs, which can, in turn, increase your risk of getting pneumonia. In addition to the increased risk of aspiration and pneumonia, severe swallowing problems may deprive you of adequate nutrition and fluids. People who find it too tiring to eat properly, or whose eating is frequently interrupted by bouts of coughing or choking, may not be able to eat or drink sufficient amounts to maintain their weight. Your doctor may recommend nonoral feedings in order to ensure that you get adequate nutrition and liquids.

There are two basic types of nonoral feeding that allow food and liquids to be taken into the body without being swallowed. A *nasogastric tube* (that goes through the nose and throat and into the esophagus and stomach) is typically used on a very temporary basis (following surgery, for example) when the person is expected to be able to resume eating by mouth within a few days or weeks. The nasogastric tube can be irritating to the nose and throat if left in for a prolonged period. A ***percutaneous endoscopic gastrostomy (PEG)*** is used if nonoral feedings are likely to be needed for a longer time. The PEG involves the insertion of a feeding tube through the abdominal wall directly into the stomach. In this relatively simple bedside procedure, an endoscope (a special instrument designed to illuminate the inside of an internal organ) guides the placement of the tube through a tiny incision in the stomach wall. The tube remains in place as long as nonoral feeding is necessary, and a special dietary formula is pumped into the tube on a scheduled basis.

Both types of nonoral feeding tubes can be removed when and if your swallowing improves. Therefore, if your doctor recommends that you begin nonoral feedings, you do not have to feel that you are making a permanent decision. You can choose to have the feeding tube removed at any time. Keep in mind that being well-nourished and getting adequate liquids are important for maintaining your strength. Losing weight and getting weaker can, by themselves, cause swallowing problems, and your chances of regaining your swallowing abilities are better when you are strong and well-nourished. So, while it can be a big decision to take some or all nutrition and fluids by tube, that decision may help you to recover improved swallowing later. Do not put off taking good nutrition and liquids by nonoral means if your physician recommends them.

If I do start nonoral feeding, does that mean that I can never eat any food by mouth?

No. Even with nonoral feeding, you may be able to take certain kinds of foods by mouth. This will generally depend on the nature of your swallowing problem and the thickness of the foods you want to eat. Many individuals take nonoral tube feeding for part of their nutritional needs and eat certain foods orally. Sometimes people can safely and efficiently swallow some types of food but not others. If you are safely able to chew and swallow foods of a certain thickness or consistency, you will be given a list of foods that are safe for you to eat by mouth and the kinds of foods you should be sure to avoid. Generally, if you are able to manage one or two consistencies of food, your speech/language pathologist or physician will try to keep you eating those types of food by mouth. However, you may need total nonoral feeding if you are having difficulty swallowing all types of foods and liquids.

If I need to have a PEG now, does that mean I will always have to have one?

No. You may only need a PEG for a few months. If your swallowing improves due to swallowing therapy or a remission in the disease, your physician will probably recommend that you resume eating by mouth at least some of the time. If you have no further difficulties with swallowing, the PEG can be removed. It is important that you pay attention to your swallowing ability and report changes or improvements to your physician and speech/language pathologist. A reevaluation of your swallowing, probably including a repeat videofluoroscopy, will indicate whether or not it is safe for the PEG to be removed.

Is there any cure for my swallowing problems or will they just keep getting worse?

Some people with MS experience swallowing problems that gradually worsen over time. Others have a temporary problem with swallowing that gradually improves to the point that they can eat efficiently and safely by mouth. Once improved, the swallowing problems may or may not return. Your best strategy is to see your physician and speech/language pathologist any

time you feel that your swallowing has changed so that they can
provide you with the best kinds of exercises and management.

Recommended Readings

Groher ME. *Dysphagia: Diagnosis and Management.* Boston:
  Butterworth Publishers, 1984.

Jone, GW, Feldmann MC, Ireland JV, Reinhart R, Yozwiak A.
  Dysphagia: A Manual for Use by Families. Austin, TX: Pro-Ed,
  1994.

Logemann JA. *Evaluation and Treatment of Swallowing
  Disorders.* Austin, TX: Pro-Ed, 1983.

Logemann JA. *Swallowing Problems: How Can They be
  Identified, Evaluated, and Treated: A Caregiver's Manual.*
  Menu Magic/ASHA, 1991.

Logemann JA. *A Professional's Guide to Swallowing Disorders.*
  Menu Magic/ASHA, 1992.

9

Cognition

Jill Fischer, Ph.D.
Nicholas G. LaRocca, Ph.D.
Pam Sorensen, M.A., C.C.C.-SLP

Cognition refers to a variety of high-level functions carried out by the human brain. These include our ability to (1) understand and use language; (2) accurately recognize objects (visual perception) and use these perceptions to draw, assemble things, and find our way around (visual construction); (3) perform calculations; (4) focus, maintain, and shift our attention as needed even when information is coming at us very rapidly (information processing); (5) learn and remember information (memory); and (6) perform complex tasks such as planning and carrying out activities in the proper order, solving problems, and monitoring our own behavior (executive functions).

It was believed for many years, even by MS specialists, that the disease rarely caused changes in cognitive function. Such changes were thought to occur only in the late stages of MS, if at all. Based on a number of research studies published since the early 1980s, however, it is clear that *cognitive impairment* is quite common in MS. The results of several large-scale, controlled studies suggest that approximately half of all people with MS experience changes in their cognitive function. Not surprisingly, cognitive impairment can have a profound effect on a person's ability to perform important daily activities related to work, social interactions, driving, preparing a simple meal, or even taking care of personal hygiene.

Just as MS can vary in terms of how it affects a person physically, there is considerable variability in the cognitive symptoms of MS. Some people experience cognitive changes as one of their earliest MS symptoms, while others who have had MS for many years may have no cognitive deficits at all. Typically, MS affects only some cognitive functions, while others remain relatively intact. Both research and clinical experience suggest that memory impairment is the most common cognitive symptom in MS. However, changes in information processing and executive functions occur nearly as often. Visuospatial deficits (i.e., impairment in visual perception and constructional abilities) are seen less frequently. Changes in calculation ability are relatively uncommon in MS, but a person may have difficulty doing activities involving calculation (such as balancing a checkbook) due to deficits in information processing or executive functions.

Although changes in the ability to comprehend or use language are less common in MS, they can result from problems with information processing and executive functions. A person with MS may have difficulty comprehending information (either heard or read) that is too complex or presented too rapidly. Distractions in the environment can also interfere with comprehension of incoming information. A person may experience difficulty formulating thoughts and retrieving specific words to express ideas either orally or in writing. While these problems are typically mild and tend to go unnoticed by most, they can at times interfere with daily life.

At present, the best predictor of cognitive status appears to be brain MRI (***magnetic resonance imaging***). In general, the greater the number and the more extensive the ***lesions*** that can be seen on a person's brain MRI, the greater the likelihood that there will be changes in his or her cognitive function. However, this "rule of thumb" is imperfect. Cognitive impairment can be present even if few lesions are visible on MRI; conversely, some people whose MRIs show many MS lesions have few measurable cognitive deficits.

The location of MS lesions is also an important predictor of their effects on a person's function. Most MS lesions tend to cluster in the white matter around the fluid-filled ventricles in the brain (the ***periventricular region***) and the bundle of fibers connecting the two cerebral hemispheres,the **corpus callosum**. This area of the brain is involved in those cognitive functions that are most susceptible to impairment in MS, including memory, information processing, and executive functions. However, isolated lesions can appear anywhere in the white matter or at the junction of the white and gray matter. Some of these may be in so-called "silent regions" of the brain and therefore have relatively little impact on cognitive function. Others may be located in very important brain regions, in which case a relatively small lesion may produce a striking cognitive deficit. Consequently, the only reliable way of determining whether a person has experienced cognitive changes due to MS is through the objective assessment of cognitive function.

Cognitive function can be assessed using an extensive "battery" of tests. This type of assessment is typically carried out by a **neuropsychologist**, a **speech/language pathologist**, or an **occupational therapist**. While these specialists have somewhat different approaches to the assessment of cognitive impairment and utilize different types of tests, their common goal is to identify changes in cognitive function that interfere with everyday life. Most major medical centers and many rehabilitation facilities have qualified specialists in these areas. Evaluations of cognitive function typically involve an interview and several hours of testing because the functions being tested are quite complex.

In order to determine whether a person's cognitive function has changed as a result of MS, the examiner compares the individual's test performance with that of healthy adults who are similar in terms of age, education, and other factors that can affect test performance. Normally, test performance should be comparable to that of this reference, or normative, group. Generally, the lower one's test performance relative to these norms, the more severe the impairment in that particular cognitive function. Unless there are other factors that could reasonably explain identified deficits, it is assumed that they are attributable to MS.

Cognitive rehabilitation refers to techniques designed to improve the functioning of people who have cognitive impairment due to MS and other central nervous system disorders. Most of these techniques were developed for patients with acute changes in their cognitive function due to traumatic brain injury or stroke, but many are applicable to MS. Cognitive rehabilitation may be offered by different types of health care professionals, including neuropsychologists, speech/language pathologists, and occupational therapists.

There are two primary types of cognitive rehabilitation strategies, one aimed at restoring a function, the other focusing on strategies to compensate for a deficit. Restorative strategies are designed to improve the impaired function directly through repetitive drills and practice. Examples of this would include memory retraining strategies based on repetitive list-learning, or attention retraining strategies based on practice and mastery of progressively more challenging exercises. In contrast, compensatory strategies assume that the impaired function will not improve. Consequently, the person is taught to compensate for identified deficits through the use of such strategies as visual imagery, techniques for minimizing distractions, or the use of a personal organizer. The ultimate aim of any cognitive rehabilitation technique is to improve a person's ability to function as independently and safely in his daily activities as possible in spite of cognitive impairment.

Assessment

My wife and children keep telling me that I'm becoming forgetful. How can I tell if MS has affected my memory?

Unfortunately, people are often inaccurate in judging their own cognitive function. Those who are extremely distressed (depressed or anxious) are more likely to believe that their memory is worse than it actually is or to believe that they are having problems with many cognitive functions when they may only have deficits in one or two areas. Conversely, others may be unable to acknowledge their cognitive deficits because it is too emotionally painful for them to accept that MS can affect cognitive as well as physical function. Finally, individuals with extensive cognitive impairment may have only limited awareness of their deficits because they have lost the ability to monitor their behavior and performance.

The perceptions of family members and close friends can also be inaccurate. To be fair, subtle cognitive deficits are often hard to detect in the course of normal social interactions, even for experts. However, relatives and friends sometimes observe cognitive symptoms and misinterpret them as indications of "depression" or "laziness." Family members may be aware of cognitive deficits but feel reluctant to acknowledge them for fear that these deficits would require changes on their part (for example, in the distribution of household responsibilities). Conversely, some relatives and friends may become overly vigilant, interpreting even the most infrequent memory lapse as something abnormal, and therefore caused by MS.

An objective assessment can help determine whether cognitive impairment is present and, if so, its nature and extent. Such an assessment can lead to recommendations regarding treatments for underlying problems, be they neuropsychological, emotional, or interpersonal.

Can I be tested for cognitive problems while I'm taking medications? Can medications affect the way my memory works and therefore alter the test results?

The interpretation of test results is simpler if a person is not taking medications because there are no medication effects to confound or confuse those results. While you do not need to stop taking most medications in order to be evaluated, it is important to tell the examiner what drugs you are on and their dosages. This knowledge will enhance the examiner's ability to interpret the test results.

Many medications, such as antibiotics and medications used to treat spasticity and bladder problems in MS, have no known effects on the *central nervous system*, and therefore do not affect a person's cognitive function. Other medications, such as some that are used to treat hypertension and depression, have subtle effects on the performance of certain neuropsychological tests. However, the effects of these medications are small relative to the effects of MS, and the conditions for which they are prescribed can affect cognitive function as well.

Medications that pose the greatest problems for test interpretation are those that have known central nervous system effects. This includes medications with sedative properties, such as tranquilizers and certain pain medications, and some treatments for MS exacerbations, such as methylprednisolone. If at all possible, a person should be tapered off these medications prior to

cognitive assessment so that they do not confound the test interpretation.

**Sometimes my memory and thinking seem much better than at
other times. When I'm tired, my memory seems even worse
than usual. Can fatigue affect cognitive function?**

Many people with MS report that memory and other cognitive
functions seem to fluctuate, getting worse in periods of increased
sleepiness, fatigue, or stress. This is true of everyone, whether or
not they have MS. However, this is a bigger issue for people with
MS since they are at greater risk for disabling fatigue. The limited research available on fatigue and cognitive function suggests
that fatigue affects cognitive test performance to a lesser extent
than even MS experts would have predicted. However, if you
find that fatigue adversely affects your memory, try to plan your
activities in such a way that you use your best times to do your
most demanding work. Place fewer demands on your memory at
times when you are most likely to be fatigued. It is also important
that you keep in mind that the adverse effects of fatigue are temporary and will reverse once you have recovered from the fatigue,
which for most people is within a few hours.

Does heat affect cognitive symptoms?

Many people with MS report that heat can adversely affect all of
their symptoms, including cognitive function. This may be due
in part to the fatigue that can result from prolonged exposure to
high temperatures. Unfortunately, there have been no research
studies on the effects of temperature changes on cognitive function in MS. However, research is currently under way to determine whether cooling suits or vests can reverse the adverse
effects of heat on a range of MS symptoms. Whatever the effects
of heat and cooling on cognitive function, these effects are transient and will pass in a few hours. You may find that you feel
better in general, and as a result think more clearly, if you stay
out of the heat.

**I know that there can be exacerbations and remissions of phys-
ical symptoms in MS. Are there exacerbations and remissions
in cognitive symptoms?**

Although there has been no formal research on cognitive ***exacerbations*** and ***remissions***, it has been observed clinically that cog-

nitive function may get worse during an exacerbation and improve during remission. In rare cases, cognitive function can become dramatically worse in a very short period of time and then may gradually improve. These dramatic changes are most likely the result of an *acute* inflammatory process. When MS is active, there is swelling in the central nervous system as the immune system attacks *myelin* and a person's symptoms are at their worst. As this acute stage nears its end, people often notice improvement in their symptoms. This process generally runs its course in a matter of weeks at most. If cognitive impairment has developed gradually and been present for months or years, it is unlikely to improve substantially on its own.

Recent tests by a neuropsychologist indicated some problems with my memory and concentration. Will my cognitive problems get worse?

Unfortunately, relatively little is known about the course of cognitive impairment in MS. Some recent research suggests that MS-related cognitive impairment may be more stable over time than physical disability, or at least may progress at a slower rate. This is one of the reasons why there is increasing interest in the use of rehabilitative strategies for improving or compensating for cognitive deficits in people with MS. If, over the course of the next year or two, you notice that you are having more problems with your memory or concentration or new cognitive problems appear, you may find it worthwhile to be reassessed neuropsychologically to determine if there have been any objective changes in your cognitive function.

Do cognitive symptoms ever occur before physical symptoms in a person with MS?

Although physical symptoms are usually the first clue that a person has MS, there have been instances in which changes in cognitive function were the first observable MS symptom. Likewise, after a person has been diagnosed with MS, cognitive changes may signal disease activity before new physical symptoms develop. To the surprise of many MS experts, there is only a weak relationship between cognitive impairment and physical disability. A person with very little physical disability may have striking cognitive deficits, while one with severe physical disability may be quite intact cognitively. Although there is some evidence to suggest that cognitive impairment may be more common in those whose MS is following a progressive course, there are many exceptions to this rule. In short, knowing the extent of someone's physical disability tells you very little about that person's cognitive status.

Why am I able to remember things that I knew a long time ago better than things that just happened recently?

People use the term *memory* to refer to a number of cognitive processes that are actually quite different. MS is much more likely to interfere with a person's ability to lay down new memories than with the ability to summon up old ones from the distant past. This is because the processing of new information is often slowed in MS, making it more difficult to consolidate the new information in a meaningful way. Thus, you may be able to recall your high school years or your first job (drawing on your **remote memory**) much more readily than what occurred in a meeting you attended yesterday (**recent memory**) or at breakfast when you agreed to stop at the grocery store on the way home from work (**prospective memory**). This can be particularly puzzling to friends and family members, who may misinterpret this as a sign that you do not care enough to remember details of shared conversations or activities. However, once these memory problems are understood as a symptom of MS, a number of strategies can be used to help manage or compensate for them.

How are MS-related cognitive problems different from those in Alzheimer's disease?

MS-related cognitive problems differ from those in Alzheimer's disease in several important respects. Cognitive impairment is the *primary* symptom in Alzheimer's disease, whereas not everyone with MS experiences changes in cognitive function. This difference results from the fact that Alzheimer's is a disease of the brain characterized by dramatic changes in, and loss of, nerve cells (**neurons**) in the "gray matter" of the brain (**cortex**), while MS is a disease involving the white matter in the brain, optic nerve, and spinal cord (central nervous system). A diagnosis of Alzheimer's disease requires impairment of at least two cognitive functions, one of which must be memory, with progressive worsening of these functions over time. Even in its early stages, Alzheimer's disease typically involves severe impairment of memory (both recent and remote) and breakdown of language (primarily comprehension and word retrieval), as well as possible visuospatial deficits.

Ultimately, a person with Alzheimer's disease loses the ability to recognize family and friends and to perform even the most basic personal care. In contrast, MS exerts selective effects on cognitive function, typically involving recent memory, information processing, and/or executive functions. Furthermore, MS-related cognitive impairment appears to be relatively stable over time, so that a person may be able to function quite effectively for many years, given appropriate cognitive rehabilitation.

Can cognitive impairment affect my driving ability?

There have been no formal studies of the effects of cognitive impairment on driving in MS. Based on clinical experience and the few studies that have been done in other patient populations, your driving ability may well be impaired if MS has affected your information processing, visuospatial abilities, and executive functions. Often, a person who is aware of having these deficits voluntarily restricts his or her driving or stops driving entirely. However, because driving is a major source of personal independence, this is often a difficult decision to make.

Unfortunately, the procedures used by the Departments of Motor Vehicles are not designed to detect driving problems related to cognitive impairment, so a person's license may be renewed even if he or she is unsafe to drive. If you are concerned about your driving, the best approach would be to obtain an objective driver's evaluation (often done by an occupational therapist with specialized training) and a cognitive assessment so that you can find out the impact of both physical and cognitive symptoms of MS on your driving. Many major medical centers and rehabilitation facilities offer these services; your local chapter of the National Multiple Sclerosis Society can help you locate the one closest to you.

I know that I have begun experiencing some changes in my thinking and memory. What is the best way to explain these changes to my family and friends? People always seem to say "Oh, the same thing happens to me all the time—I can't remember a thing!"

Well-meaning family and friends often try to reassure a person by saying that they have a similar problem with memory or word-finding. This can be frustrating when you are trying to explain your MS symptoms and request their help. You can try explaining to them that, although you may have experienced some of these problems before you had MS, your cognitive problems are different now and much worse. Explain to them that these are a direct result of your MS, much like your physical symptoms. If you have had a cognitive assessment of some kind, you may want to share the results of that assessment with them so that they can begin to understand how MS-related memory problems are different from everyday forgetting. Then you can work together to develop strategies to help you function better, such as using a family calendar to keep track of appointments and social events, designating a specific place to store commonly used household objects, and speaking one at a time so that you can take in information more effectively. If you are having difficulty getting your family and friends to understand your cognitive problems, you may want to set up a family meeting with a psychologist, social worker, or speech/language pathologist who is knowledgeable about these problems and can explain them to your family and friends.

How can I explain my cognitive problems to my children?

Children vary in their need to know about your illness, depending on their ages and the seriousness of your MS. They are usually able to take cognitive changes in stride as long as they understand that these are symptoms of MS and the changes do not interfere too drastically with the flow of everyday life. Children will probably be more upset by your distress over these problems (especially if you are angry and irritable) than by the problems themselves. A matter-of-fact explanation is probably best, using words such as "MS has affected the way my brain works, just like it has affected my walking." Children may ask if this means that you are "stupid" or "crazy." The answer, of course, is an emphatic "NO!"

Be open to questions, but avoid flooding your child with unrequested information. Younger children may need to be reassured that you are going to be okay and that what is happening is not their fault, while adolescents may need to be reminded that they should not take advantage of your memory problems (or any other symptom of your MS). If your cognitive problems are a major source of distress for your children, or if you find it too difficult to discuss these problems with them, you may want to seek professional help from a psychologist, social worker, or cognitive rehabilitation specialist. One or two family meetings is often enough to ease the way for better family communication about these problems.

Should I discuss my cognitive problems with my supervisor at work?

There is no easy answer to this question. Like the decision to disclose the diagnosis of MS, the decision to inform your supervisor that you have cognitive problems due to your MS is complex. One approach is to disclose the information on a "need to know" basis. There may be little reason to tell your supervisor if you have some mild memory problems for which you have effective compensatory strategies and which do not affect your job performance. On the other hand, if your work is beginning to suffer because of your cognitive changes, it may be to your advantage to set up a meeting to talk frankly with your supervisor. Otherwise, any problems with your performance could be misinterpreted as lack of motivation, sloppiness, or a host of other incorrect factors. Many people fear that revealing the presence of cognitive symptoms may be a "kiss of death," stigmatizing them as impaired and incompetent. Such fears are generally unfounded.

When you meet with your supervisor to discuss the cognitive changes caused by your MS, be sure to emphasize your track record and strengths. Try to engage your supervisor in problem-solving about how you and your work environment can adapt to accommodate these changes. Many people find it helpful to work with a cognitive rehabilitation specialist or *vocational rehabilitation* counselor familiar with the cognitive symptoms of MS. This counselor can meet individually with you and together with you and your supervisor to identify ways in which your job or your work environment can be modified so that you can continue to do your job effectively.

My wife, who has MS, seems to be forgetting a lot lately. What is the best way to talk to her about this?

Family members are often reluctant to bring up concerns about memory or other cognitive problems with a person who has MS for fear that it will be upsetting. Often, however, it is a great relief to the person with MS when these concerns are raised because he or she can stop pretending that everything is okay. This can also open the door to a constructive discussion of ways that the person with MS and the family can adapt so that these problems do not "snowball" and cause major disruptions in family functioning.

You should plan to raise your concerns about your wife's memory at a time of day when you and she are well-rested, will not be interrupted, and will have plenty of time to talk things over. You may want to start out by asking her how MS has been affecting her recently to see whether she brings up concerns about her memory. If so, you could offer your observations and then talk about getting an objective memory assessment and recommendations about what can be done. If she does not mention memory problems on her own, you could offer some recent examples and then ask her whether she thinks MS could be affecting her memory. You might want to add your observations about how these memory lapses have affected her, as well as how they have affected you and other family members, and suggest that she undergo cognitive assessment to sort things out.

If your wife becomes irritated or defensive when you bring this up the first time, it is probably best to drop it and try again at another time. If you get a similar response the next time, it may be wise to call and inform her physician of your concerns so that he or she can raise the issue and recommend appropriate assessment. Memory problems can have several different causes, many of them treatable or amenable to rehabilitation once they have been properly assessed.

Treatment and Rehabilitation

Are there any medications to treat cognitive deficits?

At present, there are no medications that are generally accepted as improving cognitive function in MS. Physostigmine, a medication that was originally used experimentally in Alzheimer's disease, proved to be of some benefit in a pilot study with a small number of people with MS. However, the beneficial effects were seen on only a few memory measures and were not evident to family members who rated the person's everyday memory performance. While there is a rationale in Alzheimer's disease for the use of medications such as physostigmine that increase the availability of a neurotransmitter called acetylcholine, there is no such rationale for their use in MS. Furthermore, the currently available form of this medication must be taken six times a day, making it impractical for most people with memory problems.

A different type of medication, pemoline (Cylert®), a psychostimulant that has been used to treat fatigue in MS (see Chapter 2 and Appendix B), is currently being studied to determine its effectiveness in treating MS-related information processing deficits. Results of this trial are not yet available. A medication called 4-aminopyridine (4-AP), which is thought to improve nerve conduction, has also been shown to have modest effects on some neuropsychological measures, but this medication is short-acting and has some problematic side effects (see Chapter 3). In the short run, rehabilitative strategies are the most readily available method for improving the daily functioning of a person with MS-related cognitive problems.

I would like to see if cognitive rehabilitation can help me with my memory problems. How can I find out where to get this type of treatment?

Cognitive rehabilitation by a neuropsychologist, speech/language pathologist, or occupational therapist may be offered at a comprehensive MS center or through an outpatient rehabilitation facility. Such a facility should have expertise in MS or mild cognitive impairment due to other neurologic conditions, as well as an interdisciplinary team approach. Your physician or the local chapter of the MS Society can refer you to such a facility or to individual practitioners who have had experience with MS and cognitive rehabilitation.

Depending on the cognitive rehabilitation specialist's assessment of your particular needs, one of three general approaches might be recommended: (1) a general stimulation approach, in which activities such as listening to stories and playing games encourage cognitive processing at several levels; (2) a process-specific approach, in which a specific cognitive function is targeted for intervention through a hierarchical series of successively more difficult exercises; or (3) a functional adaptation approach, in which rehabilitation is performed in your natural home or work environment. Thus, some approaches to cognitive rehabilitation are very focused while others are part of a broader rehabilitative approach that may also include psychological counseling and other types of therapies. The cognitive rehabilitation specialist should give you the rationale for the approach that he or she recommends, as well as an estimate of what kind of results to expect and how many sessions this will take. Unfortunately, there are currently no published studies of cognitive rehabilitation in MS, so the clinical experience of the cognitive rehabilitation specialist is very important.

If cognitive rehabilitation is done by neuropsychologists, speech/language pathologists, and occupational therapists, how do I know which type of professional I should see?

Neuropsychologists became involved in cognitive assessment and retraining because of their interest in brain-barrier relationships. Speech/language pathologists offer cognitive rehabilitation because of their expertise in language- and communication-related problems. Occupational therapists direct their rehabilitation efforts at reducing the impact of cognitive impairment on a person's ability to carry out the activities of daily living. While each of these professionals brings to the rehabilitation process a somewhat different set of assessment tools and treatment strategies, they share a common goal of enabling people with MS to function comfortably and successfully in everyday life.

The type of professional you see for cognitive rehabilitation will probably be determined by the availability of these service providers in your area. Your physician will be able to refer you to the nearest agencies or individuals with expertise in cognitive rehabilitation in MS. If you have the luxury of choice, you might want to discuss your situation with the available professionals and decide which individual(s) and which treatment approach(es) seem best suited to your particular needs and personality style.

How long will cognitive rehabilitation take?

There is no standard time frame for cognitive rehabilitation. Its duration will depend on the nature and severity of your cognitive problems. Cognitive rehabilitation techniques were originally developed in inpatient settings where sessions occurred daily or even more than once a day. Many of these techniques have been adapted for use in outpatient settings, with sessions occurring at least once a week (but preferably more often, to improve carryover) for several weeks.

You and your cognitive rehabilitation specialist should periodically review your progress together to determine how you are progressing toward your goals and to revise or set new goals as needed. When you have achieved the goals you set, it is a good idea to taper the frequency of cognitive rehabilitation sessions (i.e., gradually increase the length of time between sessions) rather than discontinuing them abruptly. Scheduling "booster sessions," much like dental checkups, can also help ensure that you continue to apply the techniques you have learned and identify any new problems before they become too disruptive.

Can cognitive rehabilitation help me even if my memory and concentration are slowly getting worse?

Yes. Cognitive rehabilitation is designed to maximize your cognitive function and develop long-term strategies to compensate for functions that are not likely to respond to restorative treatments. In the course of cognitive rehabilitation, you will learn skills that you can use now and in the future, even if your problems get worse. In fact, there is probably some advantage to learning these skills early on, when it may be easier to assimilate them. For example, you may learn strategies for better regulating your attention and limiting environmental distractions—techniques that you can continue to apply if your concentration problems get worse. Or you may learn how to use an organizer notebook to record appointments, phone numbers, and things you need to remember to do. If your memory problems get worse, you can still use this notebook and perhaps add new sections, such as a diary in which to record the major events of the day so that you can review them at a later time. If your cognitive problems get worse or new problems arise, you may want to return to your cognitive rehabilitation specialist to review how you can get the most out of methods you learned in the past and identify new strategies that may be useful to you.

My children keep accusing me of forgetting things that they have told me. Sometimes I remember these things once they remind me, but other times I don't recall them saying these

things at all. I'm starting to wonder if they are telling the truth. How can we deal with this problem?

The first step in coming up with effective solutions is to obtain a thorough assessment of the problem. In a situation like this, it is important not only for you to have an objective cognitive assessment, but also for your family to be evaluated by a social worker, psychologist, or other health care professional familiar with MS-related cognitive problems and their potential impact on family relationships.

If it turns out that you do have some identifiable cognitive problems, a cognitive rehabilitation specialist can work with you and your family to identify the circumstances under which these problems are most likely to occur and to modify them. For example, if your children are trying to talk with you while the television is on or while there is another conversation going on in the room, the cognitive rehabilitation specialist may suggest that the television be turned off during these discussions or that you and your child seek a quieter, less distracting place to talk. If you are having trouble remembering where your children have said they were going, the cognitive rehabilitation specialist may suggest a family "memo board" in a central location for everyone to record where they have gone and when they will be back. Often very simple changes can make a world of difference.

In some situations, however, cognitive changes are only a minor factor, and the real difficulty is an underlying family problem that has been present for some time. In such cases, working with a social worker or psychologist to address the underlying family problem is critical.

Recently I've noticed that I have a lot of trouble concentrating or following conversations, particularly when there is something else going on in the room. Is there anything that I can do about this problem?

It is not uncommon with MS to have difficulty ignoring background noise or distractions and, as a result, to have difficulty following social conversations. This ability to pay attention selectively to important information (i.e., what the person is saying to you) while ignoring unimportant information (such as other conversations in the room) is one aspect of information processing, often termed "selective attention." A cognitive rehabilitation specialist can work with you to improve this skill, teach you how to compensate for this problem, or both. For example, restorative strategies might include improving your selective attention through a series of gradually more difficult exercises in which you have to ignore competing background messages and attend only to what is important. Compensatory strategies might include learning ways to alter the environment so that it is easier for you to concentrate.

Communication is a cycle of "give and take" between speaker and listener. Some people are embarrassed when they cannot keep up with a conversation, so they nod and pretend they are following it. Others simply find excuses to avoid social situations in which they will be confronted with this problem. However, it is your responsibility and right as a listener to let others know what you need in order to participate successfully in a conversation. There are two ways to regulate input in this type of situation—quieting the background noise or moving away from it. For most people, it will take practice to learn to feel comfortable making requests such as "I'd appreciate it if you could lower the volume of the TV so that we can continue our conversation" (to quiet the background noise) or "Let's go to a quieter room so that we can talk without being interrupted" (to move away from the noise). In the long run, it is far better to learn strategies for regulating input than to allow a breakdown in communication.

I used to enjoy reading, but now I find that I have a lot of trouble remembering who the characters are and what the story line is. Are there strategies for dealing with this problem?

Problems with reading can have several different causes. First, reading requires you to see and use your eyes well. Visual problems typical of MS can interfere with the reading process, such as blurriness, double vision (**diplopia**), "jiggly eyes" (**nystagmus**), and difficulty with left-to-right scanning eye movements. Second, reading requires you to concentrate on the written material, understand what you are reading, and remember it later. People with MS report little or no difficulty understanding what they read. However, problems with concentration and memory result in frequent complaints such as "I cannot read for as long as I used to"; "I have to reread it many times"; "When I pick up a book to continue where I left off, I can't remember what I've already read."

A treatment plan can be developed following a thorough evaluation to determine the cause of your reading difficulties. If you have problems with eye movements and coordination, an occupational therapist or behavioral optometrist (an optometrist with additional expertise in eye training) can suggest eye movement exercises that may be helpful. The eye specialist will also make sure that you are fitted with the proper lenses.

If concentration and memory problems interfere with reading, a cognitive rehabilitation specialist may recommend exercises directed at the underlying attention/concentration problem, as well as specialized reading techniques such as the "four R's"—Read, Reread, Reorganize, and Review. The first phase of the "four R's" involves scanning the headings, pictures, and first and last paragraphs (of a newspaper article, for example) to get the "gist" or main idea. This builds a framework within which to organize new information as you read each paragraph. As you proceed to reread the entire article, it is helpful to highlight the key ideas, make notes, and continually relate the information in the new paragraph to the previous one. The next step is to reorganize the information by putting various elements into your own words, developing opinions, and personalizing the information. Many people find it helpful to reorganize information into a format of "Who, What, When, Where, and How" details. Finally, as you review your highlights and notes, it may be beneficial to discuss the information with another person. The goal is to involve as many language modalities as possible (seeing, saying, hearing, and writing it) in order to improve your reading ability. It may take extra time to process information in this fashion, but the likelihood of recalling it later is much greater.

Recently I'm finding that it takes me a very long time to do routine tasks like paying the bills and balancing my checkbook. I even make errors on simple calculations. I don't want to have to ask my husband to do this for me. Is there a solution to this problem?

The skills required for effective money and checkbook management are more complex than most people realize. Not only are adequate vision and hand function important, but a whole host of cognitive skills are involved (e.g., attention to detail, calculation ability, calculator use, organization, sequencing, decision-making, problem-solving, and the ability to follow through and complete an activity). If independence in money and checkbook management is a realistic goal, the cognitive rehabilitation specialist can use treatment strategies such as devising a monthly budget, developing a flow chart for bill-paying, and teaching you how to avoid checkbook errors by "talking your way through" checkbook entries and double-checking your work with a calculator. If you are comfortable with the use of a computer, you may be instructed in the use of a money management software program.

If independent money and checkbook management is not a realistic goal, the cognitive rehabilitation specialist can work with you and a family member to develop ways for you to be involved in financial decision-making without the burden of maintaining a checkbook and paying bills. In some communities, banks and special agencies can provide automatic bill-paying services and assistance in reconciling your checkbook with the bank statement on a fee-for-service basis. As always, it is important to have a thorough evaluation of the problem in order to set realistic goals and develop appropriate solutions to problems such as these.

I've been having problems with my memory, managing the household, and keeping track of things I have to do. Would an electronic organizer or computer be helpful to me?

A variety of compensatory aids can help with memory and organizational problems. These include the loose-leaf organizer books that have become so popular in recent years, pocket electronic organizers, and computers. The disadvantage of computers and electronic organizers is that learning how to use them can be somewhat complex. However, if you can master their operation, they are among the most powerful tools at your disposal. Pocket electronic organizers can keep track of names and addresses, appointments, and to-do lists. In their more expensive incarnations, they can even send faxes and do word processing. Computers do all these things and more, but are not as portable.

There are also many types of computer software that may assist your memory and organizational efforts. Personal information managers perform most of the functions that loose-leaf organizers can do, but generally also have a powerful database capability. You can type in notes on a given subject, such as "Christmas List," and later do what is called a "random search," in which all your notes on the subject are retrieved, sorted, and presented to you. Money management software can allow you to keep tabs on your checking account and reconcile your bank statement in a matter of minutes, with no need to do any arithmetical computations yourself. If you find that memory problems are requiring you to write yourself a lot of notes or lists, the computer can be a godsend. Large amounts of data can be managed and retrieved using database and/or word processing software. Sometimes relying exclusively on paper can become cumbersome as you begin to accumulate piles of notes, reminders, and other materials.

Electronic organizers and computers are not magic. Like all compensatory strategies, they require learning and practice to make best use of their potential. Working with a cognitive rehabilitation specialist can help you to develop skill and consistency in using these modern marvels. Ideally, your response to MS cognitive changes should involve a comprehensive program that includes individual, social, paper-and-pencil, and electronic strategies. A well-balanced combination of all of these approaches should enable you to deal effectively with many of the cognitive changes brought about by MS.

I have always been an organized person. Now I seem to be having a lot of trouble scheduling my time and estimating how long it will take me to get a job done. Even when I have figured out what I am going to do, I seem to have a lot of trouble getting started. Is there anything that I can do about this problem?

Organizational skills are extremely important for a person's independent functioning; these include goal setting, planning, scheduling, monitoring the progress of a task, and completing tasks in a timely fashion. MS can affect your ability to carry out activities efficiently, causing you to take "detours" along the way or to backtrack in order to take care of a step or two that you inadvertently left out. MS can also cause you to get "stuck" while trying to solve problems that come up in daily life. Problems with executive functions such as these are thought to be due to MS lesions in the white matter connecting the front portion of the brain (***frontal lobes***) with other important brain structures.

Cognitive rehabilitation for problems with executive functions typically has the dual focus of teaching compensatory strategies and identifying environmental modifications. Helpful compensatory strategies might include using structured approaches to analyzing tasks and activities, setting timetables, and problem-solving. Environmental approaches might include maintaining a consistent daily schedule and involving family members to generate alternative solutions to problems or to cue you to begin an activity. Generally, the greater your problems with executive functions, the greater the likelihood that the cognitive rehabilitation specialist will emphasize environmental approaches to these problems.

My friends and family have started to complain that I interrupt a lot and seem to have trouble waiting until they're finished before I start to speak. I've always disliked people who interrupt a lot and I don't know why I'm doing this. Can I learn to control it?

Conversational problems such as poor listening and interrupting others are referred to as "pragmatic communication deficits." They are thought to stem from executive dysfunction due to MS lesions affecting connections to the frontal lobes. Often a person who has pragmatic communication problems may not be aware of them or of subtle negative feedback from the listener. Since people tend to avoid interacting with those who dominate conversations, interrupt them when they are talking, do not listen well, or do not take turns, social isolation can be a significant consequence of these communication deficits.

A speech/language pathologist is skilled at evaluating and treating deficits in the pragmatics of communication using both individual and group therapy techniques. The first step in learning to control these problems is for you to become aware of behaviors that you or others exhibit that can disrupt communication. Watching a videotape of yourself in conversation and getting feedback from the speech/language pathologist and others are good starting points. The speech/language pathologist can then teach you ways of improving your listening skills through the use of eye contact, verbal and nonverbal acknowledgments (e.g., saying "that's interesting" or nodding), and minimizing interruptions. You may be videotaped practicing these skills so that you can monitor the reactions of others to these behaviors and chart your progress. Improving your pragmatic communication skills can make a major difference in the quality of your social interactions and the enjoyment you derive from social relationships.

I seem to have trouble coming to the point when I'm talking. Even though I know what I want to say, I seem to go off on tangents and talk too long. Is there a solution to this problem?

People tend to become "wordy" and go off on tangents when they are having trouble retrieving specific words or find it difficult to organize the complex thoughts they wish to express. "My vocabulary seems to be shrinking," "It's on the tip of my tongue," or "My thoughts and speech are out of sync" are commonly heard complaints from people with MS. While these word-finding difficulties can be quite frustrating, they are typically less noticeable to the listener than to the speaker. Evaluation and treatment by a speech/language pathologist or other cognitive rehabilitation specialist are recommended for these mild cognitive/language difficulties.

Therapy may include word association techniques and self-cuing strategies to improve specific word retrieval. Learning to "impose a delay" and quietly organize your thoughts before speaking often helps verbal expression. Concise, specific expression of ideas is possible when adequate time is allotted for pre-planning. Using a "Beginning, Middle, End" format can help you stay on the topic and teach you how to delete unnecessary, irrelevant comments. During therapy it is also important to refine your self-evaluation skills to help guard against wordiness and tangential speech.

Recommended Readings

Dohrmann V. *Treating Memory Impairments: A Memory Book and Other Strategies*. Tucson, AZ: Communication Skill Builders, 1994.

Erlich J, Sipes A. Group treatment for communication skills for head trauma patients. *Cognitive Rehabilitation* 1985;3:32-37.

Prutting C, Kirchner D. Applied pragmatics. In: Gallagher T, Prutting C (eds.). *Pragmatic Assessment and Intervention Issues in Language*. San Diego: College-Hill Press, 1983.

Rao S, Leo G, Bernardin L, Unverzagt F. Cognitive dysfunction in multiple sclerosis. I. Frequency, patterns, and prediction. *Neurology* 1991;41:685-91.

Rao S, Leo G, Ellington L, Nauertz T, Bernardin L, Unverzagt F. Cognitive dysfunction in multiple sclerosis. II. Impact on employment and social functioning. *Neurology* 1991:41:692-96.

Sohlberg M, Mateer C. *Introduction to Cognitive Rehabilitation: Theory and Practice.* New York: Guilford Press, 1989.

Booklet available from the National Multiple Sclerosis Society (Customer Service: 212-986-3240; Information: 800-344-4867)

◇ *Solving Cognitive Problems*—Nicholas G. LaRocca, Ph.D., with Martha King

10

Psychosocial Issues

Rosalind C. Kalb, Ph.D
Deborah M. Miller, Ph.D.

Multiple sclerosis has been compared to the unexpected visitor who arrives at your house, complete with bag and baggage, and never leaves (as described by Jacqueline Faffer, Ph.D.). This visitor has the tendency to spread his belongings through every room of the house, affecting the lifestyle and activities of all the members of the household. MS, with its varied symptoms and unpredictable course, is an intrusion that the whole family must learn to accommodate. While a relatively small number of people with MS experience severe disability, the uncertainty and variability of the disease create their own day-to-day stresses even for those with minimal impairment.

By necessity, the adjustment process is an ongoing one; as the symptoms of MS come and go, or come and stay, coping and adjustment ebb and flow as well. Since each family member will approach this challenge with his or her own particular coping style, effective communication will enhance the family's ability to work together to handle the day-to-day challenges of life with a chronic illness.

The questions in this chapter cover those aspects of a person's social and emotional life that are most often touched by MS, including self-esteem, coping efforts, and relationships with family members and friends. The answers also serve to highlight the role of ongoing education, effective coping strategies, and supportive counseling in each individual's and each family's efforts to live comfortably and productively with this intrusion in their lives.

Sense of Self

How do I begin to figure out who I am now that I have difficulty doing so many of the things I used to do?

Your self-image has been built up slowly over your lifetime. Your accumulated skills and life experiences all contributed to the picture you have of yourself. If MS interferes with your ability to do something that is important to you, that is a significant loss that must be grieved over. Because MS can affect a person in so many different ways, you may find that you are grieving over one loss or another much of the time. At the same time, however, you are in the process of learning new things about yourself. As you confront the challenges of everyday life with MS and learn alternative ways to do things, you will begin to identify strengths and talents you never knew you had. If you are forced to give up one or another activity that has been important in your life, try to experiment with others that may turn out to be equally satisfying. Most importantly, look for that aspect of yourself which MS is unable to touch. For one person it may be his sense of humor, for another her religious beliefs, for yet another his love of music. By identifying this "MS-free zone" within yourself, you can retain a sense of who you are even in the face of stressful changes.

I still can't bring myself to tell anyone about my diagnosis. I don't know how people will react and I'm not sure I'm ready to find out. What is the best way to talk about my MS with other people?

While it is never possible to predict exactly how another person will react to your MS, it is safe to assume that most people will take their cues from you. Be prepared to explain what MS is and to let the person know if you feel comfortable talking about it and answering questions. Some people will want to tell you about others they have known with MS; others will want to give you a lot of suggestions or advice. Most, however, will express shock and concern and then wait for you to tell them what you want or need from them. Since you will want or need different things from different people, think this through before you talk to the person. Try not to jump to conclusions about their reactions to you. Some people may seem to withdraw a bit; this is probably a reflection more of their own anxiety about how to talk to you about the MS than any lack of care or concern on their part. For more information about talking to your employer or colleagues about your MS, refer to Chapter 14.

Family, friends, and work are all important parts of my life. Now that I have MS, I don't have enough energy to deal with any of them as well as I would like. How can I learn to accept my limitations and feel less guilty?

Accepting personal limitations is always difficult, but everyone, with or without MS, experiences the frustration of overload at one time or another. Try to remember that the MS is not your fault and that doing the best you can is all that anyone can ask of you. Then take time to think through your priorities at home and at work and look at your weekly schedule to see if the way you actually spend time matches these priorities. Most people find that they spend too much time on activities that are not really necessary or important to them. Be sure to allow yourself enough time for brief rests if you need them. The time you invest in these rest periods will help you be more productive in all your activities. Talk with the significant people in your life about the ways in which MS affects you and share with them your concerns about limitations on your time and energy. They will be reassured to know that you care enough to discuss this with them and you will be relieved of some of the worry about letting people down.

What is a support group and what kinds of groups are there for people with MS?

A support group is a form of self-help in which people with a common problem get together to share information, feelings, and ideas—or just to listen. Some of the larger groups (anywhere from twenty to two hundred people) are more educational in nature, with invited speakers coming to talk about various topics of interest. Other groups, usually with a smaller, more consistent membership (eight to ten people) from one meeting to the next, place greater emphasis on mutual support and shared problem-solving. Groups can be led by trained professionals, peer-led (by someone with MS who has taken on the leadership role), or have no leader at all. Some support groups are time-limited while others continue on a regular basis until the membership decides that it is time to stop.

At the present time the National Multiple Sclerosis Society sponsors more than 1,500 support groups. Among the most common are groups for the newly diagnosed, for those with more severe disability, and for couples, spouses, or children. There are also employment groups in which people discuss problems related to job stress, disclosure, reasonable accommodations, and retirement. There are singles groups for men and women who want to meet others with MS and share some of the problems and frustrations of life with the disease. The important thing to remember about groups is that they can vary in size, structure, focus, and quality. Consult your local MS Society chapter about the groups available in your area. Ask the Patient Services Representative to help you select the group that is most suitable for you. If you try one and it does not seem to meet your needs, try another. If you try several and cannot find what you are looking for, think about starting one of your own. The MS Society is interested in your suggestions and ideas and will be very helpful in your efforts to find a support group or start one in your area.

I'm embarrassed to be seen using a cane. If I ever get to the point of needing a walker, I'm afraid I'll just lock myself in the house. What can I do about this feeling?

Some people are reluctant to be seen using a cane or walker because they are worried that other people will think less of them. Others are afraid that people will feel pity. The first step in dealing with these concerns is to look at your own feelings about the cane or walker. If you believe that you are less of a person or that you have less to offer others because of these aids, try discussing this with your spouse, a close friend, or a colleague. Let them remind you of the qualities and talents they value in you, whether or not you need a mobility aid. You might also think about joining a support group with others who use mobility aids. As you get to like and respect others in the group, you will gradually learn to see beyond their canes, walkers, or wheelchairs; you will find that you notice the people and not their hardware. As you begin to see beyond their mobility aids, you will also begin to see beyond your own.

The second step in adjusting to a cane, walker, or any other mobility aid is to begin to see it as an important energy-saving tool in your life. Rather than interfering with your ability to do your chosen activities, the mobility aid makes it possible for you to do them more safely, quickly, and effectively. As you start to view the aid as a tool for getting things done, others around you will begin to view it in the same way.

Although there are many things I'm still able to do, all I can think about is ending up in a nursing home. How can I learn to stop anticipating the worst and get back to enjoying the life I have?

For most people, "ending up in a nursing home" means totally losing control over one's life. While a small percentage of people with MS do require residential care, the reality is that the vast majority do not. Therefore, the best way to deal with the fear of loss of control is to break it down into more manageable bits. Try to identify those areas of your life in which you feel most vulnerable and least in control and tackle them one by one. There are many resources available to help you with this problem-solving effort. Your physician can help you to manage MS symptoms as effectively as possible; an occupational and/or a physical therapist can recommend tools and strategies for dealing with many aspects of daily life; a lawyer and/or accountant can help you plan effectively for the future; a support group can help you learn how to live more comfortably with the uncertainties that MS brings to your life. As you begin to tackle some of the stressful problem areas, you will find that you feel less vulnerable and therefore more able to enjoy your daily life.

I have a lot of very supportive family and friends trying to help and encourage me. But no one really understands what I'm going though with my symptoms. I feel very alone and don't know what to do about it.

Perhaps the loneliest aspect of life with MS, or any other illness, is that even the most loving and supportive friend cannot "get in your shoes" and feel what you are feeling. Because so many of the symptoms of MS are invisible, e.g., fatigue, visual problems, and sensory changes, family and friends will often have a hard time understanding what is going on with you. Let them know when you are not feeling well, explain your symptoms, and offer reading materials about the illness to those who would like them. Do not expect people to be able to read your mind. Try to remember that a person does not have to be able to understand exactly what you are experiencing in order to offer you love and support.

Sometimes the best way to feel less alone is to spend some time with others who know firsthand what it feels like to live with this disease. There are a variety of ways to share experiences with others who have MS, including reading what others have written—in books or MS publications, posting messages on computerized bulletin boards, or joining a discussion group.

MS has taken away a lot of my independence. It has been many years since I needed anyone to help me with toileting, eating, and dressing. How can I hold on to my self-respect when I need so much help with everything?

We all spend many years learning to be self-sufficient, independent adults, and it is painful to lose any aspect of this hard-earned independence. Because the symptoms of MS make it impossible for you to perform routine activities of daily living in the usual way, you need to rely on special equipment and/or the help of other people to get the job done. Part of the process of learning to cope with this change in your life is recognizing that you are still getting the job done. In the same way that you developed self-respect as a child by learning to master the environment, you can and should take satisfaction in meeting the challenges of life with MS. Your self-respect will come from finding solutions, identifying useful tools, and availing yourself of whatever resources might enable you to lead your life in the fullest way possible.

Loss of self-esteem is a central focus of many MS support group discussions. As people deal with the changes and compromises that MS sometimes forces them to make in their lives, they find that sharing these experiences and problem-solving with other adults bolsters their sense of self-worth.

I get angry at colleagues and friends who tell me, "But you look so good. . . ." How can I explain to them that I almost never feel as good as I look?

Some people say that you look good because they are trying to be supportive and encouraging. Others are asking in a roundabout way why you are not being more active or more productive. Almost everybody who says it is trying to figure out what MS is and how it affects you. Try to remember that most people's experience with illness is that it makes you feel and look sick for a few days or weeks and then you get better. It will take them quite awhile to understand that MS does not go away like the flu or the measles, and that it affects how you feel and act even when they cannot see any signs of it at all. Be patient; answer people's questions about MS; and whenever possible try to explain how you are feeling in ways that others can relate to ("Because of my optic neuritis everything looks as though I'm seeing it through a dark mesh screen." "When I walk around it feels as though I'm slogging my way through thick mud." "I constantly feel as though I just stepped off the roller coaster and haven't got my balance back."). Additionally, there are several short, easy-to-read pamphlets about MS, which you can give people if they are interested.

I used to have a pretty active social life. Now I don't even try to meet people. Why would anyone be interested in a relationship with a person who has MS?

Before you can understand why others would be interested in having a relationship with you, it is important for you to reconnect with those parts of yourself that you value. In spite of the fact that you have MS, you are still a person—complete with interests, opinions, and feelings. You may have gotten so overwhelmed by MS-related stresses and changes that you have temporarily lost sight of the rest of you. Take some time to get to know yourself again. Whether you do this in an MS support group, in psychotherapy, or with a close friend, try to identify those aspects of yourself and your life that are independent of the MS. Then leave the rest up to others. You cannot decide for another person whether he or she will want a relationship with you. All you can do is be yourself. Some people will be put off by the MS, but many others will not.

I was diagnosed with MS about a year ago and most of my symptoms are not apparent to other people. Occasionally I need to use a cane when my walking is a bit unsteady. When should I tell someone I begin to date about my MS?

As with other interpersonal issues, there is no single correct answer to this question. You need to do whatever makes you feel most comfortable, given your sense of the situation and the person with whom you are dealing. The following guidelines may be helpful:

◇ First dates are a time for deciding whether you have any interest in pursuing the relationship further. There is no need to share any personal information with someone you do not like enough to see a second time.

◇ Once you have decided that the person is someone with whom you would like to develop a longer-term friendship/romance, keep in mind that half-truths and secrets make a very shaky foundation for a healthy, comfortable relationship.

◇ Revealing information about a chronic illness does not usually get easier as a relationship progresses; the more involved you are and the more you care about a person, the greater the potential loss.

◇ In deciding when to reveal significant information about yourself, think about when you would want to know similar kinds of information about the other person.

◇ Although some people will probably be frightened or put off by the MS, many others will not. You may be better off knowing the relationship's potential sooner rather than later.

Coping

If the doctor could just tell me what was going to happen with my MS, I think I could handle it. It's never knowing what's going to happen that upsets me. Is there any way to cope with all this uncertainty?

Unfortunately, unpredictability is one of the hallmarks of MS, and you are not alone in finding this so stressful. Most people find that they gradually adjust to taking life one day at a time, making the most of good days and putting up with the bad days. If you find yourself dwelling endlessly on "what if. . .?" (. . . I get worse, . . . I can't walk, . . . I can't see, . . . I can't do my job), it may be helpful and reassuring to do some advance problem-solving. Think through how you would deal with these changes, make contingency plans, and look into available resources. Some people find it very comforting to know that they have strategies in mind to deal with possible problems. Allowing yourself to think through the unthinkable can enable you to feel more prepared and more in control whatever the future brings.

Since my diagnosis, my husband has begun to hover over me all the time. I know he's worried about me, but I feel as though I've totally lost my independence. How can I explain to him that I need to learn how to live with my MS in my own way?

Each of you will need to learn to live with MS in your own way. At the same time that you are learning to cope with varied and unpredictable symptoms of MS, your husband will be adjusting to his own feelings about the illness and its impact on your daily life. Your husband's protectiveness is a sign of his anxiety about your health and safety as well as about your future together. Describe your symptoms to him so that he can understand how you are feeling. While explaining to your husband how much you value your independence, you can assure him that you will use caution and good sense and that you will ask him for help when you need it. Invite him to come with you to visit your physician so that he can hear what the physician has to say and ask any questions about the illness. Your physician will be able to offer reassurance and reinforce your need to be as independent as possible.

You and your husband may find it helpful to join a couples' support group. In this setting each of you can learn from others how they have coped with the impact of MS on family life. Your husband might also enjoy a spouse group in which he can share his feelings and concerns with other husbands and wives whose partners have MS.

My wife was just diagnosed with MS. She keeps giving me articles to read and insists I go to the doctor with her. All her symptoms have gone away. Why can't we just forget about this for now and get on with our lives?

Being diagnosed with a chronic illness can be a very frightening and lonely experience. Your wife is trying to learn as much as she can about MS so that she will feel less afraid and more prepared to cope with it as time goes on. She may be asking you to share the learning process with her so that she does not feel so alone. Although MS is an unexpected intrusion in both of your lives, you may have very different styles of coping with it. While talking and reading a lot about MS helps her to feel better, the same strategies might make you feel worse! The more she tries to get you to talk or think about MS, the more you will struggle to put it out of your mind. It is important to talk to each other about your different coping styles. One style is not necessarily better than the other, but she may misinterpret your reluctance to read or talk about her MS as not caring about her or her feelings. Try to reassure her while at the same time explaining that you need to deal with her illness in your own way. Perhaps you can reach a compromise that satisfies both her need for your support and your need to focus on other things in your life.

I used to deal with life's frustrations by exercising and playing a lot of sports. Now that I'm not able to be as active as I used to be, I'm having trouble dealing with the pent-up feelings. How can I find other outlets that work for me?

Most people who play a lot of sports derive satisfaction from both the physical exertion and the competition. If your primary satisfaction from sports is the exertion itself, talk to your doctor about alternative forms of exercise that might be suitable for you, such as Tai-Chi, yoga, swimming, weight training, or a stationary bike (see Chapters 2 and 5). If what you miss most is the competitive aspect of sports, explore other forms of competition such as competitive bridge, chess, or computer games. Then remember that another way to release pent-up feelings is to talk about them. In the past it may never have been your style to talk about feelings, but you may find at this point in your life that talking—whether it be with a spouse, a friend, or in a support group—is a satisfying relief.

Since my husband was diagnosed with MS a few months ago, it's all he thinks and talks about. It seems as though our whole family has been taken over by this disease. Is this normal?

While each individual reacts to the MS diagnosis somewhat differently, it is not uncommon for a person to react initially by being quite preoccupied with the illness. One person might show this preoccupation by being totally unwilling to think or talk about any aspect of MS, as if ignoring it will make it go away. Another person shows the preoccupation by talking and thinking about MS to the exclusion of everything else. Whether or not they are currently experiencing symptoms, each is aware of a new and threatening problem over which he or she has very little control. Both of these individuals are trying to come to terms with a diagnosis that changes the way they think about themselves, their lives, and the future.

A newly diagnosed person's preoccupation with MS can be very difficult for family members. Your husband may be experiencing a variety of strange and uncomfortable symptoms that you are unable to see or understand. At the same time that he is trying to deal with MS, you are trying to cope with your own feelings about it as well as everything else that is going on in the household. Although his feelings and concerns may be quite normal, it is still important for him to understand how his behavior affects other family members. Try to talk to him about your feelings. Ask him about going to a support group for the newly diagnosed. If, in another month or two, your husband still seems overly preoccupied with the MS, ask him if he would go with you to a therapist to talk about the impact of MS on the entire family.

I've been having a pretty hard time adjusting to the MS and all the changes it has caused in my life. My doctor suggested that I might want to get counseling to deal with some of my feelings but I've never needed therapy before and I don't see how it could help me now.

Your physician knows that being diagnosed with a chronic disease is a stressful and bewildering intrusion in any person's life. In short-term, problem-focused psychotherapy, a therapist who is knowledgeable about MS can help you understand and cope with your reactions to this intrusion. First, the therapist can help you work through the normal grief reaction that comes from having to alter your self-image to include a chronic illness. Second, he or she can provide you with a relaxed setting in which to ask questions and explore your options; most people find it very difficult to think of all their questions and concerns in the short time spent with the physician. The therapist can help you integrate the information you are receiving from your physician and sort through the advice and reactions of well-meaning friends and relatives. Coping with MS is an ongoing process that ebbs and flows with the changes that the disease causes in your life. As the MS follows its unpredictable course, you may find it useful to maintain intermittent contact with a therapist who can serve as a familiar resource whenever new symptoms add further stress and challenge at home or at work.

Family Life

My boyfriend and I are talking about getting married next year. He knows that I have MS and he says it doesn't matter to him— he loves me anyway. He has never been to the doctor with me and seems reluctant to go. I think it's important for him to hear what the doctor has to say so that he knows what he's getting himself into. How can I explain this to him?

You might try suggesting to your boyfriend that marriage is challenging enough without going into it blindfolded. Although love is an important part of a successful marriage, the ability to talk, problem-solve, and make decisions as a couple is also essential—particularly when life involves a chronic illness. Explain to him that you would be more comfortable sharing your life with him if you were confident that he had some understanding of what that might entail. If you are concerned that your boyfriend might be frightened by what your physician has to say, tell him so and assure him that you would rather start dealing with his fears and doubts now than be overwhelmed by them later.

We have worked hard to save money for our daughter's education. Soon my husband, who is in a wheelchair, may need a van to drive himself to work. How can we possibly choose between

a college education and a van my husband needs in order to get to his job?

The heavy expenses related to chronic illness can drain family resources and necessitate compromise on the part of every family member. Before you start trying to choose between a van and a college education, however, be sure to look into possible funding sources for each. Education loans and scholarships based on financial need are often available, and chronic illness in the family is a valid and recognized financial hardship. Contact your chapter of the MS Society to ask if there are any local sources of aid toward the cost of a van. Some automobile companies also have programs to help people meet the cost of adaptive equipment. Once you have gathered all the financial information, sit down as a family to review your options and decide which choices make most sense for your family.

Our son recently told me that he didn't like to bring friends over any more because the whole house is starting to look like a surgical supply store. There's no space to "hang out" without tripping over one piece of equipment or another. How should we deal with this?

All members of the family need to feel "at home" in the house. When the needs of one person begin to crowd out everyone else, the balance is out of kilter and needs to be restored. Ideally, there should be space for all of you to relax, converse, and entertain without tripping over assistive equipment. Have a family meeting to talk over the problem and see if together you can come up with any space-saving, organizational ideas for managing the assistive equipment and creating equipment-free areas. The essential point to share with the whole family is that it is important for each of you to feel comfortable in the home.

You may also want to discuss with your son his feelings about MS. Depending on his age, he may be feeling embarrassed or self-conscious about his parent's illness and the need for assistive equipment. He may be concerned about what his friends will think and he may be uncomfortable with their questions. If he seems to have difficulty talking this over with you, you can offer him age-appropriate reading materials from the MS Society and alert him to the possibility of talking or writing to other children his own age who also have a parent with MS. Your local MS Society chapter can help him to make these kinds of connections.

Our family used to do a lot of hiking and camping. Since my wife got MS, she can't really hike for any distance and she's uncomfortable "roughing it." I don't know whether I should take the children camping without her or give up camping and try to find another kind of inexpensive family vacation.

Like many of the other questions in this chapter, there is no one correct answer. The solution lies in talking the options over with your wife (and children if they are old enough to understand and participate) and deciding what works best for all of you. Your goal should always be to try to balance the needs and wishes of all family members. One solution may be to compromise; go on occasional father-and-children camping excursions and at the same time begin investigating other, less physically strenuous, possibilities for the whole family. If you give up camping altogether, the less than desirable outcome may be that you and the children feel a bit resentful and your wife feels guilty. Consult a travel agent who is knowledgeable about vacation opportunities for the disabled (see Appendix D). There are even camping programs for mixed groups of disabled and able-bodied people.

I've had to move back in with my mother since I can no longer manage alone in my apartment. We got along fine when I was on my own, but now we're back to the old tensions from my teenage days. How do families handle this kind of problem?

Parents and children spend many years preparing to separate. By the time the children have grown up enough to leave home, they feel ready to take personal responsibility and make decisions for their own lives. Parents let them go, usually with some trepidation and a big sigh of relief. As time passes, parents and their adult children learn to relate to each other in a slightly different way, with gradually growing separateness and mutual respect. When an adult child returns home, the parent-child relationship may need to be negotiated all over again.

Your mother once again has one of her children living with her but her parenting role is different from what it was when you were younger. You have returned to your mother's house after having spent time on your own, running your own home, making your own decisions. Presumably, you want your mother to treat you like an independent adult, free to make your own decisions and come and go on your own schedule. She, on the other hand, wants to continue to feel that her home is her own, subject to her tastes and preferences. Additionally, she has always related to you as your mother and may not know how to interact with you in any other way. Particularly when illness and/or disability are part of the picture, parents often feel an increased need to help and protect. Your mother may need time to learn how to balance your needs for help and support with your needs for freedom and independence. You may need the same time to reconcile yourself to being back in your mother's home and sphere of influence.

This is not an easy situation for any parent and adult child. You and your mother need to talk about the conflicts you are having and try to renegotiate your relationship. If you and your mother find that this renegotiation process is too difficult or stressful, a family therapist can help you communicate your individual needs and mutual expectations more effectively.

My husband has had MS for several years. I know that things are very difficult for him, but the MS has made things tough for me and the children as well. How can I explain to my husband that we're all having trouble dealing with the changes and losses in our lives?

Some people have so much difficulty coming to terms with the impact of MS on their own lives that they have a hard time realizing how it affects other members of the family. Others feel so anxious and guilty about the impact of their disability on family members that they try not to think about it. Thus, there may be a variety of reasons why your husband seems insensitive to the feelings of other family members.

Presumably, you have tried to talk with him about the ways in which MS affects you and the children. If he feels that you are being selfish and unfeeling when you talk about your own needs, try communicating about them in a different way. For example, you might consult your local MS chapter about family programs that you could attend together. Share with your husband some of the literature published by the MS Society on families living with MS. Perhaps he can hear your message more clearly if it comes from someone else. Knowing that all families

living with MS find it stressful, and that family members cope
best by helping each other, may enable him to feel less alone and
more able to respond to you and the children.

**Although I need to use a wheelchair most of the time, I have
learned to be quite self-sufficient in my own apartment. My
parents want me to live with them, but I really want to stay
where I am, in a familiar neighborhood, close to my friends.
How can I convince my parents that I'm fine right where I
am?**

Your parents are probably worrying about your physical safety
and your ability to get help if and when you need it. One way to
reassure them is to create a home "safety net" for yourself. This
is a good idea for any disabled person living alone, whether or
not Mom and Dad are worried!

A portable telephone can be carried in a pouch attached to
your wheelchair. This will enable you to make and receive calls
even if you cannot get to the regular phone. You might also wish
to install a medical alert system that gives you immediate access
to emergency help (see Appendix D). This kind of system comes
in several varieties, but the general principle is that the push of
a single button (worn around your neck or attached to the wheelchair) alerts a central office that you are in some kind of trouble.
After determining the type of problem you are having, the central office calls one of the individuals on your emergency list:
neighbor, family member, physician, police, fire department,
and so on. If you were to take a bad fall, for example, and find
yourself unable to get back up or reach a telephone, you could
get immediate help simply by pressing the alert button.

The Medic-Alert identification bracelet is another useful safety precaution (see Appendix D). If you were unable for any reason to communicate clearly about your condition (following a
serious fall, for example), the bracelet would indicate that you
have MS and identify the medications you are taking. Any other
important information about your health status would be available in your Medic-Alert file.

Knowing that this kind of safety net is in place may help your
parents feel more comfortable with your independence.
Knowing that you are looking out for your own welfare and safety may make them less inclined to feel that have to do it for you.

Parenting

Now that I've been diagnosed with MS, I don't know if I should have children. I'm afraid that I won't be able to do things for a child that a father is supposed to do. What if I can't even play catch or teach the child to ride a bicycle?

Most parents, with or without MS, will tell you that their experiences with raising children were very different from what they had expected. They will also tell you that there is no single or correct way to be a "good" parent. Your decision to have children should be based on your desire to have this experience in your life as well some assessment of your ability to provide the kind of love and security that all children need.

The diagnosis of MS should not necessarily interrupt your wishes or plans for parenthood in any way. Keep in mind that it is impossible to predict with any certainty how your MS will affect you; you might not have any of the difficulties you are anticipating. You might even have a child who has no interest in playing catch! It is certainly reasonable to expect that MS will have some impact on your future family. The best way to prepare for that is for you and your wife to educate yourselves about MS, talk to the doctor about your particular symptoms and the course they are likely to take, and talk to each other about how you plan to share the parenting and breadwinning responsibilities. Ultimately, the goal is for you and your wife to feel comfortable as an effective parenting team, with consistent ideas about raising children, mutual support, and flexible ideas about what are "father jobs" and "mother jobs."

My children don't bring their friends around the house any more. Now that I'm in a wheelchair, they seem embarrassed about me. What is the best way to discuss this with them?

It is important that families living with MS do not automatically relate all of the changes they experience to the disease. Otherwise, changes that occur because of normal maturation or because of some stress other than MS could be misinterpreted. For example, it is quite typical and normal for young teenagers to begin spending less time at home and more time with their friends. Or children may bring fewer friends around if they sense that Mom or Dad is very tired or cranky a lot of the time.

Begin the conversation with your children by letting them know that you have noticed a change. It is important to do this in a very neutral way so that your children feel free to respond to the observation you have made rather than to the tone of your voice. Ask them if they have noticed that their friends are not over at the house as much as they used to be, and, if they have, ask them what they think has changed. If they do not offer any explanation, or if they offer one that you do not quite believe, let them know that you are concerned that this might be related in some way to your MS. Assure them that you want to know about any feelings or concerns that they might have because it is important to you that they and their friends are comfortable in the house. If they do voice concerns about the MS or anything else, work with them to develop strategies to make the situation more comfortable.

Now that my wife has become a bit more disabled, the children have a lot more chores to do around the house. Will this responsibility be too much for them?

Research has indicated that children who have a parent with MS are very much like children whose parents do not have any major health problems. They continue to develop and thrive in spite of the added stresses and responsibilities. Let your children know that you are aware that they have more responsibilities than their peers and that you appreciate their efforts. Offer your children choices about which chores they take on and give them some leeway in deciding when they will complete them. Reassure them with both words and actions that, in spite of their increased responsibility, you are there to parent, protect, and take charge. Try to make sure that your children have time in their lives to *be* children; they need some regular opportunities, however limited, to participate in a school activity or be with friends. If, in spite of these efforts, you notice a significant change in your children's school performance, usual moods, or social relationships, it would be best to have a consultation with a child or family therapist.

I went into the hospital for a four-day course of steroids. We told our seven- and nine-year-old children about the admission ahead of time and they seemed okay with it. But while I was

away, the older one got really upset at school and my husband had to go pick him up. How should we handle this in the future if I have to be admitted again?

Children have a difficult time with the unknown, and you and your husband were right to try to prepare them in advance for your admission. In spite of parents' best efforts, however, children are often frightened by the idea of a hospital stay (since many people who go into hospitals are sick or dying) and worried that the parent will not come home again. Having you return safely from this initial hospitalization is the first step in preparing them for any future ones that you may need. Take the time now to describe what happened to you during this hospital stay and let them talk to you about what it was like for them while you were gone.

If and when you need to be hospitalized again, ask the hospital staff if the children can accompany you during the admission process. Find out if the hospital has child life workers on staff who can talk with them about the hospital and its procedures. Make plans with your children to talk with them by phone at a scheduled time each day—or to have a visit if that is allowed. The idea is to give your children an understanding of what happens during the admission and how it will help your MS, and assure them that you are okay and available by telephone while you are gone.

We have told our parents and a few of our closest friends about my MS. I've asked them not to talk about it because I don't want my children to know yet. My husband thinks I'm wrong to try to keep this from them. I think that eight- and ten-year-old children are too young to have to worry about this. What should we be telling them?

Eight- and ten-year-olds are very observant people who generally have a sixth sense when something is not right in the family. Your children are probably aware that you are having some sort of health problems, whether or not these problems are influencing your usual activities with them. The ideas that children conjure up for themselves are almost always more frightening than the reality, particularly if they get the idea that the "something" is so terrible that Mom and Dad cannot even talk about it. In short, not discussing your MS with the children can, in the long run, cause them more worry than talking about it would. Additionally, the longer you delay talking to them, the more you increase the risk that they will hear the news from someone other than yourselves. By openly discussing an important issue like this one in your life, you also lay the groundwork for good parent-child communication about issues that will come up in their lives.

I know that all children need to test and "see who's the boss" sometimes. But since I started to use a cane, it feels as though the children are testing all the time. How can I discipline my children when I can't even keep up with them?

There are many different styles of discipline. The better your negotiation and communications skills and the more consistent you are in using them, the less you will have to depend on being mobile to provide discipline. Different approaches to parenting and discipline are described in the parenting literature (see Recommended Readings). Additionally, many community centers and schools offer parent effectiveness programs that are designed to help you build confidence and consistency in using these techniques. Keep in mind that being a good parent does not mean doing it all on your own. Enlist your spouse or other adults to help you learn and use these different approaches. In the meantime, remember also that children sometimes "test" in order to reassure themselves that the adults in their lives are still in charge and can still take care of them. Your children may be expressing their fears about MS and whatever effects it is having on you. Be alert to their questions and worries, and read or talk with them about the MS whenever it seems appropriate.

I always used to enjoy doing things with my children after school or in the evening before their bedtime. Now I'm so exhausted by the time they get home that I am either asleep or so cranky that they wish I were asleep! Is there any way to deal with this problem?

Fatigue is a common MS symptom that is usually best managed by prioritizing your activities and budgeting your energy. In some cases fatigue may also be helped with medication (see Chapter 2). At your first opportunity, discuss the fatigue with your physician, who can help sort out its cause and recommend a plan for managing it. Your best day-to-day strategy is to find a time to recoup some energy before the children come home so that you can resume some of the activities that you and they are missing. Since MS-related fatigue is most noticeable in the late afternoon, try to work in a brief rest just before the children arrive home. You may want to rearrange your daily routine so that you do more of your physically demanding chores earlier in the day and then have a chance to rest. If you are returning from work late in the day, schedule a regular rest time for yourself and make a "date" with the children for some special time together before they go to bed. Brainstorm with the children about some new "quiet time" activities that you could enjoy doing together.

Since my wife began having difficulty getting around the house and doing things for herself, she's always after the rest of us to do, or get, or go. The children and I want to be helpful but we don't like being constantly on call. How can I make her understand how we feel?

There are two very difficult aspects to the situation you are describing in your family: how frustrated and out of control your wife must be feeling; and how unappreciated and burdened you and your children are feeling. One key to making home life more satisfying and comfortable for all of you is to develop some ways of talking about what is happening so that you can start building solutions together. The best way to start talking with others about your own feelings and needs is to show some understanding of theirs. This helps to facilitate open communication and cut down on everyone's tendency to become defensive. Then you can begin to tackle specific areas of stress and conflict one at a time. Let your wife know that the family wants to meet her various needs, but that you each have needs and commitments of your own to deal with as well. Family members should speak openly about how they would like requests to be made and how they feel when their own needs and activities are ignored. If you find that these conversations become too difficult because of all the issues that seem to emerge, keep in mind that there may be a lot of emotions in the situation that need to be sorted out. You may want to enlist the help of a family therapist who is knowledgeable about chronic illness to get you started on this process.

My twelve-year-old has had to help me up from the floor a couple of times when I have fallen. Now he's afraid to be at home alone with me. How can I help him with these feelings?

Your son's feelings may be difficult for him to describe, but are probably related to a fear that he cannot do enough to help you, or that he is having to deal with a problem that is bigger and stronger than he is. For both your sakes, do everything you can to protect yourself from falls. Arrange for the two of you to have a session with an occupational therapist or physical therapist in your home. This professional can point out ways to maximize your stability and safety, perhaps by removing area rugs, installing bathroom safety equipment, or recommending a mobility aid. The therapist can also show you different ways of performing transfers and teach your son techniques for helping if you do fall. You might also consider having a medical alert system installed in your home that enables you to notify family, neighbors, or community safety officials that you need help. These steps will reduce your son's fears by demonstrating to him that you are doing everything you can to protect yourself and that you do not expect him to be solely responsible for your safety.

Our youngest daughter will graduate from high school next year. Recently she started talking about getting a job rather than applying to college. My husband and I are afraid that she feels worried about leaving me now that I've become so much more disabled. Should we push her to go to school?

Your daughter's second thoughts about college could be caused by any number of factors. As her parents, you should certainly discuss her plans with her and share your feelings about her going away to college. However, it would do little good to force her into a decision about leaving home; her reasons for deciding against college at this point could be very well thought out and unrelated to your illness. If her change in plans does seem to stem from anxiety or guilt about your MS, let her know what steps you and your husband have taken to manage your increasing disability. Remind her that just because she is the youngest child does not mean that her role in life is to take care of you. If finances are her major concern, share with her your plans for balancing medical costs and any help you plan to give her with her educational expenses. Be prepared to help her explore options for attending college away from home or locally. The goal of the conversation should be to let her know that her needs and priorities are important to you and that you can, as a family, come up with a plan that addresses the needs of all the members of the family.

Sometimes my son or daughter has to help me with getting dressed or going to the bathroom. I don't like this any more than they do and I'm worried about how this will affect them.

Your concern about having the children help with your personal care activities is very understandable and appropriate. Providing that kind of intimate assistance can be very confusing for youngsters who are developing their self-concepts and working to attain more independence from their parents. Additionally, your children's involvement in personal care sends a strong message that you would be "lost" without them—a message that could have a significant impact on their plans for the future.

Some of the tasks that you need help with happen at the same time each day. Try to develop a schedule with adults in your family to help with your morning routine. Ask to talk to a social worker about the possibility of getting help from a home health agency or, perhaps, the local chapter of the National Multiple Sclerosis Society. If, in spite of your best efforts, you can find no other helpers, consider involving your children in individual or family counseling. An opportunity to sort out their feelings about their caregiving role could relieve some of the stress on all of you.

My husband has been very upset and angry about the way his MS is getting worse, and he seems to take a lot of it out on the children. They try so hard to please him but he yells a lot and criticizes everything they do. What is the best way to talk to him about this?

While your perception is that your husband's relationship with the children is very strongly affected by his MS, he may not recognize the ways in which his reactions to the disease are spilling over onto the family. The sooner you begin to talk this over with him, the better it will be for all of you. He needs to begin to understand the impact of his behavior on the children. It is best to start this process by talking about a particular situation rather than about his general attitude or the way he is coping with MS; discussing how to improve on the outcome of a specific, recent event will be less threatening. Undoubtedly, one conversation will not reverse the pattern that has developed; it will, however, lay the groundwork for future conversations.

It is not unusual for people to take out their uncomfortable feelings on those closest to them. As MS interferes with a person's sense of independence and personal control, the natural tendency is often to try to take control in other ways—perhaps by bossing people around or "trying to organize the raindrops." Children often feel that they get the brunt of this type of behavior. The most effective way to deal with this problem is often to help the person talk about the loss of control and brainstorm about more effective ways to restore a sense of order and independence in daily life.

Keep in mind, as well, that mood swings, irritability, and depressive feelings are also fairly common in MS (see Chapter 11). While the exact relationship between these emotional changes and the illness is not well known and can certainly vary from one individual to another, the resulting behaviors can have a significant impact on family life. If you feel that your husband is behaving very differently from his "usual self," you could ask him to go with you to a psychotherapist *who is familiar with MS* to talk over these changes.

Most of my MS problems don't show on the outside; fatigue and vertigo are my worst problems. How can I help my children understand how I am feeling? They are angry about things I can't do any more and don't seem to appreciate the things I still manage to do for them.

It is difficult to describe to children symptoms that they cannot see and have probably never experienced. Try to describe your symptoms in terms that they can readily understand. For example, you might have your children experiment with ankle and wrist weights to learn how your body feels when you are fatigued. Or you might tell them to spin themselves around a bit and then try to walk from one room to another. Reading together about MS will let them see that other parents experience very similar symptoms. The National Multiple Sclerosis Society has several excellent booklets written for children in different age groups. Many chapters of the National Multiple Sclerosis Society also offer special programs to help children learn about the disease and its symptoms and provide ways for them to get in touch with other children who have a parent with MS. Contact your local chapter or the national headquarters (see Appendix D) to learn more about these services. Your physician can also be a valuable resource. For example, the children might sit in during one of your office visits to learn about the neurologic exam and the ways in which your physician tests those "invisible" symptoms. He can also refer you to a child or family therapist who can help your family develop more effective ways to talk about MS and the ways it is affecting each of you.

As you try various strategies for teaching your children about MS, keep in mind that no two children learn in exactly the same way. What seems to work with one of your children may be of no interest to the other(s). One child might be interested in reading or talking with you about MS, while another might want to attend a meeting and talk with other children who have a parent with MS. Some children want simply to be reassured that you will continue to be able to take care of them.

Should I let my children's teachers know about my MS?

Under most circumstances it is very helpful to let your children's teachers know about your diagnosis. School can be a very important source of stability and self-confidence, and the teacher is a primary player in any child's day-to-day experiences. If they are aware of the MS, teachers can be very helpful to you in gauging how your children are responding to your illness and the changes it is causing in your family. Additionally, awareness of your situation will enable the teachers to be attentive to any changes in your children's school performance and social relationships and prepared to provide help and support as needed.

The Caregiving Experience

Everyone is always asking how my husband is. How do I let them know that my life has changed almost as much as his and that I need them to ask about me too?

Your feelings are shared by many well spouses. There is no reason to feel embarrassed, selfish, or in any way inadequate because you have needs of your own. Over the course of the illness, you will need support just as much as your husband does, but you may have to look for it from different sources. Having one special friend or relative with whom you are comfortable sharing your feelings can be much more meaningful than expressions of concern from people with whom you have a more casual relationship. Many chapters of the National Multiple Sclerosis Society sponsor spouse groups that provide the opportunity to meet with others who are sharing your experiences. The National Well-Spouse Foundation (see Appendix D) is another organization that provides support to care-giving spouses through newsletters, local support groups, and annual national meetings. An increasing amount of reading matter is available to inform, support, and empower you in your role as the spouse of someone with a chronic illness (see Appendix C).

My wife can't play tennis anymore. She gets upset when I go and play and I feel guilty about wanting to play. Should I give up the active things that I like to do because she can no longer do them with me?

There are likely to be a variety of changes that you and your wife will have to face together in dealing with MS, and responding to changes in her level of disability is a very significant one. Before making any decisions about continuing to play tennis, try to talk the situation over with her. Your wife's distress may stem from feelings of loss and envy; she may simply find it very painful to know that you are doing something that she loves but can no longer do. Or she may be concerned that the two of you will have less time together if you continue to play without her. She may also worry that she will miss out on the social contacts the two of you had with other players. Identifying the sources of her distress will help the two of you decide the best way to deal with the situation. Make sure that your wife understands how important it is for you to keep playing tennis while reassuring her that you are interested in finding other activities that you can do together. Support her own efforts to find satisfying and enjoyable hobbies to replace those that she can no longer do. It is important that family members not rush to give up any and all activities that the person with MS is unable to do. The eventual cost in resentment and guilt is too great.

I've started to feel more like a caregiver than a husband. I am committed to my wife and have no wish to leave her, but I really miss the companion who shared so much with me. How do other people cope with the loneliness and loss of companionship?

The feelings of loss you are describing are particularly common for couples who have always shared many interests and activities but now increasingly spend time simply managing the consequences of MS. In the same way you have partnered each other in other aspects of your life, try to become partners in the management of MS. An important goal of this partnership is to be able to communicate effectively about ways to integrate MS-related care activities into your lives in such a way that there is still time and energy left for other enjoyable activities. This will help both of you to feel that you are managing the MS rather than the other way around. It will also help you regain your feelings of togetherness so that each feels less alone with the burdens imposed by MS. Discussing your concerns at a couples' support group could benefit you and your wife in several ways: You will be reassured to learn that other couples are living with, and finding solutions to, the kinds of stresses and strains you are describing; the group can brainstorm together on ways to solve commonly shared problems and find substitute activities for ones that you can no longer do because of the MS; and you may find that the group becomes a social outlet as well.

I feel as though my whole life is controlled by MS and I don't even have the disease. How can I regain my life and still make sure my husband has the care he needs?

When life with MS becomes so overwhelming that you feel you are losing yourself in the disease, it is time to take a step back from the situation and find ways that it can be made more manageable. The first step in this process is to begin to think of yourself as your husband's care *partner* rather than care*giver*; the responsibility for managing the MS and the needs that it generates rests on both of you.

In as objective a way as possible, the two of you should make a list of his needs and yours. Try to identify the specific ways in which the MS-related needs have infringed on yours, paying particular attention to those times when you feel especially burdened or overwhelmed. Finally, write down those activities that you personally are missing and want to regain in your life. The goal of this process is to help you think in more specific terms than "MS" and "my whole life." The more specific you are able to be, the more likely it is that you and he will be able to identify strategies for regaining a sense of independence and control in your lives.

While it will not be possible for you to free your lives totally of MS, you will be able to adopt strategies and identify resources to help both of you meet your needs. This kind of problem-solving requires good communication and a lot of creativity. Working with a family therapist can help with the process if you find that, individually or together, you are feeling too overwhelmed or emotionally overloaded to be able to discuss the issues. Also keep in mind that MS support groups can be a particularly helpful resource, particularly those designed for couples.

My wife is desperate to find a cure for her MS. Every time a new treatment is mentioned in the newspaper, she is ready to fly around the world to get it. I get angry when she is ready to spend our retirement money on every quack gimmick that comes along. How can I get her to understand that the money we saved is for both of us and that we need to agree on how to spend it?

This commitment to trying every publicized MS "cure" can be especially frustrating to family members. In addition to making them feel as if their own needs have become unimportant, it tends to keep the entire family on an uncomfortable emotional roller coaster as hope is repeatedly replaced with disappointment. Your wife may be responding more with emotion than with reason to these reported "cures." In order to give her some background on the great number of these that have turned out to have no real value, you may want to read together a book entitled *Therapeutic Claims in Multiple Sclerosis*. This book describes most of the proclaimed treatments and cures, the reported ways that each was thought to work, and the quality of the scientific research done to evaluate their effectiveness. Another way to help your wife feel satisfied that she is doing everything possible to treat her MS is to encourage her participation in a clinical trial of one of the very promising drugs that are now being scientifically tested (see Chapter 3). If your wife continues to want to use your retirement savings to pursue untested "cures," the two of you might consider a consultation with an accountant or tax attorney to determine how her spending will affect your retirement and how to establish a financial plan that will protect your retirement funds.

My husband has become quite disabled by his MS and doesn't get out of the house much any more. Friends have stopped inviting us to do things because he is no longer able. How can I let them know that I still need to see people and have a social life even though he can't come with me?

You are wise to take the initiative with your friends rather than waiting for them to take the initiative with you. Your friends may simply need to hear from you that you want to maintain your social relationships and continue to be active. You may start by inviting one friend or couple over for dinner and say-ing that your husband will join you for part of the evening but excuse himself if and when he becomes too tired. Or invite them to join you at a restaurant for dinner and let them know that although your husband won't be coming, he is pleased that you are arranging an evening out. During the evening, after you have had a chance to catch up with one another, ask your friends to tell other members of your circle that you are still looking to socialize with them. You may want to let them know, if it is indeed the case, that you and your husband have talked this over and are both comfortable with the idea that you will continue to make plans even if he is not always able to be with you. It is by your own example that your friends will become comfortable seeking you out for social engagements even if your husband cannot always participate.

My husband insists on driving a car even though some of his MS symptoms are making him an unsafe driver. We added hand controls to the car two years ago, when leg weakness was his major problem. But now his vision is very bad and I'm afraid that his concentration is just too poor for him to be safe. He has already had one accident and I'm afraid that someone will be hurt the next time.

People find it very difficult to give up driving because it repre-sents a tremendous loss of independence. However, as you have indicated, the consequences of severely impaired driving skills can be life-threatening. Trying to convince your husband by yourself that he should stop driving might be difficult. If you are uncertain about his driving competence, or if you believe that your husband will resent your suggestions, you might accompany him to his next medical appointment and raise the issue with his physician. Explain your concerns to the doctor and ask about the availability of a driver's evaluation. This kind of evaluation, which should test both physical and cognitive skills, is often available at rehabilitation facilities. With your husband present, ask about the doctor's responsibility for reporting unsafe drivers to the state bureau of motor vehicles (this responsibility varies from state to state). If your husband insists on continuing to drive, and you are certain in your own mind that he is an unsafe driver, let him know that you and your other family members will not ride in the car when he is driving it. Help him to make arrangements for rides to those places he is accustomed to going on his own. Many communities have door-to-door transportation services that can help him remain independent. You might also encourage him to consult a psychotherapist for help with the feelings of loss and helplessness that accompany this kind of major life adjustment.

My husband wants our sexual relationship to be the way it used to be. But I am exhausted after a full day of work and taking care of him. It's hard for me to feel romantic after helping him with his other personal needs. How can I discuss this without hurting his feelings?

A couple's sexual relationship is important both because of the physical pleasure it provides and because of the emotional intimacy that it expresses. At different times over the course of every marriage, the sexual relationship is influenced by how the couple is getting along, their family responsibilities, and their physical and emotional health. Remaining close and intimate with each other during these times is an important part of sustaining a good marriage. Before discussing your sexual relationship with your husband, you may want to spend some time sorting out your own feelings. As you have described, your sexual feelings for your husband have been affected by your own physical exhaustion as well as changes in how you feel emotionally. It is also possible that some of your husband's MS-related physical changes are interfering with your sexual activities or your sexual response to him. It will probably make your conversation easier if you have sorted through some of these feelings in advance and perhaps talked them over with a therapist.

The next time your husband talks about your sexual relationship, try sharing some of your feelings with him. As with any important conversation, be sure to put as much effort into hearing him as in expressing yourself. By being honest with him about the way you are feeling and open to his response, you are initiating an important and satisfying form of intimacy. The two of you might also consider talking with a therapist who specializes in sexual relationships. That person can help you talk about your feelings and concerns, explore ways of being sexual that accommodate your husband's disability, and otherwise enhance the intimacy in your relationship. The sexual relationship in MS is discussed in detail in Chapter 12.

Recommended Readings

Burnfield A. *Multiple Sclerosis: A Personal Exploration.* New York: Demos, 1985.

Garee B (ed.). *Parenting: Tips from Parents (Who Happen to Have a Disability) on Raising Children.* Bloomington, IL: Accent Press, 1989.

Halligan F. *The Art of Coping.* New York: Crossroad, 1995.

James J. *One Particular Harbor.* Chicago: Noble Press, 1993

Kalb R. Psychological counseling and the MS person. *Multiple Sclerosis Quarterly Report* 1984;3:29.

Kalb R, Scheinberg L. (eds.). *Multiple Sclerosis and the Family.* New York: Demos Vermande, 1992.

Kalb R. *Families Affected by Multiple Sclerosis: Disease Impacts and Coping Strategies.* National Multiple Sclerosis Society, January 1995.

LaRocca N, Kalb R, Foley F, McGann C. Psychosocial, affective, and behavioral consequences of multiple sclerosis: treatment of the "whole" patient. *J Neuro Rehab* 1993;3(4): 30–38.

Pitzele S. *We Are Not Alone: Learning to Live with Chronic Illness.* New York: Workman Publishing, 1986.

Selected booklets from the National Multiple Sclerosis Society (Customer Service: 212-986-3240; Information: 800-344-4867)

◇ *Living with MS*—Debra Frankel, M.S., O.T.R., with Hettie Jones

◇ *What Everyone Should Know About Multiple Sclerosis*

◇ *Things I Wish Someone Had Told Me: Practical Thoughts for People Newly Diagnosed with Multiple Sclerosis—* Suzanne Rogers

◇ *PLAINTALK: A Booklet About MS for Families*—Debra Frankel, M.S., O.T.R., and Sarah Minden, M.D.

◇ *Coping with Stress* (adapted from material by the Arthritis Foundation, Philip Smith and staff)

◇ *Someone You Know Has MS: A Book for Families*—Cyrisse Jaffee, Debra Frankel, Barbara LaRoche, and Patricia Dick

◇ *When a Parent Has MS: A Teenager's Guide*—Pamela Cavallo, M.S.W., with Martha King

◇ *Taking Care: A Guide for Well Partners*—Nancy Holland, R. N., Ed.D., with Jane Sarnoff.

11

Stress and Emotional Issues

Nicholas G. LaRocca, Ph.D.
Jill Fischer, Ph.D.

Stress is no stranger to MS. In fact, many people living with the disease believe that stress may be one of the precipitating factors in the onset of MS and its progression. While research has provided little evidence to support this belief, there is no doubt that MS *creates* significant stress in people's lives.

Life's stresses are primarily of two types. The first is caused by major events or changes that require significant adjustment. Such stressful life events might include the loss of one's job, the birth of a new child, or the diagnosis of a disabling illness. The other type of stress, aptly termed "hassles" by some, consists of the pressures of everyday life. While these daily hassles do not call upon us to make major changes in our lives, they are still emotionally taxing. Examples of this type of stress might include fighting rush hour traffic, paying bills, or dealing with children's homework. While everyone is subject to both types of stress, having MS seems to worsen the effects of both.

Since stress is so much a part of life with MS, it is not surprising that people report all sorts of emotional *dis*-stress. It is safe to say that adjusting to something as unpredictable and potentially disabling as MS may entail quite a bit of emotional turmoil. To experience such distress and turmoil from time to time is therefore a natural and normal reaction. It is important to keep this in mind because at one time it was believed that MS was the result of an emotionally weak and immature personality. Such notions have long since been abandoned, but one occasionally encounters the idea that people with MS should respond without complaint to the changes and losses imposed by this disease. Not only would such a reaction be unnatural, but it would also interfere with the normal and necessary adjustment process.

People often look for a road map to guide them in their adjustment to MS and are disappointed to find that there is none. Unlike terminal illness, in which a person's adjustment may follow a fairly consistent set of emotional "stages," adapting to life with MS follows no fixed pattern. It is impossible to map out predictable "stages" of adjustment because the disease can vary so much in the types of symptoms it presents and its speed of progression. However, significant emotional issues arise intermittently over the course of the illness:

⋄ *Uncertainty* may be the first emotional challenge facing people with MS. It begins with the initial mysterious symptom of MS, be it fleeting optic neuritis, intermittent numbness, or a fall. When symptoms first appear, the person believes that something is wrong but is uncertain what it might be. Months or years may go by before a diagnosis is established, during which time uncertainty breeds a lingering feeling of anxiety. Uncertainty remains even after the diagnosis has been made. Will the symptoms get worse? Will new symptoms appear? How long will walking be possible? Will working become impossible? Creating a sense of security in one's life in the face of such uncertainty is a significant and lifelong challenge.

⋄ *Accepting* the reality of having a chronic, disabling illness is not a simple matter. Most people with MS will say that they have never really "accepted" it, any more than they would "accept" living in the middle of a battlefield. People sometimes feel a sense of relief when the diagnosis is first pronounced, simply because some of the uncertainty is resolved and many of their questions have finally been answered. However, a sense of shock and disbelief often follows—a state that may be prolonged by a person's inability or unwillingness to acknowledge what has happened. For most, this reaction is short-lived, and the reality of the diagnosis is eventually recognized even though it may never be "accepted."

◇ *Grief* often ensues as the reality of the diagnosis sinks in. The person grieves for his or her lost sense of self. Most people think of themselves as invulnerable to disease and take for granted the physical and intellectual abilities with which they were born. A chronic, disabling illness robs people of this old sense of self and may also compromise many of those physical and intellectual abilities. As people mourn these losses, they are forced to reformulate their expectations for themselves and the future.

◇ *Self-image* is likely to go through a transition. The person slowly and painfully lets go of the old sense of self and works gradually to build a new one that incorporates the limitations and constraints brought about by the MS.

◇ *Accommodation* occurs as people with MS and their families make specific changes in their life patterns in response to the disease. Such accommodations may involve changing jobs, swapping roles within the household, making alterations in the house, and giving up certain physical activities.

◇ *Re-emergence* eventually occurs as people make the necessary changes in their lives. The disease may occupy a great deal of attention and effort at the time of diagnosis and during subsequent exacerbations. As it stabilizes somewhat, people may find that they can pay less attention to the disease and more to the business of living.

Adjustment to MS takes time. Moreover, since the disease can wax and wane, many people find that they have to adjust over and over again. They may go through a grieving process each time new disabilities appear. Because of the changeable nature of MS, people may experience dramatic fluctuations in their emotional state. They may plunge into a severe depression when a bad exacerbation occurs and experience joy and relief if remission occurs. Living through this emotional roller coaster is one of the most significant challenges of MS.

Adjustment to MS is as complex as it is slow. Many factors may influence how a person copes with the illness, including disease course, personality and coping style, the availability of social supports and financial resources, and other concurrent life stresses. A very important factor influencing adjustment is one's self-appraisal. People who view themselves as ineffectual and powerless are likely to adjust differently than those who view themselves as effective and able to manage what life brings them.

Emotional Aspects of MS

How common is depression in MS?

The answer to this question depends in part on what you mean by "depression." People tend to use the term to describe many different feelings. Everyone feels distressed, demoralized, and "down in the dumps" from time to time. When we feel that way, we say we are "depressed." However, technically, we are simply experiencing the generalized psychological distress that is a standard part of living.

If this generalized state of sadness and distress is fairly constant and continues for years, it is known as chronic dysphoria (or dysthymic disorder) and probably warrants professional treatment. A third form of "depression" is really grief, which comes about as the result of the loss of someone or something that is important to us. MS can bring about significant losses in people's lives, including the loss of certain abilities, expectations for the future, and employment. As a result, most people with MS go through a grieving process that may be repeated many times over the course of the illness as new losses occur.

The most serious form of depression is a "major depressive episode," characterized by sadness that is severe and unremitting, and accompanied by a variety of other symptoms such as low self-esteem, sleep disturbance, changes in appetite, hopelessness, and sometimes suicidal thoughts. Some people experience recurrent major depressive episodes, and others seem to alternate between episodes of major depression and periods of unusually good or "high" moods (manic episodes). Alternating episodes of depression and mania are known as "bipolar disorder" (formerly referred to as manic depression).

There is ample evidence that people with MS are at greater risk for depression in all its guises than the general population. It has been estimated that at any given point in time, one out of every seven people with MS is experiencing a major depression. Approximately 50 percent of people with MS will experience a major depressive episode during the course of their illness, compared to 5–15 percent in the general population. Bipolar disorder is less common than major depression alone, occurring in about 15 percent of people with MS.

The estimated frequency of severe depression in MS is quite controversial. The diagnosis of depression is highly technical and requires a very specific set of symptoms along with an equally specific time frame. Additionally, many of the symptoms of depression can easily be confused with MS symptoms and effects. For example, the symptoms of depression include fatigue, sleep disturbance, difficulty concentrating, and feelings of worthlessness. These symptoms are often part of the MS picture as well. It can thus be very tricky to diagnose a major depressive episode in a person with MS.

Keeping the above in mind, it is important to remember that MS is a psychologically challenging condition. People with MS are at greater risk than the general population for a variety of emotional complications. Those who deal with MS, either their own or someone else's, need to be alert to the potential need for help, especially professional help. For the sake of clarity in the remainder of the chapter, the term *depression* will be used to distinguish the more severe major depressive episode or chronic dysphoria from the relatively common, episodic feelings of distress and discouragement that most people experience from time to time.

Why do some people with MS get severely depressed while others do not?

The intensity of a person's reactions seems to depend on a variety of factors in addition to the severity of the disease itself, including personality style and coping skills, availability of social supports, financial security, and genetic predisposition to depression. Additionally, there has been some speculation among researchers that MS may cause demyelination in certain parts of the brain that play a role in the experience or expression of emotions. Therefore, disease severity is by no means the most reliable predictor of a person's emotional response. A person with less disabling disease may develop a severe depression while one with greater disability does not.

How can I tell if I'm having a normal reaction to being diagnosed with a chronic illness or if I have a serious depression?

Almost everyone reacts negatively to being diagnosed with a disabling illness. Reactions may include shock, disbelief, anger, anxiety, sadness, grief, pessimism about the future, and loss of self-esteem. These reactions can at times become fairly intense and may be difficult to distinguish from depression.

However, depression does have some distinguishing characteristics. Serious clinical depression consists of more than just feeling down in the dumps. The feeling of sadness tends to be constant, with little or no relief. People who are depressed may lose interest in most of the things that used to be enjoyable, such as hobbies, visiting friends, reading, work-related projects, and sexual activity. They may experience loss of appetite or gradually begin eating much more than usual. Sleep may be disturbed by early morning awakening or they may begin wanting to sleep longer or more frequently. Depression can include feelings of worthlessness and self-blame for everything that seems to be going wrong. Individuals who are depressed may also feel guilty without knowing why, as if they had done something horrible that must be punished. A depressed person's thoughts and actions may be slowed, and behavior may appear listless. However, unlike those who are simply suffering from MS fatigue, people who are depressed do not really care about feeling listless because they are not interested in doing anything. The person who is depressed may also be plagued by thoughts of death and even suicide.

In contrast to this devastating picture of clinical depression, the reaction to having a chronic illness tends to be less severe and not as broad in its effects. For example, individuals who are reacting to MS may also feel downhearted, blue, and pessimistic, but can still be interested in life activities and forget their troubles long enough to take care of their responsibilities and engage in enjoyable activities. The person who is learning to live with MS may struggle with an altered self-image that includes newly acquired limitations, without necessarily feeling useless or worthless. Thoughts of suicide are less likely to arise.

It is important to keep in mind that there can at times be considerable overlap between the "ordinary reaction" to chronic illness and a serious depression. Most people are likely to experience something in-between—a reaction to MS that occasionally has some of the characteristics of depression. Consultation with a psychologist or a psychiatrist can help you to clarify the issues involved and identify the most useful form of treatment.

I can't tell if I'm tired all the time because I'm depressed or depressed because I'm always tired. Who can help me find the answer to this question?

Depression is often accompanied by a feeling of listlessness and/or a lack of interest in everyday activities. On the other hand, people who experience MS fatigue often feel "down" because they are not able to do the things they would like to do. It is not always easy to separate depression from an intense feeling of fatigue; however, people who have experienced both usually report that they feel quite different. You are probably not depressed if you are frustrated because your fatigue prevents you from getting your chores done and enjoying your hobbies and social life. However, you could well be clinically depressed if you wake up in the morning feeling tired, and find you don't really care if you get anything done or not.

The difference between depression and fatigue is not just academic. It is important to have an accurate assessment because the treatments for clinical depression and fatigue are quite different. Consultation with your neurologist in conjunction with a psychiatrist or psychologist can help you to identify the exact nature of your problem. Depression should be treated with psychotherapy and/or medication. Fatigue is usually treated with drugs such as pemoline (Cylert®) or amantadine (Symmetrel®) and by energy conservation measures such as schedule changes, naps, and the use of adaptive equipment. However, keep in mind that depression and fatigue can occur in the same person and both may need to be addressed.

What is the best treatment for depression in a person who has MS?

Appropriate treatment requires identification of the exact nature and severity of the depression. The two major approaches to the treatment of depression are psychotherapy and medication. Psychotherapy is generally conducted individually (although it can be done in groups) by a qualified psychiatrist, psychologist, or social worker. Support groups and peer counseling may be a useful addition to treatment but are not a substitute for psychotherapy (see Chapter 10). Research has shown that psychotherapy can improve depression in MS, sometimes in just a few weeks. However, psychotherapy generally requires at least several months to achieve substantial results. While there are many different approaches to psychotherapy, the important factor seems to be the ability of the therapist. Many people find that a combination of psychotherapy and medication work well; the medication helps to elevate mood while the therapy provides a supportive setting in which to explore feelings and learn more effective coping strategies.

A variety of medications have been used successfully to treat depression in MS. For many years, tricyclics were the treatment of choice, e.g., imipramine (Tofranil®), amitriptyline (Elavil®), nortriptyline (Pamelor®). In recent years, however, the seratonergic antidepressants Prozac®, Zoloft®, and Paxil® have become more widely used (see Appendix B). These medications should be administered under the supervision of a psychiatrist who can monitor your progress and adjust the dosage as needed. In some instances, electroshock therapy can be very effective and extremely safe. In rare instances in which episodes of depression alternate with periods of elevated mood and hyperactivity, lithium may be used in addition to or instead of an antidepressant. Whatever you are experiencing, you need not suffer alone. Getting help is a constructive and active coping strategy. It does not imply weakness or giving up. Quite the contrary, it means that you are determined to confront the emotional challenges of life with MS.

Can any of the medications I'm taking for my MS affect my mood?

Yes, many of the medications used in MS can affect your mood. Space does not permit a discussion of all of them, but here are some of the more important ones.

◇ Antidepressants are sometimes used to treat bladder problems and unpleasant sensory symptoms, generally in doses lower than those used to treat depression. However, some people find that the antidepressants may improve their mood even in these low doses.

◇ Pemoline (Cylert®) is used to treat fatigue in MS. It is a stimulant and may in some cases make you feel more optimistic or slightly irritable.

◇ Valium® is a benzodiazepine (a class of tranquilizers) that is sometimes used to treat spasticity (see Chapter 2). Valium® may make you feel more relaxed both physically and psychologically.

◇ Baclofen (Lioresal®) is the drug most commonly used to treat spasticity. When treatment is started, many people feel drowsy until their bodies get used to the drug. However, a more dramatic side effect may occur if you abruptly stop taking it, especially if you are on a very high dose. Stopping a high dose of baclofen abruptly may cause you to experience extreme symptoms such as hallucinations (seeing or hearing things that are not there while awake), agitation or restlessness, convulsions, or mood changes. It is therefore important not to cease taking this medication abruptly, but to taper the dosage.

◇ Steroids that are used to treat MS exacerbations can produce a variety of mood alterations. Some people become depressed on steroids while others become happy, euphoric, irritable, or hyperactive. This steroid "high" is often followed by a "low" when treatment ends. Individuals react differently to steroids. Moreover, the same person may have different reactions at different times. In other words, just because steroids gave you a "high" the last time you had them does not necessarily mean that you will have the same experience the next time. People who have a history of extreme reactions to steroids are sometimes treated with mood stabilizing drugs in advance to prevent these wide and upsetting swings. It is important to work closely with your physician when you are treated with steroids and to report promptly any unusual reactions (see Appendix B).

Will I ever stop feeling angry and sad all the time?

Many people with MS go through periods when they feel acutely and persistently distressed. This often happens when the disease is first diagnosed and when symptom flare-ups cause greater disability. At times like these, the disease (and your feelings about it) seems to fill your life, crowding out other thoughts and feelings. Most people find this to be a temporary experience. You will probably find your distress becoming less acute as you begin to get used to having MS and learn how to make a place for it in your life, thus allowing more space for other emotions to return. MS will no longer occupy your total attention and you will once again become interested in your work, family, social life, and hobbies.

If you remain persistently sad and angry, despite the passage of time and despite improvement or stability in your symptoms, you probably need to seek professional help. A psychiatrist, psychologist, or social worker can help you determine whether you need some psychotherapy or medication to help you get through these feelings. If and when the MS flares up, you may find that the disease once again becomes an all encompassing emotional preoccupation. These periods of intense distress followed by relative calm are not uncommon in MS. Because of this, many people with MS find that they benefit from brief psychotherapy at several points in the course of their lives. When things get tough, they may return to therapy for a "tune-up." *Adjustment to MS is an ongoing and evolving experience, not a one-time happening.*

I have read that suicide is very common in MS. Is this true?

Although precise estimates vary, suicide is at least twice as common in MS as it is in the general population; indeed, it is one of the major causes of death among people with MS. This frequency probably stems from many roots. Suicide is most often associated with depression, and depression is more common in MS. However, suicide is generally more common among people with chronic, "incurable," debilitating illnesses. Many of the so-called "assisted suicides" that have been in the news recently have been individuals with MS. The disease can create the sorts of conditions (e.g., financial strain, family stress, isolation, overall deterioration in quality of life, and a bleak outlook for the future) in which suicide occurs. Suicide tends to result from feelings of hopelessness rather than depression per se.

At present a great ethical debate is raging in the United States concerning suicide, particularly assisted suicide. Many believe that one has the right to choose to end one's life. Others believe that the desire to take one's own life is by definition a psychiatric condition against which the person needs to be protected by society. Tragically, many individuals take their own lives while in a state of depression and hopelessness that could have been successfully treated with psychotherapy and/or medication. Depression can make a person perceive the life situation as more hopeless than it really is. However, there are people who seem to choose suicide not as a result of the distortions attending depression, but as rational adults in full command of their faculties who see clearly what they want for themselves. The debate over suicide will continue and expand during the next few years. For a variety of reasons, MS will occupy an important place in that debate.

Since my husband quit working because of MS, he seems to have lost interest in most of the things that he used to enjoy. Now he just sits in front of the TV all day doing nothing. Why is this and what can I do to help him?

Lack of motivation and failure to initiate activities can be symptoms of depression, but they can also occur when there has been extensive demyelination in important brain regions responsible for planning and initiating activities. Oftentimes, the family member is more distressed by this behavior than the person with MS. If your husband left work because of MS-related physical problems but his mind is still "sharp," he could well be depressed. Depression is fairly common following a major life change such as leaving the workforce. If, on the other hand, he was having trouble performing his job due to changes in his cognitive function, or if you know that he has had an MRI that showed a lot of MS plaques in the front part of his brain, his difficulty initiating activities may be due to structural changes in his brain rather than to a mood disorder.

In either case, you should discuss your concerns with both your husband and his neurologist. The neurologist can refer you to a neuropsychologist or neuropsychiatrist who, through a diagnostic interview and appropriate testing, can identify the likely cause of your husband's problem. If the cause is depression, treatment may involve psychotherapy, medications, or a combination of these. If the cause is demyelination, recommendations may include setting up a daily schedule with activities appropriate to his level of function and making sure that he has the help he needs to get started and continue working on activities.

Depending on your situation, this could be carried out at home, or you might want to look into having your husband get involved in a structured activity program at a clinic or community center. You will have a clearer idea of which solutions are likely to work best for both of you once you have a better sense of the cause of the problem.

My husband seems to go through a lot of mood swings lately, which make him pretty difficult to live with. Are these mood swings caused by the MS and is there anything to do about them?

The issue of mood swings is one of the most common mentioned by MS families. The disease causes structural changes in the brain that may increase the risk of abrupt changes in mood and emotional expression that can occur within minutes. This type of mood swing is often referred to as "emotional lability" to distinguish it from the longer lasting periods of depression and mania that typically alternate in bipolar disorder. Some mood swings may be caused by medications, especially high-dose steroids. Many people also use the term *mood swings* to refer to the anger and frustration felt by people who have had their lives turned upside down by MS. Regardless of the cause, abrupt changes in mood can make family life stressful and unpleasant for all concerned. It is important to seek professional consultation and treatment for this problem.

Depending on the cause, mood swings can be handled in different ways. Emotional lability may respond to low doses of tricyclic antidepressants such as amitriptyline (Elavil®). Mood swings caused by high-dose steroids should abate once the steroid treatment has ended. For someone who has reacted strongly to steroids in the past, the physician may prescribe some preventive treatment such as lithium or carbamazepine (Tegretol®) to diminish the reaction (see Chapter 3). Mood swings related to frustration may be helped by psychotherapy and/or medication. Family therapy is often extremely useful, both to help family members understand the problem and to ensure that they are not inadvertently contributing to the deteriorating emotional climate within the family. Finally, if the mood swings last significantly longer (two weeks or more) and are part of a bipolar disorder, treatment typically involves a combination of medication (usually lithium) and psychotherapy.

I find that I cry at the drop of a hat. Any time I feel the least bit emotional I start crying and can't stop. I never used to be like this and it's very embarrassing when I'm trying to talk to a colleague or have a simple disagreement with my husband. Is there anything to do about this problem?

Many people with MS find that they cry easily and have trouble stopping once they have begun. The crying is likely to be precipitated by any type of heightened emotional tension. The first step in handling this problem is to be aware that it is something that happens to you in times of tension or distress. With enhanced awareness, you are less likely to let your reactions run away with you.

For example, if you are trying to discuss something with a colleague or family member and suddenly find yourself becoming "choked up" and tearful, try to stop and take a few deep breaths. Remind yourself that you need to take the strength of your reaction with a grain of salt. You should not discount what you are feeling, just realize that the *strength* of that reaction may be out of proportion to the situation. Many people find that they can forestall the worst effects of this problem by slowing down a bit and reflecting. Self-awareness and deep breathing can help you to regain at least some of the control that has been lost. Working on this problem with a psychotherapist can be extremely helpful. In therapy you can identify those situations most likely to set you off and experiment with different types of strategies.

Sometimes my wife starts laughing or crying for no reason. Sometimes she even seems to be doing both at the same time even when there is nothing funny or sad going on. She thinks her "wires are crossed." Why is this happening to her?

Your wife is probably experiencing what is known as **affective release** (or *pseudo-bulbar affect*), a condition in which fits of laughing and crying can occur with no obvious precipitating event. This condition was formerly thought to be caused by damage to some of the nerves passing through the medulla oblongata (a structure in the **brainstem**). The current thinking is that affective release is associated with lesions in the limbic system, a group of brain structures involved in emotional feeling and expression and structures connected with it. Unlike what occurs with the mood swings discussed earlier, the person's actual mood may be totally unrelated to the emotion that is released. A fit of crying may thus begin even when the person is feeling rather content. Once these laughing or crying episodes begin, the person is often unable to stop them.

This symptom requires patience and understanding on the part of family and friends. The bouts of laughing and crying can be misunderstood by others, who may be offended by what they consider to be inappropriate or embarrassing behavior. Some types of antidepressant medications may help. One small study found some benefit from the use of amitriptyline (Elavil®). Many people find that the experience becomes somewhat less frightening once they get used to the fact that these uncontrolled bouts are going to happen from time to time. Again, the understanding of others is a key part of dealing with this problem.

My husband has gotten depressed about all the changes in our lives since the MS got worse. I've asked him to see a psychiatrist but he says he's not crazy and adamantly refuses to go. What should I do? I'm really worried about him and about our relationship.

Going to a psychiatrist or other mental health professional still carries an unjustified stigma for many. You might try pointing out to your husband that depression is one aspect of life with MS that can be effectively managed. If it's OK to seek help for problems with walking or vision, why not for the emotions? Using psychotherapy and/or medication, it is possible to come to grips with depression, feel more optimistic about things, and thus put more enjoyment back into life.

Going for psychotherapy does not mean that someone is crazy. Quite the contrary, it indicates that he or she is sharp enough to know when some assistance is needed to get through a difficult life situation. You might suggest that your husband see a therapist on a trial basis. Many people resist this sort of help until they meet a therapist who makes talking seem comfortable and enjoyable.

Since you are having a hard time with your husband's depression, you might also want to tell him about your own feelings. Ask him to see a therapist for the sake of your relationship and offer to go with him. Treatment cannot be sustained over a long period of time if it is being done only for the sake of another person, but this may be a way to get him started. If all else fails, you should consider going to see a therapist yourself for assistance in dealing with the situation. Individual therapy for the non-MS partner can be quite helpful, and in many instances the MS partner eventually agrees to join the therapeutic effort. Some adamant spouses grudgingly show up for the first session, determined never to return, and wind up staying for the duration of treatment. For you, the important thing is to get help for all who are willing to use it, even if that means only you.

I've read some older books about MS that talk about the "MS personality." What type of personality does this refer to?

At one time it was thought that certain medical conditions were caused, at least in part, by specific personality types. MS was supposed to be more likely to develop in people with emotionally immature and dependent personalities. Such archaic notions of disease were abandoned long ago. Some people still believe that MS can "produce" a specific type of personality after the disease develops, but this is not the case. People with MS may find that they share similar problems, experiences, and concerns, and so have a lot in common. However, they do not have the same personality. The personality characteristics one had before getting MS are likely (for better or worse!) to be the same ones the person has after getting MS.

What is euphoria and is this a common phenomenon in MS?

MS euphoria is an exaggerated and unrealistic state of happiness or well-being that, to the observer, seems out of keeping with an individual's life situation. People with MS are said to be euphoric when they appear blasé and lighthearted in the face of serious or life-threatening problems. Someone who is euphoric may tend to giggle inappropriately, even when nothing funny has happened. This inappropriate giggling almost always occurs in people with severe intellectual loss. Euphoria is thought to be the result of damage to parts of the brain involved in judgment and the control of emotions. It is sometimes confused with the uncontrollable laughing and crying that can affect people with MS, but these are more often precipitated by something that is emotionally charged and can occur even in the absence of significant intellectual loss.

Stress and MS

Can stress cause MS or make it worse?

There is perhaps no more controversial question in MS. Many investigators have attempted to show that stress can precipitate the onset of MS, trigger exacerbations, or hasten progression. Although some studies have found limited evidence to support one or more of these ideas, the issue of stress and MS remains largely inconclusive. Most of the studies used methods that were of poor quality, thus rendering their findings suspect. More recent studies have begun to focus on different questions such as "how does stress affect the immune system and through the immune system affect MS?" Research in a variety of medical conditions and in healthy controls has shown that the immune system is sensitive to stress in a variety of ways. By understanding the links between immune functioning and stress, we may shed light on the potential links between stress and MS.

In the meantime, we should be very cautious about attributing changes in the disease to stress. Family members sometimes feel guilty in the belief that they caused stress that worsened a loved one's MS. Such beliefs are unfounded. People with MS occasionally quit their jobs in the mistaken belief that they can slow the progression of their MS by reducing "occupational stress." Nothing is gained by such actions, and the individual loses the stimulation and satisfaction that working can provide.

Everyone is searching for explanations for this mysterious disease, and stress is one explanation that is readily available because we encounter it every day. MS adds a lot of stress to most people's lives. Thus the real issue is not whether stress is altering the course of the MS, but how we can most effectively deal with the stresses that life and MS produce.

What should I do about the stresses in my life? I don't think I can make them all go away.

Sometimes people with MS are told by well-meaning people to try to "reduce the stress in your life." Nice trick if you can do it! Most sources of stress in our lives are not under our control. Moreover, many times when people set out to "reduce stress" they do so by bailing out of important life activities such as work or family responsibilities. These activities provide much of the stimulation and inspiration that make life worth living. Do not withdraw from life on the basis of the mistaken notion that this will reduce stress. The key is to learn how to cope with stress rather than to avoid it. You can learn to deal with this problem in a variety of ways, including stress management programs, psychotherapy, counseling, support groups, peer counseling, self-help books, exercise, and developing better organizational skills. The first step is to identify the sources of stress in your life and evaluate your present coping style. Next you need to experiment with more effective coping strategies. Learning to deal more effectively with stress is probably best done with a professional who is trained in the requisite skills. Once you have mastered these skills, you should be able to cope on your own, perhaps returning from time to time for a "tune-up" to sharpen your skills or learn how to deal with new situations that have arisen.

Recommended Readings

Burnfield A. *Multiple Sclerosis: A Personal Exploration*. New York: Demos, 1985.

James J. *One Particular Harbor*. Chicago: Noble Press, 1993.

Scheinberg L, Holland N (eds.). *Multiple Sclerosis: A Guide for Patients and Their Families*. New York: Raven Press, 1987.

Pitzele S. *We Are Not Alone: Learning to Live with Chronic Illness*. New York: Workman Publishing, 1986.

Selected booklets from the National Multiple Sclerosis Society (Customer Service: 212-986-3240; Information: 800-344-4867)

◇ *Multiple Sclerosis and Your Emotions*—Mary Eve Sanford, Ph.D., and Jack H. We, M.D.

◇ *Taming Stress in Multiple Sclerosis*—Frederick Foley, Ph.D., with Jane Sarnoff.

12

Sexuality

Frederick W. Foley, Ph.D.
Michael A. Werner, M.D.

Multiple sclerosis can affect the experience of sexuality in a variety of ways. People sometimes report feeling less sexually interested or aroused, either as a direct result of neurologic changes or because of their efforts to cope with the impact of these changes on their lives. Partners often misinterpret the sexual changes they observe in the person with MS, and may also experience their own changes in sexual responsiveness in the face of the illness. Both members of the couple often find it difficult to communicate with one another about their changing sexual and intimacy needs.

The few studies on the ***prevalence*** of sexual problems in MS have relied primarily on the survey or questionnaire method. Up to 80 percent of men with MS report at least occasional sexual problems, with erectile difficulties being the most commonly reported symptom. The proportion of women reporting sexual problems ranges from 56 percent to 74 percent, with changes in sensation and vaginal lubrication being the most commonly cited problems.

The ways in which MS can affect sexuality and expressions of intimacy have been divided into primary, secondary, and tertiary sexual dysfunction. "Primary sexual dysfunction" is a direct result of neurologic changes that affect the sexual response. In both men and women, this can include a decrease or loss of sex drive, decreased or unpleasant genital sensations, and diminished capacity for orgasm. Men may experience difficulty achieving or maintaining an erection and a decrease in or loss of ejaculatory force or frequency. Women may experience decreased vaginal lubrication.

"Secondary sexual dysfunction" stems from symptoms that do not directly involve nervous pathways to the genital system, such as bladder and bowel problems, fatigue, *spasticity*, muscle weakness, body or hand tremors, impairments in attention and concentration, and non-genital sensory changes.

"Tertiary sexual dysfunction" results from disability-related psychosocial and cultural issues that can interfere with one's sexual feelings and experiences. For example, some people find it difficult to reconcile the idea of being disabled with being fully sexually expressive. Changes in self-esteem—including the way one feels about one's body, demoralization, depression, or mood swings—can all interfere with intimacy and sexuality. The sexual partnership can be severely challenged by changes within a relationship, such as one person becoming the other's caregiver. Similarly, changes in employment status or role performance within the household are often associated with emotional adjustments that can temporarily interfere with sexual expression. The strain of coping with MS challenges a couple's efforts to communicate openly about their respective experiences and their changing needs for sexual expression and fulfillment.

I've noticed a lot of changes in my body and my sexual feelings in the past few years. My doctor has never brought up the subject of sex and neither have I. Where is the best place to get information about sexual problems in MS?

Changes in sexual feelings normally occur throughout the life span. However, the experience of MS can complicate the typical changes that occur. MS affects sexual feelings both directly and indirectly, as discussed previously. Neurologists and other health care providers often do not spontaneously bring up the subject of sexuality. Physicians and nurses may ignore sexuality because they perceive this line of questioning as an unwelcome intrusion into the private lives of their patients, because of personal discomfort in asking about sexuality, or because of lack of professional training in this area. Although it can be difficult and potentially embarrassing, your sexuality is important enough to bring up with your primary MS physician. Discuss your changes in sexual feelings and ask directly about treatments that are available to enhance sexuality. Talk over with your physician the ways in which your symptoms and the medications used to treat them may be affecting your sexual responses. Although the burden of opening the door to communication about sexuality may initially fall on you, taking this step with your health care team will ensure that this frequently untreated symptom gets the attention it deserves.

To get information about literature on sexual problems in MS, begin by contacting your local chapter of the National Multiple Sclerosis Society or the NMSS headquarters in New York City. Also refer to the Readings and Resources at the end of this chapter.

My wife still seems to enjoy having sex as much as she always did, but she doesn't have an orgasm any more. She says it's not my fault but I don't understand what the problem is.

MS can interfere directly or indirectly with orgasm. "Primary orgasmic dysfunction" stems from MS lesions in the spinal cord or brain that directly interfere with orgasm. Orgasm depends on nervous system pathways originating in the brain (the center of emotion and fantasy during masturbation or intercourse) and pathways in the upper, middle, and lower parts of the spinal cord (which control sensations from erogenous zones such as lips, nipples, clitoris, and so on). Sensation and orgasmic response can be diminished or absent if these pathways are disrupted by plaques. Orgasm also can be inhibited by secondary or indirect symptoms such as sensory ***paresthesias***, cognitive problems, and other MS symptoms. Anxiety, depression, and loss of sexual self-confidence or sexual self-esteem represent tertiary symptoms that can also interfere with one's ability to enjoy the sexual experience and thus inhibit orgasm.

Treatment of orgasmic loss in MS depends on developing an understanding of what factors are contributing to the loss. If sensation is disturbed in the clitoris and lower body areas, the orgasmic response may sometimes be enhanced by increasing stimulation to other erogenous zones, such as breasts, ears, and lips. It can be both intimate and informative to develop a sensory "body map" with your partner to explore the exact locations of pleasant, decreased, or altered sensations. Sometimes stimulating the edges of body zones that are experiencing numbness or diminished sensation can feel sensually or erotically pleasing. Similarly, increasing cerebral stimulation by watching sexually oriented videos, exploring fantasies, and introducing new kinds of sexual play into sexual activities can help trigger orgasms.

Increasing stimulation through vigorous oral stimulation or via mechanical vibrators can help if decreased sensation in the genitals is a factor. Strap-on clitoral vibrators (available by mail order) do not interfere with intercourse and require little manipulation once in place. Vibrators that attach to the base of the penis provide direct clitoral stimulation when vaginal penetration is complete and can help stimulate erections in some men as well. In general, AC electric plug-in vibrators have more powerful motors and are more stimulating than DC powered battery-operated ones. However, some electric vibrators are quite powerful and can irritate vaginal or clitoral tissue if applied too vigorously.

My skin feels very tingly all the time. It used to feel good when my husband hugged me or rubbed my back, but now just being touched can feel uncomfortable. I even get pins and needles in my vaginal area. I need to do something about this problem before he gives up trying.

Painful or irritating genital or body sensations can sometimes be treated with medication. Amitriptyline (Elavil®), carbamazepine (Tegretol®), and phenytoin (Dilantin®) are sometimes prescribed to help manage this difficult symptom (see Chapter 2 and Appendix B). Even with pharmacologic management, however, conducting sensory body mapping exercises alone and with one's partner is frequently necessary to retain a sensually pleasing relationship. To conduct this exercise, set aside some time (about twenty to thirty minutes) when you will not be interrupted, and you and your partner can be relaxed and unhurried. Agree to do only the mapping exercise during this time, and not to engage in sexual activities. Be in a comfortable location where you can be undressed. Have your partner begin by gently stroking the top of your head, and slowly moving down your body from head to toe. The partner doing the stroking should vary the rhythm and pressure of touch, while the partner with MS should give frequent verbal and nonverbal feedback on the nature of sensations produced in each area. Mutually exploring alternative touches in the context of good communication can set the stage for sensual pleasure both during and independent of sexual activity. As with the treatment of all sexual symptoms in MS, sexual experimentation and communication are the keys to enhancing sexuality.

I love my husband very much but I seem to have lost all interest in having sex. He's worried that I don't love him any more but I keep telling him that I wouldn't be interested in sex with anybody right now. What's happening to my body? Will my sexual feelings ever come back?

The brain does not appear to have a specific, localized sexual center; rather, sexual interest and pleasure seem to be influenced by several different areas of the brain. Sexual interest normally waxes and wanes throughout the life span. "Libido," or sexual drive and interest, can be directly or indirectly affected by MS lesions. Changes in libido can also occur as secondary or tertiary symptoms. For example, libido will tend to decrease if fatigue is a severe MS symptom or if clinical depression or demoralization are present. When libido is compromised by MS, it is frequently a source of misunderstanding by the partner and also causes anxiety for the person with MS. The misunderstandings and anxiety associated with this problem will compound the libido loss. Assessing and treating secondary and tertiary sexual symptoms are therefore important components to restoring libido.

Increasing sexual drive that has been directly reduced by central nervous system changes is somewhat more challenging. The man or woman with MS who is involved in a sexual or intimate relationship with another person can begin by focusing on the "sensual" and the "special person" aspects of the relationship. Sensual aspects include all physically and emotionally pleasing, non-erotic contact, such as backrubs, handholding, and gentle stroking of the face, arms, and other non-genital body zones. Sex partners often neglect these sensual, non-sexual aspects to their physical relationship during periods of diminished sexual drive, in part because of the difficult emotions that may accompany loss of libido. Making a date for a non-sexual but sensual evening can enable partners to enjoy each other physically and to engage in enjoyable sensual exploration of their bodies, without the pressure of working toward sexual intercourse. In essence, sexuality has to be "relearned" when the central nervous system has compromised libido. Relearning one's *sensual* nature is a critical first step in the process.

The "special person" aspects of a relationship include all those behaviors that one engages in to show the other person that he or she is special and important. Loving gestures from an earlier, "romantic" phase of a relationship, such as unexpected flowers, a surprise note in a lunch bag, or a spontaneous affectionate hug, tend to be forgotten amidst the pressures of raising children, developing careers, and coping with MS symptoms and disabilities. Restoring or increasing these special acts toward one another other can help set the stage for increasing intimacy, which, in turn, can sometimes stimulate new libido.

Exploration of one's sensual and erotic body zones is an important step in restoring libido for the person without a current sexual partner. Combining enjoyable cerebral sexual stimulation (achieved via fantasy, sexually, explicit videos, books, and so on) with masturbation or sensual, physical self-exploration is sometimes helpful. Using vibrators or other sexual toys may complement these efforts. Although beginning to work on restoring libido may feel like an unrewarding "chore" when there is little or no intrinsic sex drive, working toward rekindling this vital aspect of "self" can be an important aspect of coping with MS.

Kegal exercises are sometimes prescribed to enhance female sexual responsiveness, although they have not been tested in a clinical trial to determine whether or not they are helpful in MS. To perform the Kegal exercise, a woman alternately tightens and releases the pubococcygeus muscle (identifiable as the muscle that starts and stops the urine flow in mid-stream). Exercising this muscle several times a day or more is recommended. The rationale for these exercises is that sensation from the muscles around the vagina is an important part of erotic sensation, and female orgasm consists of contractions in several of them. Kegal exercises are directed at strengthening their tone and responsiveness.

Sometimes I have trouble getting an erection even though I feel sexually excited. Other times, I get an erection but then lose it partially or completely while my partner and I are trying to have intercourse. Why is this happening?

The first step in understanding MS-related erectile problems and their treatment is to understand the normal erectile mechanism. Getting an erection is like filling a balloon. Two things have to happen: one has to fill the balloon with air and tie the balloon to prevent the air from coming out. The arteries that lead to the penis are lined with smooth muscle. When a man is excited, either psychologically or physically, his body releases transmitting substances that cause relaxation of the smooth muscle. As the smooth muscle relaxes, the arteries become enlarged, allowing an increased blood flow into the penis. This increased blood flow into the penis is what causes an erection. As the penis becomes erect, a trapping mechanism is activated that holds the blood in the penis until ejaculation occurs.

Normal erectile function depends on an intact nervous system. A complex series of nerve impulses must travel between the brain, spinal cord, and penis in order for an erection to be initiated and maintained. When nerve transmission is impaired at any point along the way, a man's ability to achieve or maintain an erection can be affected. The lower area of the spinal cord has nerve pathways traveling to and from the genitals, which allow for reflex erections. If these pathways are intact, reflex erections (that do not involve the middle or upper parts of the spinal cord or brain) can usually be triggered by stimulating the penis directly. Therefore, some men with impaired erectile function can obtain reflex erections by vigorously stimulating the penis with a vibrator. Reflex erections can also result from "stuffing." To engage in stuffing, the woman sits astride her partner and *gently* inserts the flaccid penis into the (well-lubricated) vagina. It is important that the stuffing be done with some care because the flaccid penis can fold back on itself and be squeezed or injured by the pressure of the partner's weight. Internal damage to the penis could go undetected in the presence of reduced sensation.

Is there anything I can do about the erection problems I am having?

Several options are available to treat erectile problems caused by MS. One noninvasive device that readily aids in erections is the vacuum tube and constriction band, which can be purchased with a prescription from a urologist or other physician. With this method, a plastic tube is fitted over the flaccid penis, and air is pumped out of the tube to create a vacuum around the penis. The pumping process may be done mechanically (via hand pump or squeeze bulb) or with a battery-operated, push-button mechanism. The vacuum draws blood into the erectile tissues and produces an erection. Once engorgement of the penis is achieved, a latex band is slipped from the base of the cylinder onto the base of the penis. Air is returned to the cylinder and the tube is removed. The band maintains engorgement of the penis by restricting venous return of blood to the body, thus allowing for intercourse or other sexual activity. However, the use of the band must be limited to thirty minutes or less to avoid any medical complications. Moderate hand sensation and dexterity are required for placing and removing the band in some models. Other models have assistor sleeves that permit hands-free placement of the constriction band. The constriction band alone can be used with satisfactory results by persons who can attain erections readily, but have difficulty maintaining them.

Perhaps the most common treatment for erectile dysfunction involves the injection into the penis of medications that activate the engorgement and trapping mechanisms. The medication stimulates relaxation of the smooth muscle of the arteries so that the penis can become erect and similarly activates the necessary trapping mechanism that keeps the penis rigid until ejaculation.

Men who are reluctant to self-inject or have been unsuccessful with this form of treatment may find the surgically implanted penile prosthesis to be a better alternative. Following a careful evaluation of your history and presenting symptoms (medical, psychological, neurologic, and sexual), your physician will work with you to determine which type of treatment would be most beneficial for you.

How would I use the penile injections to help me with my erectile problems?

Once you and your doctor have decided that penile injections are a reasonable treatment option, the doctor will teach you the injection techniques so that you can self-inject at those times when you wish to have an erection. The injection is done with a very fine needle into an area at the base of the penis, which, although somewhat sensitive to pleasure, is relatively insensitive to pain. The doctor may recommend an "auto injector" that works with a simple push-button mechanism. Most men report very little, if any, pain from this injection. The sensation is best described as similar to being flicked by a rubber band. Some men with neurologic impotence of the type caused by MS report a slight achiness caused by one of the medications that is sometimes used in these injections. If this occurs, different medications can be substituted.

When you wish to achieve an erection, you can give yourself an injection (or be given one by your partner if you are unable to do it yourself). After the injection has been given, pressure needs to be applied to the penis for three to five minutes in order to spread the medication throughout the shaft. As you initiate foreplay or self-stimulation, you will develop an erection that will last for approximately an hour. Depending on your state of sexual arousal and the amount of medication you have been given, the erection may subside when you ejaculate or continue for some period of time beyond ejaculation. *The penile injections can be used no more than once in every twenty-four hour period.*

What medications are used most commonly in penile injections?

Injections for the management of erectile dysfunction have been available for approximately fifteen years. Three different medications are currently prescribed (see Appendix B). Alprostadil (also called prostaglandin E1—Prostin VR®), which was introduced nine years ago, is both the newest and most commonly used drug in individuals with MS. Alprostadil is the natural substance released by the smooth muscle cells when a man is sexually excited. This medication has been found to have the best treatment outcome with the fewest side effects and has been approved by the Food and Drug Administration (FDA) for the management of erectile problems (and is therefore paid for by most prescription plans).

The original drug used for injections is a smooth muscle relaxant called papaverine. Its use is almost never associated with any pain, making it a good alternative for anyone who has a problem with alprostadil. Papaverine has a slightly greater tendency to cause scarring at the injection site, and it is associated with a greater risk of priapism (prolonged erection) because it also remains active in the body for a somewhat longer period of time. Papaverine has not been approved by the FDA for the treatment of erectile dysfunction.

Phentolamine (Regitine®—United States; Rogitine®—Canada) is sometimes used in combination with either alprostadil and papaverine to heighten their effectiveness. Phentolamine is not active by itself and is therefore never used independently. Depending on the type of symptoms you are experiencing, your physician may prescribe alprostadil alone, papaverine alone, papaverine with phentolamine, or papaverine with both alprostadil and phentolamine. Like papaverine, phentolamine has not been approved for this purpose by the FDA.

If only alprostadil is approved for the management of erectile dysfunction, does this mean that the other two drugs are not safe?

Medications are approved by the FDA for specific functions. They may be used for other purposes at the discretion of the physician. The fact that a drug is not FDA approved does not mean that it is not safe; it means simply that a drug company has not gone through the costly and time-consuming licensing and testing of the drug for a specific purpose. The three drugs that are currently being used in penile injections are all safe and efficacious when used properly.

Will I become dependent on the medications that are used in the penile injection?

Alprostadil, papaverine, and phentolamine are used only to potentiate the process of having an erection. No chemical dependency is associated with their use. Depending on the status of your MS symptoms, you may find that you need to use the injections at some times but not others. They can be a helpful adjunct when you are unable to achieve or maintain an adequate erection.

What side effects are associated with the use of these medications?

One possible side effect of these medications is an overly prolonged erection (priapism). In a normal erection, the penis remains rigid because the trapping mechanism keeps blood from flowing out of the penis until ejaculation occurs. Since oxygen is delivered to body tissues via the circulating blood, the penis does not receive fresh oxygen for the period of time that the penis remains erect. Therefore, a man whose penis remains erect for too long risks irrevocable damage to the erectile mechanism and to the penis itself. It is crucially important that a man never have an erection for more than four hours. If this occurs, he must see a doctor immediately for treatment, which usually involves the injection of a different medication. *Priapism almost never occurs in individuals who adhere to the prescribed dose of medication and who are properly trained in the injection procedures.*

A second potential side effect of penile injections is scarring at the injection site, experienced by approximately 7–10 percent of individuals. This problem seldom occurs in men who have been properly trained in the techniques of injection and compression of the injection site. When scarring does occur, it takes the form of a small nodule in the subcutaneous tissue of the penis. These nodules typically disappear once the injections are stopped. Any man who is self-injecting should be examined by a physician every three months for possible scarring.

What is a penile prosthesis and how does it work?

A penile prosthesis is a mechanical device designed to give a man with erectile dysfunction the option of having an erection. There are two types of penile prostheses, semi-rigid and inflatable. With the semi-rigid type, a flexible rod is surgically implanted in each of the erection chambers (corpus cavernosa) of the penis. These rods can be bent upward when an erection is desired and bent downward at other times. Following insertion of the rods, the penis remains somewhat enlarged, with a permanent semi-erection.

With the inflatable type of prosthesis, a fluid is pumped from a reservoir behind the abdominal wall into expandable cylinders inserted into the erection chambers of the penis. The fluid causes the balloons to inflate, resulting in an erection. The man pumps the fluid into the chambers when he desires an erection and transfers the fluid back into the reservoir when he no longer wants the erection. The reservoir is surgically implanted behind the abdominal wall and the pump is implanted in the scrotum. Silicon tubing is used to connect the reservoir, pump, and balloons. Since the entire device is inserted through a single, relatively invisible incision in the scrotum, this type of prosthesis is barely noticeable. However, operating the pump through the scrotum wall can be difficult for individuals with reduced hand sensation or strength.

A spouse or long-term sexual partner should be included in the decision to get an implant, as well as the selection of the type of prosthesis to be used. Extensive pre-surgery consultation with a urologist or physician familiar with MS will help to ensure that the man and his partner have realistic expectations after the surgery. Approximately 80 percent of men using these types of prostheses find them quite satisfactory. Many experience normal erectile sensations and normal orgasm. Additionally, they are able to have an erection for as long as they choose to do so.

What complications are associated with penile prostheses?

As with any surgery, there are possible complications related to anesthesia and bleeding. Infection occurs in approximately 2–8 percent of men receiving prostheses and can be quite serious. The entire device must be removed if an infection occurs. Replacement of the implant following treatment of the infection is usually feasible, but often more complicated.

How would I know if I am a suitable candidate for a penile prosthesis?

A penile prosthesis is only recommended when other efforts to manage erectile dysfunction are not feasible or are unsuccessful. In other words, you would be considered a candidate for a prosthesis only if noninvasive measures were unsuccessful, you were unable to self-inject, or an effective dosage level or combination of medications could not be found.

Are there any non-medical sexual aids available to help with erectile problems?

A number of sexual aids are available by mail order that do not require a physician's prescription (see mail order catalogues listed). Some people prefer strap-on latex penises, some of which are hollow and can hold a flaccid or semi-erect penis. Strap-on, battery-operated vibrators in the shape of a penis are also available.

Choosing a sexual device to aid with erections is best done with the advice of a urologist or sex therapist familiar with MS. If you have a long-term sex partner, it is important to include this person in the discussion. This will decrease anxiety and uncertainty when the devices are used and enhance intimacy by allowing both sex partners to explore them together. Counseling with a mental health professional who is knowledgeable about MS can facilitate the process if you have problems communicating or feel inhibited about talking through these issues.

Recently it has started to be painful for me when we have sex. My husband says I feel tight and dry. What is the best way to deal with this problem?

Similar to the erectile response in men, vaginal lubrication is controlled by two different pathways in the brain and spinal cord. "Psychogenic" lubrication typically originates in the brain and occurs through fantasy, reading erotic novels, or exposure to sexually related stimuli. Reflexogenic lubrication occurs through direct stimulation of the genitals or anus via a reflex response in the sacral (lower) part of the spinal cord. MS can affect nerve pathways that control either or both types of lubrication. Additionally, some medications used to treat bladder symptoms in MS can reduce vaginal lubrication. Psychogenic lubrication can sometimes be enhanced by establishing a relaxing, romantic, and/or sexually stimulating setting for sexual activity, incorporating relaxing massage into foreplay activities and prolonging foreplay before intercourse.

"Reflexogenic" lubrication can sometimes be increased by manually or orally stimulating the genitals prior to attempting intercourse. Vaginal dryness can also be dealt with by applying generous amounts of water-soluble lubricants such as Replens® or K-Y Jelly®, which are available over-the-counter in most pharmacies and drug stores. If condoms are used for birth control or disease prevention purposes, it is recommended that you use those that are lubricated and apply additional lubricant to the vaginal area as needed. Water-soluble lubricants that are marketed for sexual activity purposes can also be purchased by mail order via the catalogue services listed at the end of the chapter.

Health care professionals do not recommend the use of petroleum (oil) based jellies (e.g., Vaseline®) for vaginal lubrication since they are not water-soluble. Petroleum based jellies can leave residues in and around the vaginal and urethral openings, which could set the stage for bacterial infections to develop.

Spasticity in my legs sometimes makes sexual activity very uncomfortable. Is there anything I can do about this problem?

Spasticity can make straightening the legs or changing leg positions for sexual activity uncomfortable or even painful. Active symptomatic management of spasticity will minimize its impact on sexuality. Range of motion and other physical therapy exercises are commonly employed, as well as antispasticity medications such as baclofen (Lioresal®). Administering antispasticity medication prior to anticipated sexual activity can be helpful. Be sure, however, to discuss any medication changes with your physician.

Exploring alternative sexual positions for intercourse is sometimes helpful when spasticity is a problem. Women who have spasticity of the **adductor muscles** may find it difficult or painful to separate their legs. The impact of adductor spasms can be minimized by lying on your side with your partner approaching you from behind. Placing a towel between your legs while lying in this position may help you feel more comfortable. You may find that lying on your back, perpendicular to the bed, with both legs (from the knees down) hanging off the edge of the bed, makes intercourse easier and more comfortable.

A man who has difficulty straightening his legs may find that sitting upright in an armless chair allows his partner to mount his erect penis in either a face-to-face or face-to-back position. However, everyone's body is different, and the key to finding alternative sexual positions is open exploration and communication between partners.

My wife's MS makes her so tired that by the time we get the children to bed she's too worn out to want to have sex. Is there anything we can do about all this fatigue?

Energy conservation and fatigue management are important interventions to promote sexual activity and enjoyment. Fatigue is managed from physical therapy, occupational therapy, and pharmacological perspectives. It can be helpful to have consultations at an MS center that offers comprehensive care or to obtain referrals to MS experts in these areas. If stimulants such as pemoline (Cylert®) or amantadine (Symmetrel®) are prescribed for fatigue management, administration prior to anticipated sexual activity may be helpful (see Appendix B).

Even with effective symptom management, you and your wife may still want to explore other strategies to enhance your sex life and reduce the impact of her fatigue. Couples frequently engage in sexual activity in the evening, when energy is at its lowest ebb. Talk over the possibility of having sex in the morning, when fatigue is at a minimum. Although making a "date" to awaken earlier for sexual activity may initially seem undesirable, this kind of adaptation may be necessary for retaining an enjoyable sex life. Some couples are fortunate to have the flexibility in their schedules to make a periodic "lunch date" for intimate play.

Some sexual positions require less energy than others, and alternative positions that minimize weight bearing or tiring movements can minimize fatigue. As you try to initiate some of these changes in your sexual life, be aware that they require open communication and the willingness to engage in some trial-and-error exploration. Counseling may be helpful if you and your wife find it difficult to communicate about alternatives.

I've been having a lot of difficulty controlling my urine lately. I'm so worried about having an accident during sex that I keep making excuses to my husband. I want to have sex but I'm afraid that if I wet myself or him he'll never want to have sex again!

Fortunately, successful bladder management is attainable for most people (see Chapter 3). A critical first step in this process is careful bladder assessment, guided by your MS health care team or a urologist who is familiar with MS.

Try discussing your concerns about incontinence openly with your husband. Most partners are willing to "take the chance" once they are informed of the issues and assured that everything is being done to manage the bladder problems. Discussing your fears with him, and strategizing together with your health care team to minimize the risk of incontinence during sexual activity, will also give you more confidence. You may need to tailor your symptomatic management strategies a bit to allow for anticipated sexual activity. If, for example, you are taking **anticholinergic** medications for bladder storage dysfunction, you might try taking the medication thirty minutes before anticipated sexual activity in order to minimize bothersome bladder contractions. These medicines increase vaginal dryness, so you may need to compensate by using water-soluble lubricants. You can also minimize incontinence by restricting fluid intake for an hour or two before sex and doing intermittent catheterization just before sexual activity. Wearing a condom during sex is advised for men who are concerned with small amounts of urinary leakage.

A woman who has an **indwelling catheter** can manage by taping the catheter securely to the stomach, emptying the collecting bag before sexual activity, and putting additional tape around the top ring to minimize the chances of leaks. You can avoid putting pressure on the catheter or the collecting bag by lying in a "nestled spoons" position with the woman in front and using rear entry intercourse. An alternative position for a woman with a catheter is to lie on her back with her legs over the man's shoulders. He can support himself on his arms in order to reduce the weight on her. A variation of this position is for the man to sit on his knees, between the woman's legs, and position her legs over his shoulders. The latter position allows for less vigorous, more gentle "rocking" movements and allows a woman with spasticity to keep her legs closer together. These are examples of ways in which sexual activity can be modified in order to compensate for MS-related changes. Each couple will need to find the solutions that best meet their needs. Some couples will find these solutions through patient trial-and-error exploration. Others will find it useful to consult with an experienced sex therapist.

Trying new sexual positions that will compensate for MS symptoms and disabilities can be anxiety-provoking for many people. Taking the time to acquire information, explore, discuss, and obtain frequent feedback during sexual experimentation will help alleviate fears. Able-bodied partners may be fearful of causing pain, or they may feel insecure about knowing what to do and how to do it. Setting aside regular time to talk about sex gives it more importance in the relationship and sets the stage for the couple to air their fears and concerns and improve their communication.

My wife has difficulty moving very much during sex since she lost so much strength in her arms and legs. Will I hurt her if we try some different positions?

Weakness is a common MS symptom that frequently requires finding new positions for satisfactory sexual activities. Reclining

positions do not place as much strain on muscles and are therefore less tiring. Pillows can be used to improve positioning and
reduce muscle strain. Inflatable pillows specifically designed to
provide back support during sexual activity may help minimize
back strain. These wedge-shaped pillows have individually
inflatable sections that allow for firmness adjustment and do not
restrict movement. Oral sex requires less movement than intercourse, and using hand-held or strap-on vibrators can help compensate for hand weakness while providing sexual stimulation.

Anxiety about hurting your sex partner is fairly common
when significant changes in physical functioning have occurred.
Open discussions with each other before attempting new positions or sexual activities will allow your wife to educate you
about her MS symptoms and enable you both to air your concerns while planning for sexual encounters. Conducting a "positioning" exercise before sex is attempted will help you both
determine if the new positions are comfortable without introducing anxiety *during* sexual activity. If your wife has a physical
therapist who knows her body strengths and weaknesses well,
he or she may be able to advise you both about positions for sexual activity that take into account your wife's vulnerabilities.

**I find that I lose my train of thought when I have sex. My inter-
est and desire start out fine, but then my mind drifts and I lose
interest. This is very frustrating for me, and my partner frequently feels like he's not doing something right. Is there anything I can do about this problem?**

Changes in attention and concentration are common in MS and
may derail the ability to sustain sexual interest and excitement.
Partners sometimes misinterpret this symptom to mean that they
are deficient or uninteresting as lovers. The person with MS
sometimes feels guilty or deficient. These negative feelings can
increase the distractibility or lead the person to avoid sex altogether. Accepting distractibility as a valid MS symptom and discussing ways to help compensate for it are crucial steps to finding a solution. Attention/concentration problems tend to be
worse when a person is fatigued, so it is vitally important to
evaluate fatigue level and compensate accordingly. In general,
*minimizing non-romantic or non-sexual stimuli and maximizing
sensual and sexual stimulation during sex is the strategy for
compensating.* You can help minimize this problem by creating

a romantic mood/environment, using multisensory stimulation (e.g., talking in sexy ways, sensual and erotic touching, and playing music that has strong romantic associations). Developing an atmosphere of acceptance and permission for the person to "re-enter the sexual experience" after losing focus can help. Sometimes briefly switching from erotic to sensual (but non-genital) touching can facilitate interest when attention wanders. Refer to Chapter 9 for suggestions on the general management of attention/concentration problems.

My husband has changed a lot since he got MS. He grabs me a lot, even in front of other people, and seems to want to have sex all the time. We always had a comfortable sex life, but now it almost feels like he's a stranger in some ways and I'm not comfortable any more.

"Behavioral disinhibition," or acting on one's sexual impulses in an uncontrolled way, is occasionally (but rarely) reported in MS. It may be associated with MS-related cognitive impairments (see Chapter 9) or a separate and distinct type of depression that has both manic (hyperactive) and depressive features called bipolar disorder (formerly called manic depression). In general, referral to a psychiatrist who is familiar with MS is important so that an accurate understanding of the symptom can be reached. Medications can sometimes manage this symptom if the impulsive hypersexuality is part of the manic phase of bipolar disorder. Regardless of the origin of the disinhibition, counseling is important to help the person with MS and the sexual partner cope with the impulsivity. If the symptom is associated with cognitive changes or other changes in judgment, the appropriateness of cognitive rehabilitation could be explored.

I've become so discouraged lately. Nothing seems worth the effort. My wife wants to have sex with me and it's the furthest thing from my mind. I'm too angry and sad all the time to even think about sex. I know it's not fair to her but I can't seem to shake this mood.

MS is frequently associated with emotional challenges that include grief, demoralization, changes in self-esteem and body image, and sometimes clinical depression (see Chapter 11). These emotional states may temporarily dampen interest in sex or the ability to give and receive sexual pleasure. Addressing these emotional challenges in an effort to enhance sexuality has several aspects: education, assessment, professional treatment, and coping interventions.

Education about emotional challenges in MS is available through the MS Society. Additionally, groups in which people with MS and their partners can share information about MS are widely available. These resources can help you and your wife to understand the feelings you are experiencing and recognize the ways these feelings can affect your sexual relationship.

Assessment of a person's emotional responses to the stresses imposed by MS can be done by a mental health professional who is familiar with the disease. Correctly identifying the type of emotional distress a person is experiencing is a prerequisite to providing the appropriate treatment. It is necessary to find out what is causing your distress in order for you to be able to "shake this mood." A normal grief reaction to the stresses and losses imposed by the illness might be dealt with very effectively in a support group or short-term individual psychotherapy. A more acute clinical depression, however, might best be treated with some combination of psychotherapy and antidepressant medication.

As you begin to experience some relief from these distressing feelings, you and your wife may find it easier to talk about the ways in which MS and your feelings about the disease have affected your sexual relationship. One of the most important coping strategies for dealing with emotional and body image changes is ongoing, intimate communication with your long-term sexual partner. It may be particularly difficult to explore new options, discuss disappointments, and express what both of you feel and want in the face of coping with all the other changes associated with MS. MS peer groups, couples groups, and/or individual or couples counseling can facilitate this process.

My husband has become quite disabled and I am his primary caregiver. It's hard for me to think of him as my husband and my lover when I also dress, bathe, and clean him. I know he wants me to have sex with him but I just don't feel like it any more.

Changes in former sexual patterns and roles represent significant challenges to intimacy and sexuality. Perceptions of being ill or disabled may be incompatible with an image of being sexually active and vigorous. Role changes that involve the "well" partner assuming many caregiving functions may challenge that person's ability to view his or her partner as a source of sexual excitement. When caregiving becomes an extensive part of a relationship, it is difficult to relax and have sexual fun. If possible, nursing activities should be done by someone other than the sexual partner so the person with MS does not assume the role of "patient" in the intimate relationship. To the extent possible, the bedroom should be preserved as a private place for closeness and intimacy; medical equipment and other illness-related paraphernalia should be kept to one side or in another room. Ideally, time for intimate talk, cuddling, or sexual activity should be set aside, separate from the times for caregiving.

Obviously, these suggestions are not always viable. Finding "substitute" caregivers to provide nursing care is not always possible. Families do not always have the luxury of keeping medical equipment in a separate space. Additionally, some couples are unwilling to give up the caregiving and care-receiving roles since much of the closeness that remains in the relationship may be in the context of these caregiving activities.

For someone who is attempting to juggle the dual roles of nurse/caregiver and sexual partner, it is very important to be able to discuss this challenge to intimacy. You may be hesitant to discuss your feelings with your husband because you do not want to upset him. In turn, he may find it difficult to express his frustration and resentment over the change in the sexual relationship because he does not want to risk hurting or angering you—his primary caregiver. Yet this reluctance to share these difficult and painful feelings represents a further loss of intimacy. You and your husband may find it helpful to talk these issues over with a family therapist experienced in chronic illness and sexuality.

Since my wife was diagnosed with MS, it feels as though we are drifting apart. Initially we worked together to cope with the uncertainties of the diagnosis and the aftermath of her first few exacerbations. Yet we seem to be feeling less and less close over time even though she is not that physically disabled. It's harder for us to be sexual with each other and to feel close.

There is a heavy emphasis in present day Western culture on youth, beauty, health, and physical vigor. Men and women in our culture often feel burdened by the pressure to be eternally young and vigorously sexual. The experience of MS, with its associated changes in body functions, can trigger a dramatic sense of sexual or sensual inadequacy in the face of these cultural pressures. It is difficult to feel sexual with another person when one's sexual feelings and performance are being threatened. Men and women with MS may have difficulty enjoying and expressing their sensual/sexual nature because of the widening gap between culturally based ideals and their own illness experience.

Pressures also exist for the sexual partner of someone with MS. The partner may begin to think of the person with MS as too fragile to engage in sexual activity or as a "patient" who is too ill to be sexually expressive. The physical, cognitive, and emotional changes sometimes associated with MS can also strain the intimacy between two people; a partner can begin to feel as though he or she is trying to relate to a person who is somehow different or unfamiliar. Similarly, the role changes that are sometimes required in the face of MS, such as one partner becoming the other's caregiver, can drastically alter the mutual feelings and expectations within a relationship.

All of these changes can lead to an increasing sense of personal isolation within a relationship. Each partner may feel less and less able to understand the other's experience, feelings, and needs. In turn, a diminishing capacity to understand and work through these differences can create greater isolation and misunderstanding. Mutual resentment can begin to fester and grow.

Throughout this chapter we have emphasized effective communication between partners (and between partners and health care providers) as a necessary step toward restoring sexual enjoyment and intimacy. However, there are many barriers to effective communication. Images of sexuality and sensuality are rampant in Western society, yet they are not depicted in a way that provides an open and acceptable means of discussion and problem-solving. Most sexual language is either too "medicalized" or technical or considered "dirty" or unacceptable to allow for easy conversation between lovers.

Part of the solution to these barriers involves developing a more comfortable vocabulary about sexuality and intimacy. Education about MS symptoms and the anatomy and physiology of sexuality can help to provide a basis for mutual understanding and problem-solving. The organizations listed at the end of this chapter can add to the information contained in this chapter. There also are many self-help books available at most bookstores that are designed to enhance communication, sexuality, and intimacy. Reading these materials together can help you become comfortable with the vocabulary you need in order to be able to discuss personal and intimate subjects. Talk to each other about what you are reading and how it might be applied to your relationship.

Another approach involves setting aside time each week to devote exclusively to restoring intimacy and talking about sexuality. This can set the stage for a couple to begin talking more easily about their intimate needs, wants, and differences. A helpful but more challenging adjunct to this process is to make regular "dates" when you are free from caregiving, child rearing, or household tasks. This kind of opportunity to focus exclusively on one another recalls the early romantic phase of most long-term intimate relationships, that has all too often been sacrificed to the pressures or careers, parenting, and coping with MS-related tasks. Partners need to rediscover each other as their roles and expectations are updated or reconciled with the changing MS situation. Many couple's, however, become anxious or frustrated with their efforts to reconnect with one another. If you and your wife find the process to be too difficult on your own, you may find that couple's counseling can provide a safe atmosphere in which to begin exploring these aspects of your relationship.

Getting through each day has gotten very hard for me. Nothing is easy any more and nothing can ever be spontaneous. We used to have sex whenever we wanted to—just because we felt like it. Now we have to plan it all so I'll be comfortable and not too tired.

One of our common Western cultural expectations is that sex should be spontaneous and passionate, with the lovers becoming "swept away" in a torrent of romantic and intimate urges. Couples may feel disappointed if this or other internalized visions of what sex "should be" are not met—so disappointed in fact that they may fail to explore other sexual possibilities or even stop having sex altogether.

Additionally, the changes imposed by MS frequently make it necessary for there to be some preparation for sexual encounters, possibly including changing the timing of certain medications, altering the time of day for sexual activity, and learning new sexual activities that compensate for disabilities. In the face of these adjustments, some couples may decide that sex—that day, that week, or even that month—is just not worth all the trouble. When there is a major symptom flare-up or any other life situation that interferes with sexual expression, it is important to communicate with your partner about the changes and feelings you are experiencing. This will allow you to retain a sense of closeness and intimacy even in the absence of sexual activity. You can use this period of time to focus on other pleasurable aspects of the relationship, such as the sensual or "special person" aspects discussed earlier.

Failing to communicate, either verbally or nonverbally, about those times when sex "isn't worth all the effort" will put you at risk for withdrawing from each other even further. Joining together in the decision "not to have sex right now" will also enable you to ask each other "what *do* we want right now?" and "how can we go about achieving it for ourselves?"

Recommended Readings

Foley FW, Iverson J. Sexuality and MS. In: Kalb RC, Scheinberg LC (eds.). *Multiple Sclerosis and the Family*. New York: Demos Vermande, 1992.

Kaplan HS. *The Illustrated Manual of Sex Therapy (2nd edition)*. New York: Brunner Mazel Publishers, 1987.

Kroll K, Klein EL. *Enabling Romance: A Guide to Love, Sex, and Relationships for the Disabled*. New York: Harmony Books, 1992.

Mooney TO, Cole TM, Chilgren RA. *Sexual Options for Paraplegics and Quadriplegics*. Boston: Little, Brown, 1975.

Neistadt ME, Freda M. *Choices: A Guide to Sex Counseling with Physically Disabled Adults*. Malabar, FL: Robert E. Krieger Publishing, 1987.

Yaffe M, Fenwick E, Rosen R, Kellett J. *Sexual Happiness for Women: A Practical Approach*. New York: Henry Holt, 1992.

Yaffe M, Fenwick E, Rosen R, Kellett J. *Sexual Happiness for Men: A Practical Approach*. New York: Henry Holt, 1992.

Selected pamphlets from the National Multiple Sclerosis Society
(Customer Service: 212-986-3240; Information: 800-344-4867)

⬦ *Sexuality and Multiple Sclerosis (3rd edition)*—Michael
Barrett Ph.D. (available from Multiple Sclerosis Society of
Canada, 250 Bloor Street East, Suite 820, Toronto, Ontario
M4W 3P9, Phone: 416-922-6065)

Recommended Resources

⬦ The Sexuality Information and Education Council of the
United States (SIECUS) has a Resource Center and Library
located at 130 W. 42nd Street, Suite 350, N.Y., N.Y. 10036
(Phone: 212-819-9770). SIECUS publishes an annotated
bibliography on sexuality and disability, which was updated in 1994. They also run database searches for more specific topics, utilizing their own extensive reference library.

⬦ *Sexuality and Disability* is a quarterly journal that publishes scholarly articles on rehabilitation, disability, and sexuality. It also publishes guidelines for professional clinical
practice, case studies, and information for consumers. The
journal is available from Human Sciences Press, Inc., 233
Spring Street, New York, N.Y. 10013-1578 (Phone: 212-620-
8000).

⬦ The American Association of Sex Educators, Counselors,
and Therapists (AASECT) certifies professional sex therapists who can document that they have met their criteria
for minimum educational and clinical experience standards. AASECT-certified therapists also must agree to
adhere to a code of ethics. Although many highly qualified
sex therapists do not choose to join AASECT, you can
obtain a list of AASECT-certified sex therapists by writing
to AASECT, P.O. Box 238, Mount Vernon, IA 52314.

⬦ Planned Parenthood is a national organization that provides information on abortion and birth control. However,
some chapters conduct sex counseling, and the chapters
can provide competent local referrals for sex therapy and
counseling. The national office is located at 810 Seventh

Ave., New York, NY 10019. Their telephone number is 212-541-7800; 800-829-7732.

There are a number of discreet catalogue services available that sell sexually oriented materials. Most of these are not targeted toward people with disabilities, but they contain products that may be helpful to both disabled and nondisabled people. Some include:

◇ Eve's Garden International, Ltd. sells books, videos, and sexual aids/toys. Their catalogue can be ordered from their offices at 119 W. 57th Street, Suite 420, New York, N.Y. 10019-2383. (Phone: 800-848-3837).

◇ Good Vibrations, Inc. offers similar fare. Their catalogue can be ordered from 938 Howard Street, San Francisco, CA 94103 (Phone: 415-974-8990; 800-289-8423).

◇ Lawrence Research offers a catalogue full of sexual novelties and aids, videos, and books, called the Xandria Collection catalogue. They also have a small catalogue that targets those with disabilities (cost $4.00) and can be reached by mail at P.O. Box 31039, San Francisco, CA 94131 (Phone: 800-242-2823; call extension 39 for additional information).

13

Fertility, Pregnancy, Childbirth, and Gynecologic Care

Kathy Birk, M.D.
Michael A. Werner, M.D.

A person might be symptom-free and feeling fine following the diagnosis of multiple sclerosis, but he or she now has a new piece of bewildering information to add to those factors that all adults must think about when considering parenthood, such as the stability of the marriage, financial security, and the commitment to raising children. Couples in which one partner is already somewhat disabled or wheelchair-dependent may also be facing decisions about starting a family or adding another child.

Regardless of the level of disability, a joint decision by prospective parents is vital. Specific questions about conception, pregnancy, and delivery are only the beginning; parenthood's bigger picture stretches many years into the future. Important long-range considerations include the possibility of increasing physical disability, the threat to financial security if income were to be lost due to that disability, the availability of adequate support from friends and extended family, and the ease or comfort with which the mother and father could share parenting and wage earning roles if needed. No single decision is "right" for everyone, and a couple may find that agreement on family planning decisions does not come quickly or easily.

Proactive ways to become more comfortable with these decisions might include working together as a couple to make an honest assessment of your family situation, including the emotional, financial, and medical aspects of your daily life; asking your doctor to participate in a thorough discussion of present disease activity and possible disease progression; talking to other families in which one of the parents has MS; and seeking information from the MS Society.

Included in this chapter are answers to some of the most commonly asked questions about family planning, fertility, pregnancy, childbirth, and nursing, as well as suggestions about well-woman care. So often, those with a chronic condition do not receive basic screening tests, medication options, and health care practices that are routinely offered to those without an illness.

Family Planning and Fertility

I am a twenty-five-year-old woman with MS. What types of contraception are safe for me to use until my husband and I decide that it's time to start a family?

Contraceptive choices should be made after considering such factors as personal preference, manual dexterity and coordination, other medications being used, and the possible risk of infection.

The use of barrier contraceptives, such as the diaphragm, spermicides, and condoms, requires manual dexterity and control or a very able partner to provide assistance. Using a diaphragm may increase your risk of bladder infections. Additionally, the diaphragm requires application of a spermicide prior to each act of intercourse and should be removed eight hours after insertion. For maximum reliability, it is recommended that a condom be used in conjunction with the diaphragm. Some women find it easier to use a spermicidal suppository that is inserted ten minutes prior to intercourse. Used in combination with a condom, the spermicide is just as reliable as a diaphragm. The condom, alone or in combination with another birth control method, reduces the risk of sexually transmitted diseases.

Birth control pills are generally a safe and highly effective means of birth control. *However, the use of certain drugs, such as antibiotics, phenytoin, and carbamazepine, may reduce the pill's effectiveness* (see Appendix B). Women who are taking any of these medications should discuss with their physician the need for additional protection, e.g., a condom or other barrier-type contraceptive. Birth control pills should not be used by any woman with high blood pressure or by women over the age of thirty-five who smoke, due to the increased risk of heart disease (may we remind you that smoking is not good for any aspect of your health and that every effort should be made to stop).

The long-acting progesterone shot (Depo-Provera®) is effective for twelve weeks and is not known to be affected by those drugs that may alter the pill's effectiveness. Depo-Provera® is also a safer method of birth control for women who are unable to stop smoking. The long-acting, implantable progesterone (Norplant®) is effective for five years and requires no ongoing attention. Each of these methods may be associated with side effects (including weight gain and irregular bleeding) and must be carefully reviewed and understood before opting to use them.

The intrauterine device (IUD) currently in use in the United States (Paraguard®) is a safe, effective, and convenient form of birth control for women with a single sexual partner who are not planning to have any more children. Its insertion is a simple, reversible office procedure. Some concern exists that the use of antibiotics or immunosuppressive medications could decrease the effectiveness of the IUD. Women who are taking any of these medications should discuss with their physician the possible need for additional birth control protection.

Vasectomy is a safe, effective sterilization procedure for men that is usually performed in a physician's office. Since reversal of a vasectomy requires delicate microsurgery that is only sometimes successful, it should be undertaken only after careful deliberation. Tubal ligation is typically done in the hospital, using general anesthesia, as an outpatient procedure. It must also be considered irreversible.

Will my MS make it difficult for me to get pregnant?

The disease itself does not cause infertility. The lower pregnancy rates that have been reported among women with MS result from a variety of factors: some of the medications used to treat

MS may lead to problems with regular ovulation; women some-times delay becoming pregnant because they are reluctant to stop taking medications that are important in the management of their MS but are not safe for use during pregnancy; and some couples decide not to have children, or to have fewer children, because of the illness.

My husband has recently been diagnosed with MS. Will this disease make him sterile?

MS does not affect sperm production. Unless your husband had a preexisting and unrelated problem with sperm produc-tion, there is no reason why he would become sterile in the future as a result of the disease. Some medications may con-tribute to a compromise of sperm quality. Any woman who is trying to become pregnant should discuss with her physician all of the medications that her husband is taking. Additionally, some men experience difficulties with intercourse and ejacula-tion that can interfere with conception, despite having normal sperm counts.

Sometimes I have difficulty getting or keeping an erection dur-ing intercourse. Will this problem prevent me from being able to father a child?

It is important to distinguish between the ability to have inter-course and the ability to ejaculate sperm and ultimately father a child. Many men who have difficulty maintaining an adequate erection for neurologic or non-neurologic reasons are still able to ejaculate. If you are able to ejaculate, even though you some-times have difficulty maintaining an erection that is firm enough for intercourse, your doctor can teach you how to use a syringe to collect your ejaculate and place it directly into your wife's vagina. There is no truth to the commonly held belief that ejac-ulation outside the woman's vagina in any way affects the qual-ity of the sperm or their ability to fertilize an egg. Refer to Chapter 12 for a discussion of MS-related erectile problems and available treatments.

I am a twenty-eight-year-old man with MS. For the past several months I have had difficulty ejaculating during intercourse. My wife and I have been trying to have a baby for several months without any luck. How will we be able to have a child if I can't ejaculate?

If you are able to ejaculate on some occasions but not others, you have the option of banking your sperm for insemination during your wife's fertile period. The disadvantage of this type of banking is that the quality of the sperm does deteriorate somewhat when frozen and thawed. If you are unable to ejaculate even intermittently, there are medications that can be used to try to stimulate you to ejaculate. The most commonly used drugs are pseudoephedrine and imipramine. These are prescribed by a fertility specialist who will closely monitor your ejaculation in order to adjust dosage levels. Some men who seem to have no ejaculation actually experience a "retrograde" or backward ejaculation. These same medications can convert a backward ejaculation to a forward ejaculation.

If you are unable to ejaculate even with the use of these medications, a reflex ejaculation can sometimes be induced through vibratory stimulation of the underside of the penis. This technique is effective for those individuals whose ejaculatory mechanism is impaired because of faulty nerve transmissions between the brain and spinal cord. Your doctor can show you how to use a vibrator effectively to achieve a sufficient level of stimulation. The ejaculate can be placed in your wife's vagina for attempted fertilization, if the timing is appropriate, or stored for insemination at a later time.

Some men are unable to ejaculate with either medications or vibratory stimulation. A third technique, which completely bypasses the spinal cord and directly stimulates the nerves that release the ejaculate, is called electroejaculation. During a day hospital admission, under general anesthesia, the man is given a brief series of electric shocks through a probe placed into the rectum. The electric stimulation produces an ejaculation that can then be used for insemination. This technique has been used for some time in men with spinal cord injury, but has also been used successfully in individuals with MS.

My doctor has told me that there are various kinds of treatments for impotence caused by MS, including medications and surgical implants. Would I be able to father a child using any of these treatments?

Impotence does not lead to infertility. As long as you are able to ejaculate, at least intermittently (with or without the medical interventions described in the previous answer), none of the treatments for erectile dysfunction will interfere with your ability to conceive (see Chapter 12).

Pregnancy, Labor, and Delivery

Do I need to stop the medications I am taking before I start trying to get pregnant? I'm worried that my MS will get worse if I'm off the medications for too long.

As a general rule, *the use of any medications while a woman is pregnant or trying to become pregnant, including ones that are bought over-the-counter, must be done with caution and under the advice of a physician who is familiar with their use during pregnancy.*

Medications used to treat MS fall into two groups—those that treat symptoms and those that are used to reduce disease activity. In many cases, the medications used to treat symptoms or occasional medical problems (such as bladder infections) are safe to continue. This is not the case for most of the drugs used to treat the disease itself. Many of the latter are immunosuppressive drugs, most of which have not been studied sufficiently during pregnancy to show whether or not they cause problems for the baby. None of the newer drugs, including Betaseron®, Avonex®, or Copaxone®, have been studied in pregnancy. While you might wish to continue taking a drug that holds promise for slowing the progression of MS, the health of your unborn baby must be a primary concern. It is important to stop these medications as soon as you begin trying to conceive because the fertilized egg will begin to develop a few weeks before you know that you are pregnant. You can resume your medications immediately after delivery if you choose not to breast-feed your baby.

I am afraid to tell my gynecologist that I have MS. I don't want anyone to tell me that I shouldn't have a baby. What should I do?

There is now ample evidence that a woman should not be discouraged from becoming pregnant simply because she has been diagnosed with MS. The major factor in the decision to become pregnant for couples affected by the disease is the same as for most other couples: how will adding a child to their lives work for them, and is this the right time?

Historically (and occasionally even now), couples have found that some members of the medical profession discourage pregnancy, and even parenting, for a woman who has MS. It was often suggested to women who became pregnant that they abort. These women were even encouraged to be sterilized. We now know that there is no medical reason for women with MS to avoid pregnancy. There is less risk of relapse during pregnancy itself, followed by an increased possibility of relapse in the immediate postpartum months. Most importantly, research has shown that women who do choose to become pregnant and deliver a child do not develop more disability over their lifetime than women who never become pregnant.

In spite of these changes in medical opinion about pregnancy in women with MS, many couples find that they are discouraged from becoming pregnant by their physicians or well-meaning friends and family members. Women who are considering becoming pregnant should seek information and support from the MS Society and consult a physician who is knowledgeable and willing to discuss their questions and concerns in a supportive manner. The decision to start a family or add additional children is a very personal one that needs to be made with careful attention to current and future emotional, medical, and financial factors. If you do not feel that you can discuss this subject comfortably with your present physician, perhaps you should find another with whom you are more at ease. An open and trusting relationship with your doctor is vital to your pregnancy and childbirth experience.

I recently found out that I am pregnant. My husband thinks we should terminate the pregnancy because of my MS. I can't make him understand how much I want this baby. How do I decide what is the right thing to do?

As discussed previously, pregnancy itself will not contribute to long-term disability in most women. The strength of the desire to raise and share life with a child should be the major factor in the decision for both you and your husband. As a couple, you need to weigh your feelings about parenting against a thoughtful assessment of your existing disability and possible future limitations that the disease might impose. Encourage your husband to think about his own desire for fatherhood and perhaps contact the MS Society to talk with others who have faced the fear of future parenting when MS is part of the picture.

The decision to have a child, as well as the lifetime of parenting that follows, should be a team effort. You and your husband both need to be comfortable with the decisions that you make. If the two of you are finding it difficult to communicate openly and effectively about this important life decision, you might consider talking together with your physician or with a knowledgeable psychotherapist.

Can a woman who has MS have a normal pregnancy?

MS does not appear to affect the course of pregnancy, labor, or delivery. Studies reviewing hundreds of pregnancies have found no evidence of an MS-related threat to the fetus. For many women, the risk of relapse or worsening of MS is lower during pregnancy, with the result that many women feel particularly well during this period. Problems with weakness or *flexor spasms* in the legs are manageable with assisted deliveries (forceps or with a vacuum device) and with an epidural type of anesthesia during the labor and delivery.

I recently had a miscarriage in my second month. Will this make my MS worse?

Some disease worsening may occur in the months following any pregnancy, whether the pregnancy ends in delivery or earlier because of spontaneous abortion (miscarriage) or elective termination. This possible disease worsening is likely to be temporary; studies have found no differences in long-term disability in women having no pregnancies, one pregnancy, or two or more pregnancies. Miscarriage during the first trimester of pregnancy is more common than most realize (up to 30 percent of all pregnancies end in spontaneous abortion) and is not caused by MS.

My MS symptoms seem to get so much better when I'm pregnant that I wish I could just stay pregnant all the time. What is the reason for this?

There is something about the condition of pregnancy that causes a woman's body to be in a mildly immunosuppressed state. During pregnancy, you experience naturally the *immunosuppression* that certain medications can provide artificially for people with MS and other **autoimmune diseases** (like rheumatoid arthritis or lupus). This natural immunosuppression is probably the cause of reduced disease activity during pregnancy.

The precise reason for this helpful reduction in **immune system** activity is not clear. Research has not been able to identify a specific, pregnancy-related hormone or protein that is present at higher levels in women who have less disease activity as compared with women who have greater disease activity. Research has shown that one of the pregnancy hormones (AFP) does successfully prevent the animal model of MS (**experimental allergic encephalomyelitis**) in the guinea pig.

What drugs are safe for me to take while I am pregnant?

As discussed, *one should assume that all drugs could impact the fetus*. Notable exceptions include certain antibiotics used to treat bladder infections. This is important because bladder infections are fairly common in individuals with MS and are also more likely to occur during pregnancy. Ampicillin is commonly used to treat these infections and is very safe during pregnancy and for nursing mothers. Increasingly, however, some of the infections are found to be resistant to ampicillin and other safe alternatives will be utilized by the doctor.

Steroid medications are often used during acute **exacerbations** of MS. Fortunately, as noted previously, such disease activity is decreased during pregnancy. Prednisone is a steroid that has been used fairly commonly in pregnant women with a variety of illnesses, including MS, asthma, and arthritis. Women with a history of steroid use (particularly within the past twelve months) need to be provided with a fairly high dose of steroids (called a "boost") during labor because the labor process may stress the adrenal gland beyond its ability to respond.

If new drugs for MS become available while I am trying to get pregnant, is it safe for me to take them?

No. Extreme caution is necessary when new drugs are approved before any research has been done on their use during pregnancy. The impact of a new drug on the newborn is often learned gradually, as women who are using the medication become pregnant and choose not to terminate the pregnancy. The long-term effect on an infant's development, function, and cancer risk are not clear at the time of birth or for many years to come.

How will my labor and delivery be affected by my MS? Is there anything specific my doctor needs to know to help me have a safe delivery?

Your labor is unlikely to be significantly different from what other women experience. Although MS does not increase the chance of having your delivery by caesarean section, you should be aware that all women face a 15–20 percent possibility of delivery by C section. Take advantage of available prenatal classes that will take you and your partner through the stages of labor, teach you about helpful positions and delivery routes, and acquaint you with birthing alternatives available at the hospital.

Try to meet with someone from the anesthesia department to discuss your MS and the options (e.g., epidural) for pain control during labor. An epidural can also be beneficial for women who have difficulty with leg control and spasms caused by *spasticity*. If fatigue or muscle weakness occurs after two hours of pushing to deliver the baby, the delivery may be assisted using forceps or a suction cup on the baby's head.

As mentioned previously, be sure to let your doctor know your history of steroid use, particularly during the past twelve months. If you have taken steroids during that time, you will need an extra "boost" of steroid medication during labor.

Which types of anesthesia are recommended for labor and delivery in a woman with MS?

The use of epidural anesthesia for pain relief during labor has become increasingly popular. An epidural during labor or for a caesarean section is acceptable for those who have MS, particularly when it is provided by a skilled, experienced person. An epidural is different from spinal anesthesia, which has traditionally been avoided in patients with neurologic diseases, including MS. General anesthesia is also considered safe for patients having caesarean sections.

Postpartum and Beyond

What is the likelihood that the MS will get worse after my baby is born? Is there anything that I can do to decrease this likelihood?

While virtually all the studies have found that women with MS are less likely to experience relapse or worsening during the nine months of pregnancy, the disease does tend to be more active following delivery. About 10 percent of women experience relapses during the nine months of pregnancy, and 29 percent may have an exacerbation during the first six months after delivery.

For many women, a more significant concern than the experience they might have during pregnancy or postpartum is whether the decision to have a child will increase their long-term disability. Most research has found no difference in long-term disability between women with MS who had pregnancies and those who chose to remain childless. A recent, long-term study in Sweden even suggests that women who become pregnant after being diagnosed with MS may be less likely to develop a progressive course than women who do not become pregnant after the diagnosis.

No specific treatment has been advocated to reduce the risk of postpartum relapse. Given the increased risk of disease activity in the postpartum period, you and your doctor may decide to start one of the newly available treatments to control disease activity as soon as you have delivered.

While the extreme exhaustion that characterizes new motherhood may mimic the fatigue so common in MS, that symptom alone should not warrant new medication use. Your postpartum lifestyle should allow you to focus on caring for yourself, resting, and feeding the infant. This will require that other household tasks be attended to by others, including some of the infant care, shopping, and social events. If you are employed, find out now how much maternity leave your employer will allow. Six to eight weeks of leave time is typical in the United States. Ideally, women with MS should have a longer leave since any disease relapse that occurs is likely to have its onset in the fourth to eighth week postpartum.

I always hoped to breast-feed my babies. Now that I have MS, would nursing be safe for me and the baby?

Historically, neurologists have discourged women with MS from nursing, feling that it posed an additional physical burden to a woman already at increased risk for an *exacerbation*. However, nursing is now widely encouraged if you have adequate dexterity, strength, and stamina. It eliminates the effort involved in bottle preparations and privides your baby with the best possible food.

Certain medications are absolutely unsafe for a nursing infant. Because of the increased risk of relapse postpartum, some women may consider using medications that are secreted in breast milk and may affect the baby. You should not breast-feed your infant if you opt to begin using immunosuppressive drugs postpartum. The high doses of prednisone that are prescribed for exacerbations of MS do result in significant concentrations of the steroid being present in breast milk. Since any postpartum relapse is likely to resolve spontaneously, the decision you might make to use steroids must include the possible risk to the nursing baby. Because both the immunosuppressive drugs and the high doses of steroids prescribed for exacerbations do raise concerns about suppression of the newborn's immune system (as well as the mother's), nursing should be stopped if these drugs become necessary.

The new mother's postpartum lifestyle, as well as the care and support available to her, may help to avoid disease worsening. Caring for a newborn is an exhausting experience for all new parents. In an effort to assure yourself adequate, uninterrupted sleep, try to have someone else do at least one of the night feedings. If you are breast-feeding, do all of the feedings yourself during the first two weeks in order to build up steady and sufficient milk production. After that initial two-week period, someone else can take over the nighttime feedings with formula or pumped and stored breast milk.

Can I start taking my regular MS medications as soon as my baby is born?

As discussed previously, the only limitation to medication use is whether a woman is nursing. If you are not planning to breast-feed, you may resume whatever medications you and your physician feel are best.

What is the likelihood that I will pass my MS on to my children?

The lifetime risk of MS in a child born to a person with MS has been estimated to be as high as 5 percent, much higher than the lifetime risk for the general population of 0.1 percent. While there is some increase in the risk to children with a family history of the disease, the actual risk is small (95 percent chance that MS will not occur). At the present time there is no way to diagnose MS or assess the MS risk in a particular infant prenatally.

I was able to get pregnant with no difficulty. Now I'm worried about how I'll be able to take care of my baby once it's born. I'm exhausted all the time as it is. What should I do?

Planning ahead is essential to a successful start at parenting. If you are employed, start by trying to arrange time off from work after your delivery. Maternity leave for at least eight weeks is in your best interest and your child's. The new father should also look into the possibility of family-leave time or temporarily arrange his schedule to be home somewhat earlier in the day. The exhaustion of new motherhood, coupled with the possible worsening of MS symptoms postpartum, will gradually increase throughout the day. Good parental teamwork will make these early days go more enjoyably and comfortably.

As you shop for baby furniture and equipment, look for things that are easy and convenient to manipulate. Choose such items as a highchair, car seat, and bath equipment with an eye to both safety for your baby and energy conservation for yourself. Create child-friendly play areas in your home where you can watch and interact with your baby as easily and comfortably as possible. Try to arrange for some hours of babycare each day so that you can get uninterrupted rest.

Of course, couples who are planning a family can never know for sure what might happen to impact their parenting abilities. To the extent that you can brainstorm ahead of time about possible problems that might arise, you will feel more confident of your ability to manage in the days ahead.

Gynecologic Care

Do I need any special care from my gynecologist when I am not pregnant?

All women, including those with MS, need to be educated about their contraceptive options and knowledgeable about sexually transmitted diseases. Women who are managing the problems associated with a chronic illness sometimes neglect their routine medical care; regular checkups, Pap tests, and mammograms are as essential for those with MS as they are for anyone else.

Women who have used any immunosuppressive medications (including prednisone and beta-interferon) should have a Pap test every six months because abnormal results on tests that screen for pre-cancerous changes in the cervix are more common when the immune system is less able to discourage the formation of abnormal cells in general, including those on the cervix. All women should have a mammogram on the schedule recommended by the American Cancer Society: an initial screening mammogram between thirty-five and forty years of age; every one to two years until the age of fifty; annually after age fifty.

My friends who do not have MS are all talking about the use of hormones now that we are at menopause. I have just had a few hot flashes and I know that feeling warm sometimes makes my symptoms of weakness and numbness worse. Is it advisable for me to use the hormones?

Yes. Not only will hormones successfully relieve hot flashes, but also the overall benefit to your health of hormone replacement therapy has been clearly demonstrated, MS or not. The most obvious advantage to some women with MS is for those with compromised balance or walking who have a greater risk of falling; the hormones dramatically reduce the risk of osteoporosis and the fractures of the hip, wrist, and spine that can result. All women, starting when they are very young, should be certain they are getting at least 1000 mg. of calcium every day. Dairy products (milk, yogurt, and cheese) are the easiest way to get this amount via diet (three servings every day of a dairy product). If one does not eat a lot of dairy products, calcium-fortified orange juice is a good substitute and calcium supplements are also acceptable. Once postmenopausal, women who are not using hormones should try to increase the calcium intake to 1500 mg. every day.

Studies indicate that hormone replacement may offer additional benefits, including possible help with incontinence, a decrease in vaginal dryness, reduced risk for colon cancer and Alzheimer's disease, a favorable effect on cholesterol and heart disease risk, and improvement in hormone-related memory and cognitive function.

The disadvantages of hormone replacement include the addition of another drug for women who are already taking several; the possible continuation of (hopefully light and predictable) periods, depending on how the hormone is prescribed; and some unresolved questions about the degree to which hormone replacement might increase the risk of breast cancer. You will need to discuss with your own physician the relative benefits and risks of hormone replacement so that you can make an informed decision.

Recommended Readings

Birk K, et al. The clinical course of multiple sclerosis during pregnancy and the puerperium. *Archives of Neurology* 1990:47:738–42.

Birk K. Reproductive issues in multiple sclerosis. In: *Multiple Sclerosis: Clinical Issues*. To be published by PRO/HEALTH, Volume 2, Issue 3.

Carroll D, Dorman J. *Living Well with MS*. New York: HarperCollins, 1993.

Kalb R, Scheinberg L. *Multiple Sclerosis and the Family*. New York: Demos Vermande, 1992.

Resources for Rehabilitation. *A Woman's Guide to Coping with Disability*. Lexington, MA: Resources for Rehabilitation, 1994.

Rogers J, Matsumura, M. *Mother to Be: A Guide to Pregnancy and Birth for Women with Disabilities*. New York: Demos, 1991.

Smeltzer S. The concerns of pregnant women with multiple sclerosis. *Qualitative Health Research* 1994;4:(4):480-502.

14

Employment

Donna Kulha

In a society that values the "work ethic" and "upward mobility," most people define themselves, at least in part, by the type of work they do. The average employee spends approximately one half of his or her waking hours on work-related activities. In addition to producing income, these activities also identify your role in the community and offer an important source of personal pride and satisfaction. When the symptoms of multiple sclerosis interfere with participation in the labor force, the disease threatens not only economic well-being, but also your self-image and personal pride. Redefining one's "self" in the face of role changes precipitated by MS-related symptoms therefore plays a significant part in efforts to cope with the disease.

More than 90 percent of Americans with MS have worked at some point in their lives, and more than 60 percent continue to work after the initial diagnosis. However, only 20–30 percent remain in the work force ten to fifteen years after diagnosis. We still do not adequately understand why one person with MS remains productively employed while another similarly disabled person does not. Although further research is warranted, it is clear that several features of the disease can affect job retention, including impaired mobility, older age at diagnosis, progressive disease course, and invisible symptoms like fatigue and cognitive impairment.

Given the significant negative impact of job loss on the individual's (and family's) economic and emotional well-being, it is important to identify ways to help people with MS continue working as long as they wish to do so. Comprehensive psychosocial services, occupational therapies, job retention programs, and empowerment models have been developed to support people's efforts to continue on the job. Education for people with MS and their employers and co-workers, increased employer liaison, proactive approaches to legal rights, and legislative initiatives to improve disability regulation and work incentives are all vital to keeping those with MS in the work force.

The Americans with Disabilities Act (ADA), which became law in July of 1990, is the first comprehensive legislation passed by any country in the world to prohibit discrimination on the basis of disability. One can hope that similar laws will be enacted in other countries in the not-too-distant future. The ADA guarantees full participation in society for all people with disabilities in much the same way as the Civil Rights Act of 1964 guaranteed the rights of all people regardless of race, sex, national origin, or religion. Previous federal, state, and local laws continue to provide other protections for people who are disabled. Keep in mind as you read this chapter that the word *disabled* has different meanings within different contexts. The law, private insurance companies, and government insurance companies all define this concept somewhat differently. Suffice it to say here that the ADA definition of disability covers everyone with multiple sclerosis.

As it pertains directly to employment, the ADA requires employers with fifteen or more employees to provide accommodations for individuals with disabilities. What does this mean for people with multiple sclerosis? For some, accommodations to invisible symptoms like fatigue and heat sensitivity are sufficient to keep them productively employed in line with their age, training, and vocational choices. For others, job retention is made possible by structural accommodations (e.g., ramps, railings, widened doorways), equipment modifications, or mobility enhancement on the job site. It is important to remember that an employer is only required to provide accommodation to qualified individuals who can perform the essential functions of the job.

As guaranteed by the ADA, accommodation depends on many factors. It is not spelled out definitively by the law and must be determined on a case-by-case basis. It is the responsibility of the employee to make the request for accommodation. However, such requests require that one disclose the diagnosis and related disability, a step that must be considered carefully as it could be interpreted by the employer as an indication that a person is not qualified for the position held or sought. For more information on the ADA, call the Job Accommodation Network, a service of the President's Committee on Employment of People with Disabilities, 800-526-7234.

Disclosure is a major concern throughout the span of working life, from the interviewing process through employee supervision and disciplinary measures, to decisions about seeking alternatives to full-time employment. There is evidence that early disclosure and requests for accommodations may be the best strategy for employees, but the proper timing for disclosure is an individual decision that requires much thought. In some work settings and with some employers, the best protection is an open and honest discussion with the employer *before* there are major performance issues. Requesting an accommodation that will enhance your job performance can be a good starting point. It offers the promise of a positive outcome for both you and your employer, which, in turn, fosters a spirit of cooperation that may prove beneficial if and when additional accommodations are needed. The National Multiple Sclerosis Society pamphlet entitled "The Win-Win Approach to Reasonable Accommodations" describes a positive and effective strategy for requesting accommodations.

Keep in mind that some employers will not feel the need to cooperate or support a person's efforts to continue working. Without being overtly discriminatory in their policies, they might simply decide to make it very unpleasant for a disabled employee to stay on the job. Therefore, you must make decisions about your particular job situation (preferably in consultation with an attorney knowledgeable in this area), with careful attention to both the provisions of the ADA and the personalities with whom you are dealing.

The following terms are important when addressing employment issues and chronic illness:

◇ *ADA.* The Americans with Disabilities Act of 1990 is the federal law that prohibits discrimination against people with disabilities in employment, transportation, public accommodation, communications, and activities of state and local government.

◇ *Title I of the ADA.* States that an employer with fifteen or more employees cannot discriminate against qualified applicants and employees on the basis of disability.

◇ *Qualified individuals with disabilities.* Under Title I of the ADA, the term applies to an individual with a disability who meets the skill, experience, education, and other job-related requirements of a position held or desired and who, with or without reasonable accommodation, can perform the essential functions of the job.

◇ *Individuals with a disability.* Individuals with a mental or physical impairment that limits one or more life functions or who have a history of such an impairment or who are perceived (even erroneously) as having such an impairment.

◇ *Essential job function.* Essential functions are narrowly defined to include fundamental job duties, as opposed to marginal ones. A job function is more likely to be "essential" if it requires special expertise, if a large amount of time is spent on that function, and/or if that function was listed in the written job description prepared before the employer advertised for or interviewed job applicants.

◇ *Reasonable accommodation.* Refers to an employment-related modification that an employer must make in order to ensure equal opportunity for an individual with a disability to (1) apply for or test for a job; (2) perform essential functions; (3) receive the same benefits and privileges as other employees. The employer is only required to provide a reasonable accommodation for known disabilities (i.e., where the disability is obvious or the applicant/employee informs the employer of the disability). Although each case must be evaluated individually, some common examples of accommodation include job restructuring (to eliminate non-essential tasks); changes in job schedules; relocation of assigned desk in order conserve energy or put the person closer to a restroom; reassignment to a vacant position;

physical alteration to the existing facilities; provision of qualified readers or interpreters; and modification of qualifying examinations and/or training materials.

◇ *Undue hardship.* An accommodation might prove to be an undue hardship for the employer if its implementation resulted in "significant difficulty or expense." Factors to be considered in making this determination include (1) the nature and net cost of the accommodation; (2) the impact of the accommodation on the operation of the facility involved, taking into account the facility's overall resources and the number of its employees; (3) the manner in which the employer's business operates, taking into account its size and financial resources. In asserting that an accommodation is an "undue hardship," an employer must rely on actual, not hypothetical, costs and burdens.

The following questions illustrate some of the important employment issues faced by people with MS. Although the chapter discusses the relevance of the Americans with Disabilities Act to various employment-related problems and concerns, *the information in the chapter should not be used as personal legal advice.* These questions and answers can only provide a background for your own personal planning and problem-solving. If and when you have questions about your particular employment situation, your best strategy will be to consult the literature and other resources listed at the end of the chapter, consult with your local chapter of the National Multiple Sclerosis Society, and perhaps review your personal situation with an attorney who specializes in labor law. Canadians can obtain information related to employment policies in the various provinces by contacting the National Multiple Sclerosis Society of Canada (see Recommended Resources).

I'm interviewing for a new job. Do I need to tell a potential employer about my diagnosis? If I do need to disclose, what am I required to say?

An individual with a diagnosis of a disabling condition is under no legal obligation to disclose the disability to an employer or potential employer. Whether the disability is visible or not makes no difference. You will only need to say that you have MS if the employer requires a medical exam *of any person who fills the position for which you are applying.* You are required to discuss your limitations, but not your diagnosis, if you need accommodations for the job interview itself or will need them in order to perform the essential functions of the job. Practically speaking, however, it can be difficult and awkward to have a discussion about the limitations that necessitate accommodation without talking about the disease that causes those limitations. This is one of those situations in which the law states one thing, but the reality of the situation is not quite as simple or clear-cut as the law makes it sound.

Disclosure of your diagnosis in a job interview is not advised, particularly if your symptoms are invisible. If, however, you need to disclose your diagnosis and related disability because your symptoms are apparent, or in order to request an immediate accommodation (e.g., a desk near a bathroom or a parking space near the entrance), it is important to have a rehearsed disclosure statement that does not over-embellish the disease or the disability. Your local MS Society chapter may be able to assist you with such a disclosure statement. Consulting a lawyer who specializes in labor law is another effective way to educate and prepare yourself for this type of situation. Even if you never encounter job discrimination or disability-related employment problems, you will feel confident that you are knowledgeable about the best strategies for avoiding unnecessary problems in the future.

When checking my references, can a potential employer ask how MS has affected my work in the past?

The ADA prohibits any pre-employment inquiries about a disability or about the nature or severity of a disability on application forms, in job interviews, or in background or reference checks. Information may be obtained on the application form, in the interview, or in reference checks about previous work attendance, job functions, or the quality and quantity of work performed. Other job-related issues that do not relate to disability may be obtained, but the questions should not refer to illness or disability.

If an applicant has a known disability and has indicated that he could perform a job with a reasonable accommodation, a previous employer may be asked about accommodations made.

After being offered a job, I was told that I need to pass a physical examination. What should I do?

According to the ADA, you can only be required to pass a physical examination if the exam is required of *all* candidates and if the exam requirements accurately reflect the skills needed for the job. For example, an employer cannot require you to pass a test of physical endurance for an office job that requires no strength. Your employer cannot require you to have an exam merely because of suspicions about your health, nor can the employer deny you the job based on your diagnosis or speculation about future impairments. In order for an employer to deny you employment based on any current impairments, he or she must be able to demonstrate that no reasonable accommodations are available or that the accommodations would impose undue hardship on the company.

The results of a physical examination need not be feared; according to the ADA, employers are generally forbidden from considering medical diagnosis in either pre- or post-employment decision-making. A diagnosis of MS cannot, by itself, disqualify you from getting, keeping, or being promoted to a job for which you are qualified. Of course, an employer who is familiar with the provisions of the law may attempt to disqualify you on other grounds without ever mentioning your disability. Again, this is the type of situation for which some advance consultation with a labor lawyer can help you feel more prepared.

I use a cane on bad days and I may need one on the day of my job interview. Should I tell the interviewer that I have MS?

You are under no legal obligation to disclose your diagnosis to a potential employer. However you may need to address your limitation and possible accommodations if the essential functions of the position would be impacted by your disability. Once again, your personal, on-the-spot assessment of the immediate situation and the person with whom you are speaking may be that complete frankness is in your best interests—in other words, that the potential employer would be more put off by evasiveness than by the MS. Unfortunately, the law can only tell you what your rights are; it is no substitute for your personal judgment or insight into a given situation.

I have been offered a job, and the question of medical benefits arises. Can I be denied coverage under my employer's health insurance because of a diagnosis of MS?

One of the stipulations of the ADA is that an employer cannot make a contract that has the effect of discriminating against a person with a disability, before or after being hired. This would include using a health insurance company that refuses to cover a person with MS. Employees with disabilities must be given the same coverage as all other employees.

Additionally, an employer cannot refuse to hire you because the company's insurance will not cover someone with MS, or because providing you with proper coverage might increase the company's future health care costs. However, an employer may continue to offer health insurance that contains preexisting condition exclusions or limits coverage for certain procedures or treatments, even if this adversely affects individuals with disabilities. For example, an employer may offer a health insurance plan that limits or excludes coverage for long-term rehabilitation or physical therapy to *all* his employees, even though an employee with MS may require these courses of treatment. These exclusions, however, must comply with federal and state insurance requirements and cannot exist merely as a way to evade the purpose of the ADA.

People sometimes wonder whether to conceal their MS when filling out employment-related medical plan applications. The simplest answer to this question is that a person should answer honestly any questions about present or past medical history. Any insurer who subsequently discovers that a person has concealed information about an illness or medical condition has the right to cancel that person's health insurance policy (see Chapter 15). You are not required to volunteer the information if you join a new company and are automatically entered into their medical plan without any questions about your medical history being asked.

My wife has had MS for many years. Am I required to disclose this information if I am offered a job at a company that will be providing my family's health insurance coverage? Will my wife's medical costs be covered by this new coverage?

Some companies provide a grace period during which you can enroll a spouse or other family members in the company health plan without providing any medical information about them. Once the grace period passes, however, medical information would be required about any family member you wish to enroll.

The ADA provides some protection for individuals who provide care for relatives and friends with disabilities. Employers cannot exclude or deny an equal job or benefits to a qualified individual because of a relationship or association with an individual with a disability. It is important to remember, however, that the ADA requires the employer to provide an accommodation to an employee with a disability, but not to a disabled family member.

I've just been told that I have a definite diagnosis of MS. Should I quit my job?

There is no reason to stop working because you have been diagnosed with MS, and there is no evidence that continuing to work will in any way affect the progression of the disease. Many people with MS remain active and productive on the job until regular retirement age. In addition to the income and benefits that your job provides, there are a variety of other, less tangible rewards related to employment. Leaving the work force will deprive you of an important social role and the satisfactions that the role has provided you in the past. Additionally, people often report that they are viewed and treated differently by others around them (including family, friends, and society in general) once they have left the work force. Even more importantly, perhaps, is the possibility that you will prematurely and unnecessarily begin to view yourself as a "patient" or "sick person," especially if you stop working before there is any real reason or need for you to do so. Remaining independent, active, and self-supporting are reasonable goals for every person, with or without a chronic illness.

Obviously, a person's ability to continue working at a particular job will depend on the requirements of that job and the kinds of impairments that the MS is causing. If you are having difficulty performing any or all aspects of your job, your best course of action is to determine whether any kinds of accommodations at your place of work would enable you to perform your job more easily and effectively. If MS makes it impossible for you to perform your essential job functions in spite of your best efforts and the efforts of your employer to accommodate your disability, your next best course of action is to look into the possibility of being trained for another type of work (refer to the questions pertaining to reasonable job accommodations and job retraining).

I have been with the same company for three years and have recently been diagnosed with MS. How do I decide whether or not I need to disclose this information?

You are under no legal obligation to disclose your diagnosis to your employer. If, however, your job performance becomes adversely affected by your symptoms, you may want or need to seek accommodations. ADA protections only apply once the employee discloses disability-related problems on the job. In other words, if you need accommodations to perform your job, you will need to disclose your diagnosis and related disabilities to your employer. The ADA holds the employee responsible for making the request for accommodation.

It is important to weigh your decision to disclose carefully, particularly if your symptoms are invisible. If you do decide to disclose, be prepared, write out your disclosure statement, and give your employer ideas about accommodations that will be helpful. It is best to seek advice from the National Multiple Sclerosis Society or an experienced labor lawyer before writing this statement.

If I decide to disclose, who at work should be the first to know and how much information should I be prepared to offer?

Your immediate supervisor is usually the person to whom you should first disclose. The supervisor may wish to involve others, particularly a human resources specialist or a department manager. If you do not want this information to be shared with anyone else, you need to ask those in whom you have confided to respect that request. You can do this by saying, "I do not want my diagnosis shared with anyone at this time. Please keep this information confidential."

When deciding to disclose your MS diagnosis, you must also decide how much information to share. Focus on the symptoms that are affecting your job performance and require accommodation. Avoid being too clinical or too detailed, and stay away from such words as "exacerbation," "attack," "progressive," and "disease." Write out your disclosure statement and rehearse it with a friend or an advisor; your local National Multiple Sclerosis Society Chapter staff can also help you. Try to focus the discussion on enhancing your job performance rather than on the reasonable accommodation. An early request and successful implementation of an accommodation will open communication between you and your employer and make future discussions and requests easier.

All my MS symptoms are "invisible." Do I have to tell my employer that I have been diagnosed with MS?

You do not have to disclose your diagnosis and you should carefully consider the pros and cons before you do so. You may find that even the most caring and supportive supervisor may put concerns about his or her own job performance and the company's welfare and productivity ahead of your needs.

The people in my office know about my MS. My symptoms are not very visible and my colleagues and supervisor have trouble understanding about my good days and bad days. I'm happy to work long hours when I am feeling good but sometimes I'm just not able to. How much am I required to explain to them about my condition?

You are not required to explain your disability to anyone. However, it may be helpful to educate your co-workers and supervisors about the invisible symptoms of MS. The National Multiple Sclerosis Society has educational brochures to assist you. Co-workers and supervisors are as concerned about their own job performance and reputation as you are about yours; they do not want anyone else's difficulties to have a negative impact on their own productivity. They will gradually come to understand that you need to work fewer hours on some days but will pull your own weight by putting in extra time and effort on other days.

Most of my symptoms are not visible to others. Fatigue and memory problems pose the greatest problems at work for me. Are these invisible impairments covered by the ADA?

Although the legal definition of "disabled" under the ADA is complex, it clearly protects even people with MS who have never had any visible, disabling symptoms or major changes in physical, cognitive, or emotional function. Employers cannot discriminate against "qualified individuals with disabilities."

The ADA defines "individual with a disability" as a person who has a physical or mental impairment that substantially limits one or more major life activities, or has a record of such an impairment. Thus, for example, you might want to request a change to the morning shift if MS-related fatigue interferes with your ability to work an evening shift. If memory problems interfere with your ability to remember verbal instructions given by your supervisor, you might request that your instructions be given to you in writing.

A "qualified" individual with a disability is one who meets legitimate skill, experience, education, or other requirements for an employment position that he or she holds or seeks, and who can perform the "essential functions" of that position with or without reasonable accommodation. Requiring performance of "essential" functions assures that an individual will not be considered unqualified simply because of inability to perform marginal or incidental job functions. Therefore, if you are trained and qualified to perform your essential job functions and are restricted only by the limitations caused by your disability, your employer will need to consider whether you could perform your job functions if given a reasonable accommodation. If you were given a written job description prior to being hired for your job, this description would probably be considered as evidence, although not necessarily conclusive evidence, of the essential functions of your job.

Is every employee covered under the ADA?

The ADA covers all individuals working for employers with fifteen or more employees. The only employers not covered are private employers with fewer than fifteen employees, the federal government, native American tribes, and tax-exempt private membership clubs (Sections 501-504 of the Rehabilitation Act prevent the federal government, federal contractors, and educational programs receiving federal funds from discriminating against people with disabilities). Additionally, Section 108 of the ADA permits religious organizations to give employment preference to individuals of that particular religion.

Who is responsible for deciding what accommodations I need: my doctor, my employer, my union, my lawyer, or myself?

An employer is required to make a reasonable effort to accommodate a known disability of a qualified applicant or employee.

The process is generally triggered by a request from an individual with a disability who suggests an appropriate accommodation. Accommodations must be made on an individual basis because the nature and extent of a disabling condition and the requirements of the job will vary in each case. If the individual does not request an accommodation, the employer is under no obligation to provide one. If a disabled person requests an accommodation but is not able to suggest an appropriate one, the employer and the individual (perhaps in consultation with the individual's physician) should work together to identify one.

Your best strategy is to analyze the problems you are having at work and attempt to identify solutions that would increase your efficiency and productivity. If you are having difficulty thinking of workable solutions, you can consult your local MS Society Chapter or your state vocational rehabilitation office for recommendations. Once you have created your list of possible solutions, make an appointment to talk with with your supervisor or someone in the personnel department. The purpose of this meeting is to share your ideas for enhancing your job performance and to work with your employer to identify accommodations that will work both for you and for the company.

If you have not previously consulted with an attorney who has expertise in the area of labor law for informational or educational purposes, it would certainly be in your best interests to do so before requesting accommodations. The reason for consulting an attorney is not necessarily because you are expecting conflict or controversy. It is simply the most effective way of ensuring that you have an accurate understanding of your rights, that you know all of your available options, and that you are following whatever course is best for you. The attorney may also be able to instruct you in effective ways to communicate with your employer as well as ways to document your efforts to obtain accommodations.

Who decides if a requested accommodation is reasonable?

When a qualified individual with a disability requests an accommodation, the employer must make a reasonable effort to provide an accommodation that is effective for that individual. An accommodation does not have to be made if it presents an "undue hardship" to the employer. Undue hardship refers to accommodations that would be too expensive or disruptive for a particular business to handle. The determination of undue hardship can be challenged in court or before the Equal Employment Opportunity Commission (EEOC).

Who pays for the accommodations that are made (e.g., adaptive equipment, building renovations, schedule changes)?

In most cases, the employer will be required to pay the cost of the accommodation unless it presents an undue hardship. In determining whether an accommodation represents an undue hardship, the cost that will be considered is the actual cost to the employer. Specific federal tax credits and deductions are available to employers who make accommodations required by the ADA. A vocational rehabilitation counselor in your area can tell you about local funding sources that might help pay for some accommodations.

My boss says that the accommodations I have requested are too expensive. What should I do now?

An accommodation may be labeled an undue hardship if it goes beyond the bounds of practicality. For example, does the accommodation cost more than alternative measures that would be equally effective in solving the problem? Does it require extensive renovations that will disrupt the business? Will it affect other employees or customers in a negative way? If the answer is "yes," an employer is not required to provide the requested accommodation.

A consultation with an attorney will help you to identify the next steps to follow. The determination of undue hardship can be challenged in court or before the Equal Employment Opportunity Commission (EEOC). Undue hardship is decided on a case-by-case basis. Decisions on "undue hardship" are influenced by such factors as the size of the business and the availability of resources to reduce the net cost of the accommodation to the employer. An undue hardship for one business might not be an undue hardship for another.

I have requested several accommodations that have been denied on the basis that these changes would substantially alter my job description. What recourse do I have?

The ADA requires your employer to respond to your request in a timely manner. If your employer does not respond within ten days, make a follow-up telephone call or personal contact to arrange a meeting. If you cannot negotiate a satisfactory solution with your employer, you may choose to consult an attorney with expertise in the area of labor law and the ADA and/or file a formal complaint with the Equal Employment Opportunity Commission (EEOC). You can find this number in the telephone directory under the U.S. Government heading (see Equal Employment Opportunity Commission). You can also call 800-669-4000 for information on the EEOC. In many cases, you have about six months from the time your employer fails to address your on-the-job needs to file a formal complaint. An attorney can advise you about filing a formal complaint with the EEOC while simultaneously advising you how to proceed on a day-to-day basis with appropriately worded letters or other strategies. These are two separate types of recourse, and you may not want to wait idly while the more bureaucratic procedures of the EEOC run their course.

For more information on legal help or advocacy, contact your local National Multiple Sclerosis Society chapter, state or local bar associations, state or local advocates for people with disabilities, and other voluntary health agencies or client assistance projects in your area. Do not assume that legal help will be too expensive for you without investigating these resources.

I feel that I need further advice at this point, from either a lawyer, a union representative, or the National Multiple Sclerosis Society. Can I be fired from my job for seeking outside advice or support?

Discrimination, intimidation, or retaliation of any kind because of your efforts to seek help or file a discrimination charge is illegal. Discrimination, intimidation, or retaliation against any person who might assist you would also be illegal.

My co-workers resent the accommodations that have been made for my disability. How can I improve the situation?

The best way to address resentment of co-workers is to educate them about MS. Since many of the symptoms of MS can ebb and flow and are not readily apparent (e.g., fatigue, optic neuritis, bladder problems), co-workers need to understand that the accommodations help you to work effectively and productively in spite of your symptoms. Most people will be supportive and accepting of the accommodations as long as they can rest assured that you are not getting preferential treatment and that their own work load will not be increased.

I have requested a promotion at work, but I was told that they are hesitant to put me in a more responsible position because I could have an exacerbation. Is a company allowed to take that position with me?

An employer can not limit, segregate, or classify a person with a disability in any way that negatively affects him in terms of job opportunity and advancement. Decisions must be based on factual evidence about the individual's disability—not on any assumption, speculation, or stereotype. Your best strategy in this situation may be to try to alleviate your supervisor's concerns about your job performance. The supervisor has a responsibility to the company to ensure that any position is filled by a person who is capable of handling the work. If he or she is concerned about your missing work because of exacerbations, review your prior work history and attendance record. If your MS is of the exacerbating-remitting type, discuss with your supervisor how you would plan to handle the workload during a period of disease flare-up. If you have not experienced frequent exacerbations in the past, your supervisor may be basing his or her judgment about you on inaccurate information about MS. You might want to ask your physician to write a letter on your behalf explaining that exacerbations are not necessarily part of the MS picture. Additionally, the National Multiple Sclerosis Society has literature designed to answer employers' questions about the disease.

If the company continues to deny you a promotion based on assumptions about you or the disease, which you believe to be false, you might want to contact the EEOC or consult a labor lawyer about other possible strategies.

My employer has accommodated all my requests, but I am still having difficulty doing my job. I have been offered a position in another department, but it would mean a demotion and a cut in pay. Do I have to take this position? If I don't, can my employer fire me from my present position?

According to the law, a person can be reassigned to a different position that is equivalent in terms of pay and job status, assuming that he or she is qualified for the position and that such a position is vacant or will be vacant within a reasonable amount of time. If no such position is available, and if no accommodations would enable you to remain in the current position, your employer can reassign you to a "lower-graded" position. In such a situation your employer does not have to maintain your salary at the level of the "higher graded" position unless it also does so for other employees who are reassigned to "lower graded" positions. Finally, your employment can be terminated if all requested accommodations have been provided, no equivalent position is available, and you can not perform the essential functions of the job.

Under what circumstances can I be fired from a job because of my MS?

You can be terminated from your job if you can no longer perform the essential job functions even with the help of suitable accommodations. You can also be terminated if the accommodations you need in order to perform essential job functions are too expensive or would pose too great a hardship for the employer. However, the employer is required to have made an effort to find more suitable, alternative positions for you within the company. In other words, you cannot be terminated because of your inability to perform essential job functions until every reasonable effort has been made to accommodate your limitations.

I feel that I can no longer do my job the way I used to do it. How will I know if and when it's time for me to retire?

It is time for you to look into other options if you have researched and requested all possible accommodations to assist you in doing your job yet still feel you can not adequately perform the essential job functions. Be sure to investigate other positions that may be available within your company. Other options include job-retraining that would enable you to continue working in some other field, or long-term disability.

How do I figure out if I am eligible for Social Security Disability Insurance (SSDI) or Supplemental Security Income (SSI)?

Both SSDI and SSI are programs run by the Social Security Administration. The medical requirements for disability payments are the same under both programs and disability is determined by the same process. For a person with MS, the recognized areas of impairment include gait, vision, cognition, and fatigue. Eligibility for SSDI (Social Security Disability Insurance) is based on prior work history, while SSI (Supplemental Security Income) disability payments are made solely on the basis of financial need. Applications for SSDI require a five-month waiting period from the determination of disability to the start of benefits. Twenty-four months after the initial five-month waiting period, the person becomes eligible for Medicare coverage (see Chapter 15). There is no similar waiting period for SSI benefits. Individuals eligible for SSI benefits based on financial need are covered by Medicaid (see Chapter 15).

To be eligible for SSDI, a person must:

(1) have worked and paid social security taxes (FICA) for enough years to be covered under Social Security, and to have paid at least some of these taxes in recent years;
(2) be considered medically disabled;
(3) not be working, or working but earning less than the substantial gainful activity (SGA) level of $500 per month ($810 for beneficiaries who are blind). In determining a person's gross earnings, certain *employment-related* expenses will be deducted from the calculation if the person is paying expenses out-of-pocket and not otherwise being reimbursed for them. These deducted expenses include some types of attendant care services, transportation-related costs, medical and non-medical equipment costs, medication costs, and some types of residential modifications.

The SSDI payment amount is based on a worker's lifetime average earnings covered by Social Security. The payment amount will be reduced by worker's compensation payments and/or public disability payments. Those individuals who are receiving payments from private disability insurance companies may find that these payments are reduced by whatever amount they subsequently receive from SSDI. The SSDI payment amount is not affected by other income or resources.

To be eligible for SSI based on a medical condition, a person must:

(1) have little or no income or resources;
(2) be considered medically disabled;

(3) initially not be working or be working but earning less than the substantial gainful activity (SGA) level of $500 per month (this restriction does not apply to beneficiaries who are blind). As with SSDI, certain out-of-pocket *employment-related* expenses will be deducted from the calculation of the person's gross earnings.

Once you begin to receive SSI benefits, work activity will not bring an end to SSI eligibility as long as you remain disabled. Even if you cannot receive SSI checks because the amount of money exceeds the SGA, eligibility for Medicaid may continue indefinitely. The SSI payment amount is based on the amount of other income, your living arrangements, and the state in which you live. The basic payment is known as the federal benefit rate. This rate is adjusted each year to compensate for cost-of-living increases. Most states pay an additional amount known as a state supplement. The amount and qualifications for these supplements vary from state to state.

What happens if I retire on disability and then find in six months or a year that I feel able to go back to work? Would that jeopardize my chances of getting disability in the future?

There are many work incentives available if you decide to return to work while receiving SSDI benefits. These incentives provide support over a period of years to allow any disability beneficiary to test his or her ability to work and gradually become self-supporting and independent. You have at least four years to test your ability to work. During the first twelve months (trial work period) you will receive full SSDI payments. Following the initial nine of these twelve months, you begin a three-year extended period of eligibility. If you stop working any time during this period, you can restart your cash benefits without a new application, demonstration of disability, or waiting period. Your Medicare benefits will also continue during this three-year period. Once Medicare stops due to renewed work activity, you can elect to buy coverage as long as you remain disabled. If you become disabled again within five years after the prior period of disability ended, you do not have to go through another five-month waiting period to get benefits, nor do you have to wait to become re-eligible for Medicare.

I can no longer work full-time and am receiving SSDI. What would happen to my SSDI if I returned to work on a part-time basis?

As long as you earn under $500 per month (the established cut-off for substantial gainful activity), you will continue to receive SSDI. However, if your earnings are greater than SGA, you will be considered gainfully employed and your SSDI payments will be stopped following your trial work period. Keep in mind that in calculating your gross income, the Social Security Administration will deduct certain types of employment-related expenses that directly affect your ability to get to and perform your job and that you have personally paid for without other reimbursement.

What is vocational rehabilitation and how do I find out if I am eligible for this type of program?

The Rehabilitation Act of 1973 provides for services designed to enable people with disabilities to become or remain employed. Although this is a program mandated by federal law, it is carried out by individually created state agencies. Each state agency has its own name and slightly different program. Vocational rehabilitation services are defined as an "eligibility" program rather than an "entitlement" program. This means that you must demonstrate eligibility by having a physical or mental disability that results in a substantial handicap to employment. There must also be a reasonable expectation that vocational rehabilitation services might help you to become more employable. As can be seen in the wording of these criteria, there will obviously be some variation from agency to agency in determining any one person's eligibility. Your first step is to contact the vocational rehabilitation program in your state to ask for information about eligibility and application procedures.

An important work incentive provided by the Social Security Administration is called Continued Payment Under a Vocational Rehabilitation Program. This incentive provides that people receiving SSI or SSDI who improve medically to the point that they are able to return to work can continue to receive their benefits if they are participating in *any* approved vocational rehabilitation program whose services are likely to enable them to resume working.

What types of services might be provided by my state's vocational rehabilitation program?

The state's VR services might include a thorough rehabilitation evaluation to determine extent of disability and need for treatment to correct or reduce the disability; vocational guidance and counseling; medical appliances and prosthetic devices if needed to increase your ability to work; vocational training to prepare you for gainful employment; provision of occupational equipment and tools; job placement and follow-up; and post-employment services. Keep in mind that although these programs are mandated by federal law, they tend to vary considerably from state to state.

What is a PASS Plan?

The Plan for Achieving Self Support is a work incentive available for people who are receiving SSI. It allows them to design individualized plans to achieve specified work goals. Under the plan, a disabled person is allowed to set aside income and/or resources for a specified period of time in order to obtain education or training, purchase work-related equipment, set up a business, or for any other reasonable expense related to becoming financially self-supporting. During this period, the income and resources set aside for the plan are excluded from the SSI income and resource restrictions.

Recommended Readings

Bowe F. *Reasonable Accommodation Handbook.* Parsippany, NJ: American Telephone and Telegraph Corp., 1983.

Dejong GB. The Americans with Disabilities Act and the current state of U.S. disability policy. *Journal of Disability Policy Studies* 1990;1:3.

LaRocca NG. *Employment and Multiple Sclerosis.* National Multiple Sclerosis Society, 1995.

Mancuso LL The ADA and employment accommodation: what now? *American Rehabilitation,* Winter 1990-1991.

National Multiple Sclerosis Society. *Employment Initiatives for People with Multiple Sclerosis,* 1992.

Ostberg K. *Using a Lawyer . . . What to Do If Things Go Wrong: A Step-by-Step Guide.* New York: Random House, 1990.

President's Committee on Employment of People with Disabilities. Arkansas Research and Training Center in Vocational Rehabilitation. *Applying Technology in the Work Environment*, 1990.

Rao S. Cognitive function in MS. II: impact on employment and social functioning. *Neurology* 1991;41:692-96.

Rumrill P. *Employment Issues and Multiple Sclerosis*. New York: Demos Vermande, 1996.

Selected booklets from the National Multiple Sclerosis Society (Customer Service: 212-986-3240; Information: 800-344-4867)

◇ *ADA and People with Multiple Sclerosis*—Laura Cooper, Esq., and Nancy Law, L.S.W., with Jane Sarnoff.

◇ *The Win-Win Approach to Reasonable Accommodations: Enhancing Productivity on Your Job*—Richard Roessler, Ph.D., and Phillip Rumrill, Ph.D.

◇ *Living with Multiple Sclerosis*—Debra Frankel, M.S., O.T.R., with Hettie Jones

Recommended Resources

A selected list of publications that address issues related to employment and individuals with disabilities:

President's Committee on Employment of People With Disabilities

1331 F Street NW
Washington, DC 20004-1107
202-376-6200 (voice)

◇ *Americans with Disabilities Act, A Summary*
◇ *Employer Incentives When Hiring People with Disabilities*
◇ *Ready, Willing And Available*
◇ Job Accommodation Network—A service of the President's Committee of People with Disabilities (800-526-7234) (Voice/TDD)

Equal Employment Opportunity Commission
1801 L Street NW
Washington, DC 20507
202-663-4264 (Voice)

◇ *The Americans with Disabilities Act: Your Employment Rights as an Individual with a Disability*
◇ *The Americans With Disabilities Act: Your Responsibilities as an Employer*
◇ *ADA: Question and Answers*
◇ *Facts About the American Disability Act*
◇ *Facts About Disability-Related Tax Provisions*

Multiple Sclerosis Society of Canada
250 Bloor Street East, Suite 1000
Toronto, Ontario M4W 3P9
416-922-6065 (800-268-7582 Division Offices)

Canadian Council on Rehabilitation and Work
410-167 Lombard Avenue
Winnipeg, Manitoba R3B OT6
204-942-4862

JANCANA—The Job Accommodation Network in Canada
c/o 410-167 Lombard Avenue
Winnipeg, Manitoba R3B OT6
800-526-2262

Canadian Rehabilitation Council for the Disabled
45 Sheppard Avenue East, Suite 801
Toronto, Ontario M2N 5W9
416-250-7490 (Voice and TDD)

15

Insurance Issues

Robert Enteen, Ph.D.

Obtaining insurance can be a complex and stressful process, particularly for people who are dealing with the added uncertainties of multiple sclerosis. But the effort you make to examine your insurance needs and explore the available options is well worth your while, because insurance can provide vitally important financial protection for you and your family. The aim of this chapter is to simplify the process for you.

While there are many types of insurance, the four that are usually most important to people affected by MS or other disabling conditions are *health* (including hospitalization and major medical coverage), *disability*, *long-term care*, and *life* insurance. Although this chapter addresses all of these, particular emphasis is given to health insurance. This should not be surprising in view of the lifelong, unpredictable, and varying medical and allied health needs that confront many people with MS. Disability insurance—whether government or private—is also extremely important since it provides income to replace the wages lost when one must leave the workforce because of a disability. Long-term care insurance, which covers an array of home, community, and nursing home services, is important for selected segments of the MS population. Life insurance is less frequently and urgently sought by most people with MS, because it generally has less relevance for one's day-to-day needs.

The following commonly asked questions and answers provide a simple, useful overview of insurance. Because insurance is complex, and because insurance planning is such a central component of financial and "life" planning, you are urged to use the chapter as a starting point, rather than as a complete and sufficient guide to making insurance decisions. At the end of the chapter, several sources are listed to which you can later turn for additional, comprehensive information and advice.

What are the different types of health insurance I need to know about?

There are more than a dozen different types or "categories" of health insurance plans and a tremendous number of variations among plans within each category. Fortunately, three very simple distinctions take us a long way toward understanding health insurance options. They are "government" vs. "private" options; "fee-for-service" plans vs. "managed care" plans; and "group" vs. "individual" coverage. Virtually any plan you select will reflect some combination of these; for example, it may be a government-provided, group, managed care plan; or a private, fee-for-service plan, purchased on an individual basis.

◇ *Government options.* Millions of Americans are eligible for government insurance programs based on their current or past employment in a government agency or program; because they meet legally mandated benefit "entitlement" requirements; or because they are the family members of living or deceased people who are or were eligible for these insurance programs. The chief types of government health insurance are Medicare, Medicaid, VA (veterans) benefits, CHAMPUS, CHAMPVA, the Federal Employee Health Benefits Program (FEHB), and state or local government employee insurance programs.

◇ *Private options.* The chief types of private health insurance include group coverage provided by an employer or membership organization, individual (or individual and family) plans, risk pools, Blue Cross and Blue Shield "Open

Enrollment" Plans, and Medicare Supplement (or "Medigap") insurance.

◇ *"Fee-for-service" plans.* In general, if you are covered under a fee-for-service plan, you may use the services of any appropriately credentialed physician or allied health provider you wish. To the extent that you use "covered" services—that is, services that are eligible for coverage under your particular contract—and so long as you meet all of the policy and procedural requirements for using such a service, your plan will either pay a specific sum (a part or the total cost of your care) to your provider or reimburse some or all of your costs directly to you if you pay the provider.

◇ *"Managed care" plans.* In contrast, a managed care plan generally combines the financing and delivery of appropriate care for covered individuals by prior arrangements with *selected* providers. Currently, the chief forms of managed care are HMOs (health maintenance organizations), PPOs (preferred provider organizations), and POS (point-of-service) plans.

How do I know which types of health insurance I'm eligible for?

Every health insurance plan has its own eligibility requirements. Because they can be complicated, some basics of eligibility for each type are presented here.

◇ *Medicare.* Medicare is the largest federal health insurance program. It is the chief source of coverage for the elderly and for certain people with disabilities, including at least 40,000 people with multiple sclerosis. Medicare's coverage is fairly comprehensive, providing both hospital ("Part A") and medical ("Part B") protection. Regrettably, its coverage is quite limited for long-term care services such as nursing home stays.

Many people are surprised to learn that Medicare is not limited to people aged 65 or above. A person who has MS (or any other disabling condition) and is under age 65 may qualify for Medicare benefits if he or she meets the eligibility requirements for Social Security Disability Insurance (SSDI) benefits (see Chapter 14 for a discussion of SSDI eligibility). Applications for SSDI generally require a five-

month waiting period from the date of the disability determination to the start of SSDI benefits. Twenty-four months
after this initial waiting period, the individual becomes eligible for Medicare coverage.

◇ *Medicaid.* Medicaid is a medical assistance program for
certain individuals and families with low incomes and
assets. In addition to offering comprehensive hospital and
medical protection, Medicaid also provides coverage for an
array of long-term care services, including nursing home
stays. Far fewer people with MS are eligible for Medicaid
than for Medicare because their family income and assets
are usually too high to meet the Medicaid requirements.

Medicaid is a joint program of the federal government
and each state government. Although the federal government contributes money to the Medicaid program, each
state administers its own Medicaid program. Medicaid differs from Medicare in another key respect: Medicaid coverage varies from state to state save for certain core (Medicaid
"mandated") benefits available in every state's program.
Thus, it is important to learn the specifics of Medicaid coverage in your own state.

◇ *Veterans' benefits.* The U.S. Department of Veterans Affairs
offers comprehensive "VA" health care to veterans with
"service-connected" disabilities and to disabled veterans
whose disabilities are not service-connected who meet certain eligibility criteria. Of particular relevance to readers of
this book, onset of multiple sclerosis in a veteran may be
considered to be service-connected under specified conditions (referred to as the "7-Year Rule").

◇ "CHAMPUS"—the Civilian Health and Medical Program of
the Uniformed Services—is a health benefit program for all
seven uniformed services: the Air Force, Army, Navy,
Marine Corps, Coast Guard, Public Health Service, and the
National Oceanic and Atmospheric Administration.
CHAMPUS does *not* cover active duty service members
(the "sponsors"), but only their families, as well as retired
service members and their families.

◇ "CHAMPVA"—the Civilian Health and Medical Program,
Department of Veterans Affairs—is a federal program providing medical care to certain eligible survivors and dependents of veterans. These include the following, provided

they are *not* eligible for Medicare Part A or CHAMPUS: the spouse or children of a veteran if the veteran has been judged by the VA to have a permanent and total service-connected disability; the surviving spouse or children of a veteran who died as a result of a service-connected condition, or who, at the time of death, was judged permanently and totally disabled from a service-connected condition; the surviving spouse or children of a person who died while on active duty.

◇ *Federal Employee Health Benefits Program (FEHB).* The Federal Employee Health Benefits program provides a choice of health plans for federal civilian employees. There is a federal government contribution toward the cost of premiums. FEHB coverage is available immediately, from the date of enrollment, without a medical examination or restrictions due to the subscriber's age or physical condition. If certain conditions are met, the FEHB offers continued protection for the subscriber and eligible family members after the subscriber's retirement from federal service, and for eligible family members after the enrollee's death.

◇ *State and local government employee programs.* In general, state and municipal governments offer health benefit plans to their employees and eligible family members. Although the choice of options is typically not as broad as the FEHB program offerings, it is not uncommon for employees and their families to have a choice of two or more options.

◇ *Employer, membership, or other group health plans.* Group coverage is typically offered by an employer to its employees, and often to the employees' families as well. Group coverage is also offered by many membership organizations, including labor unions, trade associations, professional societies, and fraternal organizations. Additionally, group coverage can be obtained on the basis of a shared characteristic other than "membership" as, for example, through a church group, college alumni association, or credit card holder group. Ordinarily these "sponsors" contract with an insurance company or managed care organization to provide a specific combination of benefits for all enrollees. In recent years, sponsoring organizations have increasingly begun to offer a choice of plans, each with special features, so that a prospective enrollee can choose the plan best suited to his or her own and family member needs.

In general, group health insurance is less costly than individual or individual and family coverage. This is because the insurer can "share" or "spread" the risk of paying out money for services across a number of enrollees. While some enrollees will prove to be relatively heavy users of care, and therefore will be costly to the insurer (costing more than the premiums paid by them or on their behalf), others will use little or no care, and therefore will be less costly enrollees (the premiums paid for their enrollment will be greater than the amount the insurer has to pay out for their care). In contrast, there is less opportunity for the insurer to spread risk and offset or limit its potential payout in individual or individual and family plans (see following); thus, higher premiums are usually charged.

◇ *Individual and family plans.* Individual and family plans, as the names suggest, are purchased by individuals to cover themselves or themselves and their family members. In general, purchase is made either through an insurance agent or broker, or directly from the insurance company or managed care organization. As the individual owns and pays directly for the coverage, it is "portable." Therefore, in contrast to most employer group coverage, the individual can retain the plan even if he or she changes employment or becomes disabled and has to leave the place of employment. While the cost of premiums for this type of insurance may be higher than employment-based coverage, it may be less expensive in the long run because continuity of coverage is assured.

◇ *Blue Cross and Blue Shield "open enrollment" plans.* Blue Cross and Blue Shield is not a single company. Rather, it is a nationwide federation of local, independent community health services corporations. In most cases, these operate under state laws as not-for-profit service organizations. The plans contract with physicians, hospitals, and other health care facilities and providers to offer health care to "subscribers" (insureds).

In return for their not-for-profit status (they are allowed to operate under special state laws and regulations, and with a special tax exemption), the "Blues" accept special responsibility for addressing needs of the public. Traditionally, they have acted as the "insurers of last resort" for people who could not obtain or afford insurance through commercial plans. Most importantly for readers with MS or other disabilities, some Blues organizations offer "open enrollment" hospital coverage, or hospital and medical coverage, to anyone in their territory, even if an applicant has a preexisting condition. (Typically, open enrollment plans include waiting periods before benefits are paid for services needed by subscribers for their preexisting conditions.)

Policies available under open enrollment vary among the Blues. They range greatly in price, coverage, and other features. There is also variation in *when* open enrollments are available and in how well they are advertised. For example, some Blues have continuous open enrollment throughout the year. Others only open their doors to all applicants during specified times of the year (often only in June and December). Thus, readers who want to investigate this option need to call their local Blue Cross and Blue Shield organization and learn whether and when open enrollment is possible, along with the details of the plan(s) offered.

◇ *Medicare supplement (or "Medigap") plans.* Medicare pays a large part of the health care costs of its insureds, but the insured individual remains responsible for Medicare deductibles and co-insurance, and for services and excess provider charges not covered under Medicare. These additional costs can be substantial. In response to these unpaid costs, many private insurers offer Medicare Supplement (also called "Medigap") plans to supplement Medicare services and to cover Medicare beneficiary costs.

Initially, there was a bewildering array of Medigap plans on the market and many questionable marketing practices, such as companies selling several overlapping plans to the same individual. To address these problems, the National Association of Insurance Commissioners developed ten standardized Medigap plans, called "A," "B," "C," and so on through plan "J." While each plan differs in the specific coverage offered, a given plan is always the same wherever it is sold in the United States (thus, if you purchase plan B in New York, it will be identical to a plan B purchased in California, Nebraska, or elsewhere). It is important to note, however, that individual companies charge different amounts for the same plan. Thus, insurance company X may charge substantially more for plan B than the insurance company Y does for an identical plan B. So it pays to shop around.

◇ *"Risk pools."* Over the past twenty years, a number of states have created "risk pools" to provide protection for state residents who are otherwise uninsurable. The pools offer guaranteed availability of health insurance to individuals regardless of their health status. A common eligibility requirement is that an applicant prove that he or she has been denied coverage by at least two commercial insurers. Among people in need of risk pools are those who have been denied coverage by private (for-profit) insurers because of a preexisting condition such as multiple sclerosis.

The costs and coverage within pools vary greatly among states that have them, but there is a fairly standard design. In general, the state legislature enacts a law requiring that all commercial insurers doing business in the state join together to create an insurance association or pool to offer insurance to individuals who meet eligibility requirements. One member insurer serves as the administrator of the pool, managing the plan under guidelines for benefits, premiums, deductibles, and other matters established in the state's law.

◇ *COBRA.* Health benefit provisions in the Consolidated Omnibus Budget Reconciliation Act of 1985 are designed in part to ensure that people who lose employment-related group health insurance benefits because of job termination or reduction in job hours can buy group coverage for themselves and their families for limited periods of time. The law generally covers group health plans maintained by employers with twenty or more employees. It applies to plans in the private sector as well as those sponsored by state and local governments. COBRA does not apply to plans sponsored by the federal government and certain church-related organizations.

If the employee has worked for a company subject to the federal COBRA law and must leave work for almost any reason, that individual (and covered family members) will be able to maintain the same coverage as under the group, for eighteen months, at only 2 percent above the group premium. If an employed person leaves work, and in the first eighteen months establishes eligibility for Social Security Disability Insurance, then the group coverage can be extended to a total of twenty-nine months, although there may be an increase in premiums from months nineteen to twenty-nine.

For companies that are not subject to COBRA, a standard conversion to another health plan may be offered. This coverage will generally be less comprehensive than in the employer group plan and will likely cost more than the premium charged within the group.

To find out if you and your family members are eligible for COBRA, ask the employee benefits manager at your company and read the plan booklet. As there are deadlines for gaining COBRA coverage, it is up to you to learn what they are and apply in a timely manner if a relevant life event occurs to you or others in your family.

What is a "preexisting condition" and what implications does such a condition have for access to insurance?

Within the insurance industry, a preexisting condition, whether due to illness (such as MS) or injury, is defined as "a physical or mental condition of an individual which (1) first manifested itself prior to the application for, or issuance of, his or her insurance policy; or (2) existed prior to application or issuance and for which treatment was received." In other words, a preexisting condition is one that began before the insurance was applied for and continues to exist; or began and was treated before the time that the application for insurance is made. While the wording may differ from one insurer or policy to another, the effects are generally the same: your application will either be denied or you will receive coverage, but it will contain various limitations and exclusions that temporarily or permanently reduce the protection your policy provides.

The basis of the restrictions concerning preexisting conditions lies in the concept of "risk." In the world of insurance, risk means chance of loss. Insurance companies base their approval of an application, the coverage they offer, and the premiums they charge on a calculation of the financial risk they take on by covering a particular individual or group. Risk is a measure of the likelihood that the insurer will have to pay out some of the money it collects in premiums, in the form of direct payments to providers, reimbursement of insured individuals who themselves pay the providers, or direct provision of care (as in the case of some HMOs).

The main insurance difficulty confronting people with preexisting conditions such as multiple sclerosis is that they are typically viewed by insurers as presenting a higher than standard risk. This explains why individuals with MS encounter difficulty obtaining affordable coverage that is adequate for their current or expected medical needs, particularly relating to their preexisting condition. Some conditions are viewed by insurers as presenting a higher risk than others. While the understanding and medical management of MS have improved in recent years, most insurers continue to view all people with MS as "high risk." The National Multiple Sclerosis Society and other MS advocates work continuously to improve insurer understanding of MS and to improve insurance options for people affected by this disease.

Which type of health insurance is best for me?

Your health insurance should cover (1) standard risks of illness and injury for yourself and your family; and (2) special needs if any member of your family has a condition such as multiple sclerosis that may require special, major, costly, and/or continuing or long-term medical attention. It is up to you to identify and become familiar with your health insurance options. In the end, you must make the decision based on your own and your family's estimated present and future needs (and associated future financial risk) and the adequacy and cost of various coverage plans.

Most people try to identify one health insurance plan that will meet all of their needs now and in the future. An alternative (and perhaps more realistic) approach is to identify your present and potential health insurance needs and then find a combination of plans or policies to address them. A person with MS should probably think in terms of the following personal and family health insurance needs:

1. hospitalization for MS and other preexisting conditions;
2. hospitalization for all other conditions;
3. major medical for MS and other preexisting conditions;
4. major medical for all other conditions;
5. long-term care.

How do I begin to identify my present and future needs?

Start by considering the key components of standard coverage. A "typical" adequate plan will include both (1) hospitalization (hospital, surgical, and medical) coverage, and (2) major medical insurance. Hospitalization insurance is the most essential and common type of health insurance because it offers protection against the enormous costs that can be incurred by even a brief hospital stay and related in-hospital medical services. Hospitalization coverage is available to individuals, families, and group members. Typically, it involves either a small deductible or no deductible at all.

In view of the rapid increase in costs of health care in recent years and the wide and increasing range of out-of-hospital services available, "major medical" insurance is an important complement to hospitalization coverage. Major medical typically involves a deductible that the insured person must pay without any reimbursement. After the deductible is met, the insurer generally pays a percentage (e.g., 80 percent) of covered expenses; the insured pays the remaining portion of the expense (e.g., 20 percent), called "co-insurance." Many major medical policies include an annual individual and family out-of-pocket maximum—a dollar limit on how much the insured(s) must pay in combined deductibles and co-insurance before the insurer assumes responsibility for 100 percent of any additional covered expenses.

Once these essential insurance protections have been determined, consideration should be given to any significant medical condition that you or your family members have (or are at significant risk for in the future), your/their past health care utilization due to the condition(s), and the prognosis—that is, the likely future course of the condition and consequent likely future use of services. In regard to future service need and use, your best source of advice is your (or your family member's) primary care physician. When there is a major preexisting condition, a specialist often fills the role of primary physician. For example, neurologists often serve as the primary physicians for people with multiple sclerosis. In such cases, it is the specialist who should be consulted about likely future medical care needs.

If you determine that certain types of services will likely be especially important to you or your family member (e.g., physical therapy, psychotherapy, inpatient rehabilitation, nursing care), you should seek out plans that provide appropriate levels of coverage for these needs, without imposing problematic limitations on use of relevant services.

How do I identify my options?

Once you have determined your own needs and those of your family members, you must begin to identify the relevant options available to you. Because many insurance plans exclude people with MS and other preexisting conditions, this process can be difficult, time-consuming, and frustrating. Following is a checklist of avenues you should explore:

√ Are you employed? If so, are you eligible for coverage under your employer's plan? If you are a fairly new employee, is there a grace period during which you (or your family) can enroll automatically, without being questioned and chosen based on your (and their) health status? If your employer does not have a plan, or if you cannot be covered under it due to MS, will your employer pick up some or all of the cost of insurance you purchase elsewhere?

√ Are you taking a new job or considering a change in employers? If so, does your prospective employer offer a health insurance plan in which you can enroll?

√ Are you married? If so, does your spouse have an employer group plan under which you might be insured? If your spouse is a new or recent employee, is there a grace period during which you can enroll automatically with no reference to the fact that you have MS? If you are rejected on first try, can you reapply at some future date? What new documentation should you submit at that time (e.g., medical support indicating that you have had few or no MS symptoms and related services during the interim)?

√ If you have left employment due to disability or some other reason, are you eligible for COBRA or another "continuation or conversion" option?

√ Does your state insurance law include provision for a COBRA-like policy? Contact your state insurance department to find out.

√ If you are close to exhausting your COBRA coverage, will you now have an opportunity for a "standard conversion," even if it means less coverage at higher cost?

√ If you have established eligibility for Social Security Disability Insurance (SSDI) (see Chapter 14), are you aware that after twenty-four months on SSDI you become automatically eligible for Medicare?

√ If you are leaving SSDI and returning to work, are you aware that you may be able to continue or repurchase your Medicare coverage? Will your new employer offer a group plan in which you can enroll despite your MS?

√ Are your family's combined income and assets low enough that you might qualify for your state's Medicaid program? The formula excludes such items as the value of your house or your first car.

√ Are you on active duty or a veteran? Are you the family member of an active duty, retired, or deceased veteran? If so, have you checked with the U.S. Department of Veterans Affairs? CHAMPUS? CHAMPVA?

√ Does the Blue Cross and Blue Shield organization serving the community in which you live offer an "open enrollment," either year-round or at certain times of the year?

√ Have you contacted your state insurance department to learn whether your state has a "risk pool" for otherwise uninsurable state residents?

√ Are you (or is your spouse) a member of any professional societies or fraternal organizations? Have you checked with them to see if they offer health insurance options to members (and perhaps to their families). Have you looked into health insurance programs through your credit cards, church, alumni association, or any other group that is offering such a program?

√ Have you contacted your state insurance department to learn whether there are any other, or "special," or "recently enacted" programs for state residents that increase the number of health insurance options, including those for people with multiple sclerosis or other disabling conditions?

√ Have you contacted the insurance committees of your state legislature to learn whether there are any bills pending that might increase your options if enacted?

√ If you are in crisis and lack health insurance, have you contacted your local or state health department to learn about free or low-cost services for which you might be eligible?

√ If you are a student, have you checked to see whether you are eligible for coverage under your parents' insurance? If you are a college student, does your college or university offer a plan you can afford and for which you are eligible?

√ If you are a recent graduate, looking forward to employment in the near future, or a working person temporarily between jobs, have you contacted insurance companies to learn whether they offer short-term plans for which you would be eligible?

√ If you are frequently hospitalized, or hospitalized for a substantial number of days each year, have you received mail offers of "hospital indemnity" insurance for which you would be eligible without reference to your multiple sclerosis? Does your professional or fraternal organization offer such coverage?

√ Have you contacted insurers to learn whether you would be eligible for a catastrophic excess plan through your professional or fraternal organizations?

√ If any sources tell you they would not cover you because of your MS, and you deem it in your interest to buy partial coverage, even if it is not optimal for needs related to your MS, have you asked whether they will sell you a plan that excludes or limits coverage for your MS, but which provides protection for the range of standard health needs?

√ Have you contacted local HMOs and physician networks in your area to see whether they will enroll you despite your multiple sclerosis?

Once I've identified one or more options, on what basis should I make my choice?

Insurance plans are complex. The complexity of your decision increases dramatically when you identify two or more plan options and try to compare them. Following is a fairly simple grid (see Figure 15.1) that you can use to analyze a single plan or to compare plans. Listed down the left are factors you should consider when choosing health insurance. If you are comparing plans, list each one across the top of the page. In this way, you can "break the plans down" into their components and judge or compare them on those factors of greatest interest to you.

Figure 15-1   Plan Comparison Grid

Factor	Plan		
	1	*2*	*3*
Plan Coverage in Relation to Your/Your Family's General Medical Needs (list specific services here, and rate)			
Plan Coverage in Relation to Your/Your Family's Special (e.g., MS-related) Medical Needs (list specific services here, and rate)			
Coverage Limitations and Exclusions			
Preexisting Condition Waiting Period			
Choice of Providers			
Access to Neurologist Expert in MS Care			
Cost			
—premiums			
—individual and family deductibles			
—% co-insurance for key services			
—out-of-pocket maximum			
—(for managed care plans) cost to you if you use non-plan providers			
Premium Rate Guaranteed?			
Policy Renewal Guaranteed?			
Yearly and Lifetime Maximums on $ of Coverage			
Company Reputation/Financial Rating			

Remember as you review your options that not all of your coverage has to come from a single source—you can distribute your insurance needs over several plans. For example, one plan that will not cover preexisting conditions may provide excellent and inexpensive coverage for other hospitalizations. Another may cover preexisting conditions but charge a higher premium.

Do I need to tell an insurance company that I have MS when I apply to join their plan?

You should respond honestly and fully to any questions asked of you by a broker, by an insurer through its agent, or on an application form. Both you and the insurer have legal rights, responsibilities, and duties in contracting for health insurance. Your duties and responsibilities include communicating facts (for example, about your health history and current health) that are relevant to the insurer's decision whether to accept you for coverage, and on what terms. The insurer is entitled to cancel your contract if you either intentionally or unintentionally fail to provide information that would have influenced the insurer's decision when it considered whether to cover you. The same is true if you falsely present relevant information, including facts about your health history or current status. In health insurance applications, all facts relating to your current or past health are considered relevant. In short, you should avoid any false representations of facts, and any omissions, on relevant matters.

In general, insurers will ask about your past and current health, often including a checklist of conditions; if you check any conditions, the insurer may ask for explanations of these. Moreover, insurers will typically ask a "blanket" additional question such as "Have you had/do you have any other health conditions not indicated above?"

The key exception to the foregoing is where the insurer simply does not ask directly *or by implication* for such information. For example, when you join a new company and are offered entry into their plan, the card you fill out may have no health-related questions; this is because employees in that company are automatically permitted entry into the plan, regardless of their health. Similarly, there is often a grace period during which your spouse can enroll without providing medical information; after the grace period, if he or she wishes to join, medical information may be required.

Are new treatments for MS such as Betaseron® covered by health insurance?

Here, as in other insurance matters, plans vary greatly in their coverage. In the end, you must investigate coverage under any plan you have or are considering. Many private insurance companies cover Betaseron® as part of their prescription drug coverage provisions. Many others do not. Among those that do cover the drug, coverage varies; many impose deductibles (generally modest ones), co-insurance (ranging from nominal, e.g., $5.00, to substantial, e.g., 30 percent of the total yearly cost), and/or yearly caps on the total amount they will pay (for example, $2,000); require submission of some documentation of "medical necessity" from your neurologist and then undertake a prior authorization review, or require that you purchase the Betaseron® at designated pharmacies.

Virtually all state Medicaid programs cover Betaseron®, but you must contact the agency in your state to confirm this and to learn the specifics of the coverage they offer (how much, with what co-pays or dispensing fees, and so on).

Currently, Medicare does not cover Betaseron®. However, many states have special drug assistance programs that will help to cover the cost for state residents who are Medicare beneficiaries. Call your state insurance department and ask whether such a program exists in your state. Additionally, some Medicare managed care plans will cover Betaseron®. If you are enrolled in a Medicare managed care plan, call the appropriate plan administrator to learn about your eligibility for coverage.

If you have problems or questions regarding Betaseron® coverage, call the Betaseron® Hotline (800-788-1467). Explain the situation and request their assistance. Ask as well if you qualify for a subsidy from them to cover the costs of the drug, and how you should apply.

. Regarding coverage of other new MS treatments, nearly all insurers require that a treatment has been approved for prescription use by the U.S. *Food and Drug Administration (FDA)* before they will even consider paying for it. A drug that has not been FDA-approved will likely not be covered. Even if a drug is FDA-approved, it may only be approved for particular uses or patients. For example, currently Betaseron® has only been approved for use by people with exacerbating-remitting MS who are ambulatory. If you do not meet these criteria, you may not be able to obtain coverage for Betaseron®, even if your insurer covers the drug for other plan enrollees (who do meet the FDA approval criteria).

People participating in clinical trials of an experimental treatment may receive coverage through the research administrators or clinicians conducting the trials. If you are considering entering a trial, ask if they will have to pay some or all of the cost of the experimental agents you will receive.

Our twenty-one-year-old daughter has recently been diagnosed with MS. She is about to graduate from college and become ineligible for coverage under our family health insurance policy. Will she be able to get health insurance of her own?

While there is no assurance that she can get coverage, there are many options for her to explore. In most parts of the country, her surest route to coverage may be to take a job with a large company that offers a group health insurance plan to its employees. Large companies often pay some or all of their employees' insurance premiums. If she lives in or moves to one of the several states that have enacted "open enrollment" legislation in recent years, she will also be assured of the opportunity to buy individual coverage, as long as she can pay the relatively high premiums. She should call the insurance departments in those states in which she has an interest to learn whether they have enacted open enrollment legislation. For additional ideas, refer to the list of possible avenues for obtaining insurance on pages 300–302.

What is managed care and how does it work for someone with MS?

Managed care is a form of organizing health care that integrates the financing and delivery of health care to covered individuals by arrangement with selected providers. The providers are available to furnish a relatively comprehensive array of health services (although many plans lack coverage for durable medical equipment such as wheelchairs or for care in the home). Explicit standards are used by the managed care organization to select health providers for participation in the plan. Formal policies and procedures exist for ongoing quality assurance and utilization review in the provision of care to enrolled individuals.

There are generally significant financial incentives for enrollees to use providers and procedures associated with the plan, rather than using "out-of-plan" providers.

The most common and best known form of managed care is the "health maintenance organization" (or HMO). In return for a fixed, periodic payment, the HMO providers offer a wide range of health care services, including preventive care. The HMO may have a single central facility, several branch sites, or may exist as an array of individual providers and facility locations that have contracted to provide service for the HMO. Two common forms of HMO are the "staff model," in which physicians and other providers are employees of the HMO; and the "individual practice association" (or IPA), in which physicians and other providers maintain their personal practices but agree to serve as HMO providers, under the terms of the HMO, when caring for an HMO enrollee. In the traditional HMO, an enrollee who goes "out-of-plan" does not receive coverage for those outside services (save in special cases such as emergencies).

The second most common managed care arrangement is the "preferred provider organization" (or PPO). In this arrangement, physicians and other providers contract with the PPO sponsor to reduce their fees when a member of the PPO comes to them for service. Plan members choosing to use out-of-plan providers receive *some* coverage, but less than if they had used one of the "preferred providers."

A new and increasingly popular hybrid, aimed at controlling costs while retaining consumer choice of providers, is the "point-of-service" HMO. Combining aspects of HMOs and PPOs, the point-of-service plan functions as an HMO, but provides some (limited) coverage for out-of-plan providers. Thus, a person who chooses to consult an out-of plan provider will generally receive coverage, but less than if he or she had stayed within the HMO for that care.

Managed care organizations work the same way for people with MS as they do for other enrollees. However, some studies and individual anecdotes raise some concerns. These concerns relate primarily to the inadequacy of access to MS experts. For example, the managed care organization may have very few (or no) providers (neurologists or others) who are expert in caring for people with multiple sclerosis. Or they may have such specialists, but the enrollee can only receive a referral to one if his primary care provider ("PCP"—generally a family physician or internist) chooses to make the referral. Because the managed care organization places great emphasis on saving money, the PCP may have major financial or other incentives to limit referrals to specialists. Informal surveys suggest that MS enrollees who have adequate access to MS specialists are generally pleased with their managed care experience. When they have inadequate access, they are usually dissatisfied with the managed care organization. PPOs try to address this problem by offering some coverage for out-of-plan consultations or treatment, but they are often more costly than HMOs. Point-of-service HMOs attempt to address this problem by combining the key features of HMOs (comprehensive care and low cost) with that of PPOs (covered access to out-of-plan providers, although typically at higher cost than staying in-plan).

In short, people with MS may fare well in managed care organizations—especially point-of-service HMOs—*if* the plan they choose is a comprehensive one and, most importantly, provides ready access to MS specialists. When considering a managed care plan, one should make sure to ask about access to providers with expertise in MS care and about coverage for the kinds of equipment or home care that are sometimes needed by a person with MS.

If my company switches over to one of the new managed care plans, will I be denied coverage because of my MS?

You should have the same rights to enrollment under the managed care plan as you had when the employer group coverage was a fee-for-service plan. If you do not, ask your employer (generally the benefits manager) about this and appeal the decision. If unsuccessful, contact your state insurance department to determine whether the employer has acted legally in excluding you from transferring to the new plan, while allowing other employees to make the transfer. This problem is more likely to arise in very small companies than among large ones.

What is long-term care insurance (LTCI) and will I be eligible for it now that I have MS?

Long-term care includes a wide range of medical, social, and support services. These services are designed for elderly people and chronically ill or disabled individuals who live in the community or in extended care facilities, and need ongoing or periodic assistance throughout their lives. Long-term care services are generally categorized as in-home assistance, community care, or institutional care.

In evaluating a person's dependence on others for assistance with everyday activities, insurance companies usually divide personal functioning into two categories: *activities of daily living* (ADLs) such as feeding, bathing, dressing, toileting, bowel and bladder continence, and getting into and out of a chair; and "instrumental activities of daily living" (IADLs), including household and community activities such as meal preparation, doing laundry, grocery shopping, managing money, making telephone calls, doing light work, getting around outside, and going places that are beyond walking distance.

Most standard health insurance plans of the sort described previously in this chapter provide only very limited or no long-term care coverage. However, many private insurance companies market long-term care insurance policies that cover some, many, or all of these services. Moreover, government programs such as Medicaid (and Medicare for certain situations) cover some or many such services.

Private long-term care insurance is not appropriate for everyone. Its main purpose is to protect against catastrophic costs associated with expensive services over a long period. In view of the risk to insurers, these policies are often costly. Thus, you may be well-advised not to use the coverage unless you have more than modest family assets to protect, as well as a sufficient income that you can readily afford the high premiums for good long-term care insurance. Of course, if you do have sufficient income and assets, this insurance may be extremely valuable to you and your family. To determine if it is right for you, contact any of the following and ask for their booklets advising consumers about long-term care insurance: your state insurance department (generally located in the state's capital city); National Association of Insurance Commissioners (NAIC) at 816-842-3600; Health Insurance Association of America (HIAA) at 800-277-4486 or 202-223-7780; American Association of Retired Persons (AARP) at 202-434-2230.

Experience suggests that relatively few insurers offering LTCI will sell to people with MS. The few in each state that do offer it tend not to advertise this fact. Moreover, they will generally decide only on a case-by-case basis. Some preliminary research suggests that they will consider people (1) whose initial MS diagnosis was made at least five but preferably ten years ago or more; (2) who currently exhibit no significant disabling MS symptoms—who have no ADL deficiencies and function independently; (3) whose "recent" medical records are free from evidence of recurrent need to treat MS generated symptoms; and (4) who are in good general health.

To find coverage, three approaches appear to be most useful:

◇ a comprehensive survey of companies listed by the National Association of Insurance Commissioners and your state insurance department;

◇ a focused search concentrating on companies that have publicly announced that they are willing to consider applications from people with MS (good sources are your friends and acquaintances with MS who have themselves purchased this coverage from certain companies); and

◇ consultation with specialized brokers who handle the policies of several companies selling LTCI.

What is disability insurance and am I eligible for it now that I have MS?

Disability insurance is more aptly called "disability income insurance." It is a form of health insurance that provides periodic payments to replace your regular income when you cannot work as a result of illness, injury, or disease. Generally, a minimum number of days when you are unable to work is required before your "sick pay" ends and your disability insurance begins. "Short-term disability insurance" typically provides partial coverage (e.g., 60 percent) of your lost earnings for a period of about six months. If your inability to work extends beyond that period and you continue to be eligible, you begin to receive "long-term disability benefits."

There are both private (including employer-provided) and government forms of disability insurance. The most common and important form of government disability insurance for people with multiple sclerosis is Social Security Disability Insurance

(SSDI), as described in Chapter 14. A person may be found eligible for SSDI who has worked and paid social security taxes (FICA) for at least ten years (five of which must be in the ten years prior to leaving the workforce), and meets the criteria for medical and vocational disability.

If you are employed by a company that has a group disability insurance plan for its employees, you should be eligible for this coverage. If you have the opportunity to purchase disability insurance through your employer or any professional or fraternal organization to which you belong (or would be willing to join), you should try to do so. By virtue of your membership in one of these groups, you may automatically be entitled to the basic amount of disability insurance that is offered to the entire group, regardless of your MS diagnosis or other medical history. This basic coverage is called "guaranteed-issue coverage." Your MS diagnosis would prevent you from buying coverage over and above this basic amount, but you would still be assured of some basic coverage. Since organizations may offer this type of group coverage only as a one-time incentive for membership, one strategy is to join as many organizations as you can that offer this type of group disability coverage. These multiple group memberships would thus enable you to piece together adequate coverage. It is certainly in your best interest to obtain disability coverage while you are actively working; it is virtually impossible to obtain disability coverage once a person leaves work due to disability.

How will the fact that I have MS affect my ability to obtain life insurance?

Life insurance is typically a less urgent matter for people with MS than is health insurance. The reason seems clear: life insurance is protection against a future (perhaps very distant) eventuality. In contrast, health insurance may be vitally important any or every day in protecting you against the substantial costs that you may incur, unpredictably, due to multiple sclerosis or any other medical problem.

For those who want to obtain life insurance, there are companies that will sell it to you. You must shop around to find them since many will refuse coverage for a person with MS. Often the amounts of life coverage they will sell to you are less than standard, and you may be charged higher premiums than non-disabled applicants.

How does the Americans with Disabilities Act (ADA) deal with the insurance questions of someone with chronic illness and/or disability?

In June 1993, the U.S. Equal Employment Opportunity Commission (EEOC) ruled that under the Americans with Disabilities Act (ADA): (1) employers cannot refuse to hire people with disabilities due to concern over the effects on the employer's health insurance costs; and (2) employees with disabilities must generally be given "equal access" to any employer health insurance. That is, the ADA prohibits employers from limiting benefits that single out a particular disability, a discrete group of disabilities such as cancers, or disability in general. Additionally, the ADA requires that these rules apply both to employers that buy commercial insurance *and* to self-insured employers (even though this group is free from certain other insurance laws and regulations). Moreover, the burden is on the challenged employer, rather than the employee, to prove that differential treatment of an employee with a disability was not "subterfuge."

Much remains to be done to test the full implications of the ADA in protecting the insurance rights of individuals with MS and other disabilities. While many law suits have been launched, at this writing the number of case law rulings remains fairly limited.

Recommended Readings

Enteen R. *Health Insurance: How to Get It, Keep It, or Improve What You've Got (2nd edition).* New York: Demos Vermande, 1996.

This book is the most comprehensive introduction available on health insurance. It includes health insurance basics, techniques for determining your health insurance needs, descriptions of nearly two dozen options, what to do when something goes wrong, and many state-by-state listings of where to turn for advice or assistance.

Isaacs SL, Swartz AC. *The Consumer's Legal Guide to Today's Health Care: Your Medical Rights and How to Assert Them.* Boston: Houghton Mifflin, 1992.

Recommended Resources

Government Agencies and Private Organizations:

Many organizations and government agencies can provide you with useful information and advice, generally at no cost. For information and assistance about virtually any insurance matter, contact your state insurance department. Other useful government agencies include your state office on aging, the agency on developmental disabilities, health department, Medicaid, workers' compensation agencies, and veterans' affairs agencies. These can be located by calling telephone information in your state's capital city. Or check the Appendixes in Robert Enteen's book, *Health Insurance* (listed previously) for numerous listings with addresses and phone numbers.

Private organizations also listed in *Health Insurance* include state pools, Blue Cross and Blue Shield organizations, veterans advocacy branches of Paralyzed Veterans of America, Medicare carriers, and Medicare Peer Review Organizations.

For information about health maintenance organizations, contact the American Association of Health Plans, 1129 20th St., N.W., Suite 600, Washington, DC 20038.

For information about Preferred Provider Organizations, contact the Association of Managed Healthcare Organizations, 601 13th St., N.W., Suite 370 South, Washington, D.C. 20005.

The chief private source of information about health, disability, and long-term care insurance is the Health Insurance Association of America, (202) 223-7780.

16

Life Planning

Laura Cooper, Esq.

The purpose of this chapter is to highlight some of the ways in which individuals with multiple sclerosis and their family members can take action and problem-solve *now* in an effort to safeguard the family's well-being *in the future.* Of all the topics in the book, this may be the one that people are most reluctant to explore. The questions touch on topics relating to severe or incapacitating disability, long-term care, financial security, and self-determination in regard to medical decisions and treatment. Although most people with MS will never have to deal with many of the questions that are raised here, there is no way to predict exactly who will be confronted with severe disability and who will not. Therefore, the chapter is designed to help you think about ways to safeguard the future for yourself and your family in the event that the MS becomes severely disabling. Having engaged in this type of long-range thinking and planning, you can feel more secure no matter what the future brings.

The legal and financial questions raised here are meant to provide you with some basic information about these complicated issues. Complete, in-depth answers would necessarily be more complex than could be dealt with in a single chapter. Not only are each family's circumstances unique, but also the laws governing many of these issues differ somewhat from state to state, and from country to country. Therefore, the chapter is designed to help you identify questions you might want to raise with an attorney and/or certified financial planner who is familiar with the laws of the state (or province) in which you live. The type of attorney to consult about this type of disability-related planning is one who specializes in "elder law" or in disability planning (see Recommended Resources). Your local chapter of the National Multiple Sclerosis Society can help you locate a qualified professional in your area to help you with life planning.

What is the difference between a living will and a health care proxy and why do I need to have one or both of them?

Every competent person has the right to accept or refuse medical care. Unfortunately, illness or injury can intrude on the decision-making process, limiting a person's ability to communicate or carry out his or her wishes when the time for a decision arrives. What actually happens is that although the person retains the *right* to make a decision, the *legal ability* to exercise the right may be lost due to the incapacity to make such decisions. When an individual is judged legally incompetent (through unconsciousness or severe cognitive impairment, for example), health care providers do not need to abide by the person's choices if those choices conflict with medical judgments. If, however, personal choices about medical treatment have been made in advance and incorporated into a legally enforceable **advance directive**, the legal ability to make decisions is protected even after the person becomes incapacitated. Health care providers can then be directed by the wishes that the person made clear in advance, even if those wishes conflict with medical judgments.

Advance medical directives take the form of written documents in which competent persons state their medical decisions for the future. This can be accomplished in two ways: (1) via a **living will**, in which you outline specific instructions for your health care providers; or (2) by a **health care proxy** (also known as a power of attorney for health-care decision-making), in which you designate another person, who knows and would be sympathetic to your desires, to make medical decisions for you in the event that you become too incapacitated to make them for yourself.

Although the living will and health care proxy are both known as advance directives, they differ in the type of directive that is involved. A living will establishes certain treatment guidelines that are to be followed in the future (e.g., an instruction that no "extraordinary measures" are to be used to prolong life in the event of permanent unconsciousness). A health care proxy does not establish treatment guidelines directly. Instead, it appoints a trusted individual to act as your agent and make any necessary decisions in the event that you cannot act for yourself. A health care proxy can incorporate provisions of a living will by requiring that the health care proxy follow any directives that you have included in your living will. Because it is almost impossible to predict all the circumstances that might arise during an illness, it would be difficult for you to include an exhaustive list of advance directives in a living will. Hence, a health care proxy is necessary, in addition to a living will, if you wish to preserve completely the right to self-determination; any decision that is not determined by the directives in your living will would then be made by the person you have entrusted to speak for you. Consequently, a good set of advance directives will include both a living will and a health care proxy, or a single document incorporating both items.

Advance medical directives are recommended for all adults, with or without chronic illness or disability. In fact, many hospitals now routinely ask any person being admitted whether he or she has made an advance directive. Once you have written your directives, be sure to give copies to your health care providers and close family members so that they can be informed of your wishes.

If my husband does not execute an advance directive, how will medical decisions be made for him if he becomes unable to make those decisions for himself?

Once it has been determined that an incapacitated person cannot make decisions and has not left specific directives, family members are usually considered to be the appropriate decision-makers. In theory, most courts agree that even in the absence of a proxy, family members are the appropriate decision-makers. In practice, however, health care providers are not required to follow the family's decisions (to withhold or remove life support, for example) if the providers question the good faith or the medical advisability of those decisions. Therefore, appointing a proxy would provide a safeguard in the event that health care providers hesitate to follow the requests of the incapacitated person as understood or interpreted by family members. Since proxies are considered to directly exercise the wishes of the incapacitated person, health care providers cannot disregard any proxy decisions that conform to the terms of the advance directive.

It is precisely because of this issue that an important legal distinction must be made between a "proxy" and a "surrogate." A proxy is named in the advance directive and is therefore chosen directly by the incapacitated individual. A surrogate is someone who is legally appointed by the court and is *not*, therefore, considered to be directly exercising the wishes of the incapacitated person. For example, if no valid health care proxy exists, a surrogate may be appointed to make the incapacitated person's decisions. This surrogate may be empowered to make these decision in one of two ways: (1) by virtue of a legal relationship (e.g., spouse, parent, or adult child) that automatically gives the person the authority to make surrogate decisions; or (2) by court-appointment as a guardian.

The extent to which you can enforce decisions concerning your husband's future care will depend on whether you are acting as his proxy or as his surrogate. If your husband named you as his proxy, you are acting for him and have the same authority as if he were making his own decisions. If you were named his surrogate decision-maker by some other process of law, your decisions will only be honored if you are thought to be acting in good faith, and if his health care providers think your decisions are medically advisable.

My wife has experienced significant cognitive changes as a result of her MS. Her memory, judgment, and decision-making abilities are severely impaired. How can we make sure that she will get proper care if I die before she does?

Assuming that your wife executed a health care proxy naming you as her proxy prior to her severe cognitive impairment, and also designated your successor, this successor could take over if you were to die or become legally incapacitated and unable to make decisions for her. However, if your wife executed a proxy without designating your successor, your death would leave her in the same position as if she had not designated a proxy at all. If your wife did not execute a health care proxy, the court will generally appoint surrogate (substitute) decision-makers according to a hierarchy established by state law, with close relatives being given priority over more distant relatives. Thus, if no valid proxy exists, you would probably be appointed her surrogate decision-maker and then replaced by another surrogate if you became incapacitated or died.

A surrogate chosen by the court does not have the power to delegate his or her surrogate decision-making authority to other persons. Therefore, if you acquired your ability to make medical decisions for your wife as a court-appointed surrogate rather than as her designated proxy, the court will simply appoint another surrogate in the event that you die or become incapacitated. As a surrogate, you cannot control in any legal or formal way who this successor will be. However, there are steps that you can take to try to assist the court to make an appropriate decision in such a matter. The best strategy is to define her wishes, as you understand them, in a "values history" form. The purpose of such a form is to assist you in describing your wife's feelings and preferences concerning her health as you understand them. Values history forms are usually available from elder law attorneys.

In addition to making decisions about your wife's medical care, you will also want to try to ensure that sufficient resources will be available after your death (or during your life if you are also incapacitated and are using substantial resources for your own care) to provide for that care. The best way to do this is to develop plans to increase, protect, and preserve your assets.

The medical expenses related to my husband's MS are already pretty high. If he should need nursing care in the future, we would be unable to afford it. We earn salaries, but nowhere near enough to cover nursing care in addition to our living expenses. Are there any ways to handle this problem?

The first step in assessing what money is available for long-term care is to identify all of your joint income and assets. Once you have a complete picture of income and assets, you need to take steps to protect as many of those assets as possible against the expense of long-term care or other extraordinary costs. For example, you want to make sure that you have adequate insurance to protect against catastrophic losses, that you make careful investments, and that you protect your credit rating. If regular in-home or outside care does become necessary, try to determine which of the necessary services might be at least partially covered by government programs or private insurance, and which are available at low cost. Finally, extended family members should begin to think about their financial contributions. While there may be no immediate need for money from relatives, planning for possible long-term care expenses will allow you to determine when financial assistance from relatives might be required. The earlier the possibility is discussed, the easier it will be for people to plan and provide for it.

If you do not have enough resources to pay for long-term services, you will need to try to create a source of money to cover the costs. People with a significant amount of "whole life" insurance, or a home with a significant amount of equity in it, have two possible avenues for raising the necessary cash. The whole life insurance policy may have a high enough cash value to provide you with a lump sum of cash via a policy loan that does not have to be repaid until the death of the insured person. You would probably, however, be required to make annual interest-only payments on the loan. You might also be able to convert home equity into cash while continuing to live in the home. The mechanism for doing this is called a "reverse mortgage," which is basically a loan against the value of a home that does not require repayment until the borrower sells or otherwise (permanently) leaves the home. For information about reverse mortgages, contact the National Center for Home Equity Conversion (see Recommended Resources).

If you find that you still cannot obtain the resources necessary to pay for your husband's long-term care, your only realistic, available option is for your husband to become eligible for Medicaid, the state health care program for low-income individuals (see Chapter 15). The amount of your joint income and assets, in conjunction with the requirements of your state Medicaid program, will determine whether Medicaid would provide care at-home or would only cover your husband's care in a residential nursing facility. Since at-home care is more expensive than residential nursing care in many states,

Medicaid will refuse to pay for a person to receive nursing care at home if the family's assets or income are above a certain level.

I need to apply for Medicaid if my wife and I are going to be able to pay for my nursing home care. How do I go about becoming eligible for Medicaid coverage?

You need to be very careful when trying to make your income and assets low enough to qualify for Medicaid coverage (see Chapter 15). Medicaid rules severely restrict protective transfers of income and assets. In other words, the rules prohibit you from reducing your assets simply by taking them out of your own name and "giving" them to children or other relatives. To understand how complex these issues are, it helps to understand the basic rules. Any assets transferred out of a person's name during the thirty-month period prior to entering a nursing facility or applying for Medicaid is generally considered a non-valid transfer and will delay eligibility for Medicaid.

There are, however, certain exceptions to this thirty-month rule. Medicaid rules allow a couple to change the title on their home when one partner enters a nursing facility and permit the at-home spouse to keep some assets and income. The family may also keep a low-value car and some personal belongings. Additionally, there are certain individuals to whom a person is permitted to transfer anything at any time, including a minor child who is blind or disabled. The person applying for Medicaid may transfer any assets to his or her at-home spouse as long as the spouse does not transfer it to anyone else within thirty months for less than its true value. A couple is also permitted to invest liquid assets in their home by paying off an outstanding mortgage, making home improvements, or buying a new home for more money than the present home is worth. Of course, an additional benefit of paying off the mortgage or increasing the value of the home is to make more equity available in case a reverse mortgage might be useful at a later time. Whatever you do, however, must result in a home in which the at-home spouse actually resides.

In addition to reducing your assets in order to qualify for Medicaid, it will be necessary to deal with your various income sources. If your wife, as the well spouse, has enough independent income (from her own employment, for example) to support herself, and if you receive your care in a skilled nursing facility, you may be able to set up an income-cap trust (also known as a "Miller" trust) for any personal income you personally receive over the Medicaid qualifying amount. The essential problem here is that all of one spouse's income and assets are deemed to be available to the other spouse if they are living together (but not if they are divorced).

However, if you move into a nursing facility for more than a month, most states have income eligibility limits that use a "name-on-the-check" rule. (Since individual states may have their own versions of this rule that place other restrictions or limits on exempt income, you should check with your state Medicaid agency for more specific information.) Essentially, after the first month in the nursing facility, any income that is received in your wife's name is generally not counted toward the state's maximum income limit for your own Medicaid eligibility. Therefore, the only income that remains at issue after your first month in the facility is income received in your name. If that income is still too high for you to be eligible for Medicaid, a trust can be set up to divert that income so that you can still become Medicaid-eligible.

The main function of an income-cap trust is to change the way that Medicaid measures your available income. In this type of trust, any income over the Medicaid limit is sheltered for special needs. The money in trust cannot be used for basic support or for services that are covered by Medicaid. The trust will have a "trustee" who administers any income of yours that goes into the trust, and the trustee can use the funds only to pay for items or services, not covered by Medicaid, that would provide you with some benefit. Money in the trust cannot be used for your wife, and the state will be entitled to the proceeds of the trust after your death (up to the total amount already spent by Medicaid on your care). It is important to keep in mind that each state's Medicaid agency may impose different requirements on the trust. If you are considering an income-cap trust, you should contact your state Medicaid agency for information about the specific requirements for this type of trust, and consult with an attorney familiar with your state's laws.

If, after examining your income and assets, you and your wife determine that Medicaid would be your only option to pay for nursing care, you should start as quickly as possible to arrange the "ownership" of your funds so that you will be immediately eligible for Medicaid when the time comes. This not only includes transferring assets in acceptable ways (taking into account the ineligibility period or transfer restrictions), but also arranging your income sources, to the extent possible, so that income is in your wife's name. While it is not usually possible to put your own pension or Social Security checks in your wife's name, it may be possible to put other sources of income such as investments in her name.

If you desire to have your nursing care at home rather than in a nursing facility, and you are not able to make yourself eligible under your state's income limitations, a last resort may be to obtain a divorce that divides your income and assets in such a way that you are left with transferable assets and no disqualifying income sources. While this may be a distressing option to consider, it might make it possible for you to live together and yet redistribute your assets in order to make yourself eligible for Medicaid. Since some state Medicaid programs do not recognize divorce settlements for Medicaid-qualification purposes, be sure to consult your state Medicaid agency about its restrictions.

Our forty-six-year-old daughter has chronic progressive MS. She is fairly well at the present time, but we would like to make financial provision for her in our estate planning. What is the best way for us to do this?

You need to develop a cohesive estate plan in which you accomplish the following: (1) decide who will get your property when you die; (2) set up procedures to make sure that your property passes to others free from probate or with the lowest possible probate fees; (3) set up ways to pass your property to others while reducing or avoiding taxes; and (4) set up a mechanism to manage property you are leaving to others who might be unable to manage it themselves, including your disabled daughter.

In general, the method you choose to distribute your assets will involve either a will, a trust, or both. In using estate planning tools to protect your daughter, it would be advisable to consult an experienced attorney; the law is quite complex and mistakes in planning could have unfortunate consequences. For example, a problem that is commonly overlooked in estate planning is the effect that inheritances or gifts can have on a person's eligibility for public benefits such as Medicaid. Under certain circumstances, it might be preferable to limit or eliminate the transfer of assets to your daughter so that she is not put in the position of missing out on valuable (government) social services (see Recommended Readings).

A written will probably will serve as the cornerstone of your financial estate plan. A will is a binding legal document that determines how your estate should be distributed after you die. In addition to distributing property, wills may be used to handle certain personal affairs such as ensuring that your disabled daughter is cared for properly in the event that she becomes legally incompetent. Parents and guardians may use wills to name their successors. Such designations, depending on the state in which they are made, may be legally binding or of invaluable assistance to a court in any necessary guardianship proceedings. These designees are known either as "successor" or "testamentary" guardians.

A trust is a binding legal arrangement in which a person transfers assets to another person, known as a trustee, who manages it for the named beneficiary. This arrangement may be made as part of a will, in which case it is called a "testamentary" trust, or it may become effective during your lifetime, in which case it is called a "living" trust. Additionally, a living trust may be changeable during your lifetime ("revocable") or it may be fixed ("irrevocable"). A trust can be used to select a trustee who will look out for the financial and personal interests of your daughter without the need for a guardian, and it may result in substantial tax savings. The disadvantages of a trust may include complexity, cost, and the possibility that changing circumstances will leave the trustee without the most appropriate options. Although trusts may come in many forms, the most important for this purpose include:

◇ *Contingent testamentary trusts*—proceeds of an estate go first to the surviving spouse and then are held in trust for your daughter after the spouse's death;

◇ *Living trust with a pour-over provision*—allows property to be added to the trust for your daughter after your death;

◇ *Discretionary trust*—carefully defines the amount and kind of discretion that the trustee will have in distributing or withholding benefits;

◇ *Sprinkling trust*—allows you to instruct the trustee, in the event that the trust has more than one beneficiary, to distribute the benefits unequally according to the unique needs of each of those beneficiaries;

◇ *Life insurance trust*—ensures that the benefits of a life insurance policy will be managed properly.

It is advisable to consult with an estate planning attorney in order to make sure, given your financial and social circumstances, that the best strategies are used to ensure that your daughter will be protected both financially and socially once you pass away. In many states there are experts in estate planning for families with children who have disabilities. You can obtain current information about such experts by contacting the National Information Center for Children and Youth with Disabilities as well as the September 1996 issue of *Exceptional Parent* (see Recommended Resources).

My husband has recently been diagnosed with MS. He is the primary breadwinner right now while I am home with our young children. Should we be doing any kind of special planning, financial or otherwise, now that he has MS?

Most definitely. You and your husband should create a financial plan that includes insurance and other protection planning, as well as a comprehensive estate plan that also includes the advance directives discussed previously. Financial planning is the methodical process of assessing your total assets and liabilities, as well as future income potential and anticipated expenses, and then using that information to determine your best options for meeting future needs and wants. Planning should be done as soon as possible and then revised periodically or as new circumstances dictate.

The planning process may include the assessment of a myriad of financial options, including insurance plans, annuities, pensions, home equity, and availability of government benefits. Certified financial planners and lawyers may be valuable in sorting though the options and identifying the possible legal and tax consequences of various choices and choice combinations. Because your husband is the primary breadwinner, you will need to pay special attention to disability, life, health insurance, and long-term care issues so that your income stream will be protected if his disease progresses and he becomes unable to work. You might also want to be thinking about the type of

employment you would seek in the event that you need to provide additional income for the family. If you would need further
training in a particular area in order to become employed, you
might want to think about taking some courses now. Then, in the
event that your husband becomes unable to continue working,
you would feel less financially vulnerable and more prepared to
take on the breadwinner role.

**Saving for the future was hard enough before I got MS. How can
my wife and I plan for our financial future now that I have such
an unpredictable illness?**

Your first priority should be to increase the rate of retirement
savings as much as you possibly can, since MS may shorten the
time you have before retirement. You should also make sure that
your financial plan includes consideration of the potential
future need for government benefits, as described previously.

Next, it is important for you to safeguard yourself and your
family from the potential extraordinary costs of the unpredictable illness. When you are planning for such risk, the sensi-
ble approach is to assume that the worst will happen, and assess
what your needs would be if the worst were to occur. You should
never plan for the best; such a strategy is doomed to fail in all
but the most ideal and infrequent circumstances. By planning
for the worst, even though the best is what you hope for, you will
feel pleasantly surprised and adequately prepared if less than
the worst comes your way.

Consider, for example, the following grim scenario. If you, as
your family's primary breadwinner, become disabled, the continuation of your family's entire health insurance package
might be jeopardized. Additionally, you would need to provide
income replacement for any time that you were not working,
including finding income supplements for added expenses
attributable to any disability you might incur. You might find it
difficult or impossible to increase your life insurance to provide financial security for your family members in the event of
your death. And, even upon returning to work (assuming that
you were able to do so, and that you could obtain adequate
health insurance coverage from your employer following a period of disability), you might find that you were no longer as productive as you were before your disability occurred, and therefore could not earn as much money. You might even lose your

job altogether. All of these possibilities are frightening, to say the least. If you planned for all of them, you might be able to preserve whatever lifestyle you had before your disability occurred. If you adequately planned for none or only part of them, and you were handed a significant disability for a substantial period of time, your family's quality of life would no doubt be negatively affected.

The ultimate question in this circumstance is how can a person deal with the financial risks attributable to ill health but still maintain adequate income and savings? The answer to this question lies mostly in devising a strategy of protection planning for the risk of ill health. The object of this kind of protection planning is to find ways to lessen the risks—e.g., to make yourself and your loved ones as "bullet-proof" as possible, given whatever unpleasant surprises your MS or other health conditions might bring your way. As described in Chapter 15, your best strategy is to devise an insurance package that covers your family's five separate elements of health risk: (1) major medical coverage for any preexisting conditions such as the MS that may be excluded from your primary policy; (2) major medical coverage for all other conditions; (3) hospitalization for the excluded health condition(s); (4) hospitalization for all other conditions; and (5) some provisions for long-term services. You should also make special efforts to obtain adequate life and disability insurance (see Chapter 15 for a discussion of ways to obtain these types of insurance after you have been diagnosed with MS). Once your savings rate is on target, and your assets are protected from depletion with sufficient insurance, you are well on your way to financial security despite the potential intrusion of disability.

I have progressive MS and seem to be slowly getting more disabled. My husband and I want to protect the money we have saved toward our children's educations and our own retirement but we both know that my medical expenses may grow considerably if my MS gets much worse. Are there any strategies to deal with this?

The most important strategy is to maintain a "stop-loss" in insurance coverage. This refers to the maximum out-of-pocket expense you will have to absorb before you are completely insured for the medical costs. There are two basic elements to this strategy. The first is to obtain adequate basic major medical and hospitalization coverage that has a built-in "stop-loss" provision that limits your maximum out-of-pocket expenses in any calendar year. The second element is to obtain a good "catastrophic" or "excess" major medical policy. These policies are usually available to members of large organizational groups, and your diagnosis will not necessarily exclude you from eligibility for these group policies. Although you will be excluded from some, others will only impose a waiting period (perhaps a year or two) before you can claim benefits for your preexisting condition. The benefit of such a policy is that it provides an additional measure of protection by increasing the maximum lifetime benefits available, as well as enlarging the scope of expenses that may be covered for your illness. For example, many of these policies expressly provide for custodial (as opposed to skilled nursing) long-term care, a benefit that is specifically excluded in most major medical policies. Additionally, these policies are relatively inexpensive, so they are usually manageable in addition to your usual major medical coverage.

Another strategy you might consider if you find that you are spending a significant amount of time in the hospital is to collect multiple hospital indemnity insurance policies. These policies will pay you a specific indemnity—or dollar amount—for every day that you are in the hospital. These can be real money-makers if you are hospitalized with any frequency due to your MS or related conditions. Additionally, many of these policies can be obtained without preexisting condition exclusions (usually only with waiting periods). These policies can be obtained from many organizational groups and are fairly inexpensive. Unless you find yourself having more than sporadic, brief hospitalizations, you might only want to carry a single good policy of this type to help pay for the deductibles and co-payments you may have when you are hospitalized. Keep information on other available indemnity policies for which you qualify in a file. Then, if your amount of hospitalization increases to a point that justifies the cost of multiple premiums, you can sign up for additional policies.

A good certified financial planner who is well-versed in disability issues should be able to assist you in putting together an adequate insurance portfolio for your needs.

Although this chapter comes at the end of the book, its more suitable placement might well be at the very beginning. Effective planning means looking ahead in an effort to make the future as workable and predictable as it can possibly be in the face of life's uncertainties. MS only adds to those uncertainties. Every chapter in this book is designed to help you familiarize yourself and your family members with the possibilities inherent in living with this type of unpredictable chronic illness. While many people will never experience much of what is described in these pages, being educated about the disease and the resources that are available to help you will enable you to feel more prepared to deal with whatever the future brings.

Recommended Readings

Garner RJ, Coplan RB, Raasch BJ, Ratner CL . *Ernst & Young's Personal Financial Planning Guide*. New York: John Wiley & Sons, 1995.

Isaacs SL, Swartz AC. *The Consumer's Guide to Today's Health Care*. New York: Houghton Mifflin, 1992.

Matthews J. *Beat the Nursing Home Trap: A Consumer's Guide to Choosing & Financing Long-Term Care (2nd edition)*. Berkeley, CA: Nolo Press, 1993.

Mendelsohn S. *Tax Options and Strategies for People with Disabilities (2nd edition)*. New York: Demos Vermande, 1996.

Pond JD. *The New Century Family Money Book*. New York: Dell Publishing, 1993.

Roberts R. *The Veteran's Guide to Benefits*. New York: Signet, 1989.

Russell LM, Grant AE, Joseph SM, Fee RW. *Planning for the Future: Providing a Meaningful Life for a Child with a Disability After Your Death (2nd edition)*. Evanston, IL: American Publishing, 1993.

Recommended Resources

National Academy of Elder Law Attorneys, Inc. (1604 N. Country Club Road, Tucson, AZ 85716; tel: 602-881-4005). If you send them a stamped, self-addressed, legal-sized envelope, they will send you a brochure entitled "Questions and Answers When Looking for an Elder Law Attorney."

National Association of Personal Financial Advisors (800-366-2732). They will send you names of association members in your area.

National Center for Home Equity Conversion (Reverse Mortgage Locator, National Center for Home Equity Conversion, 7373 147th Street, Suite 115, Apple Valley, MN 66124; tel: 612-953-4474).

National Information Center for Children and Youth with Disabilities (P.O. Box 1492, Washington, D.C. 20013; tel: 800-695-0285; 202-884-8200).

Resource directory in the September 1996 issue of *Exceptional Parent*.

Appendix A

Glossary

Abductor muscle A muscle used to pull a body part away from the midline of the body (e.g., the abductor leg muscles are used to spread the legs).

ACTH (adrenocorticotropic hormone) ACTH is extracted from the pituitary glands of animals or made synthetically. ACTH stimulates the adrenal glands to release glucocorticoid hormones. These hormones are anti-inflammatory in nature, reducing edema and other aspects of inflammation. Data from the early 1970s indicate that ACTH may reduce the duration of MS exacerbations. In recent years it has been determined that synthetically produced glucocorticoid hormones (e.g., cortisone, prednisone, prednisolone, methylprednisolone, betamethasone, dexamethasone), which can be directly administered without the use of ACTH, are more potent, cause less sodium retention and less potassium loss, and are longer-acting than ACTH.

Activities of daily living (ADLs) Activities of daily living include any daily activity a person performs for self-care (feeding, grooming, bathing, dressing), work, homemaking, and leisure. The ability to perform ADLs is often used as a measure of ability/disability in MS.

Acute   Having rapid onset, usually with recovery; not chronic or long-lasting.

Adductor muscle   A muscle that pulls inward toward the midline of the body (e.g., the adductor leg muscles are used to pull the legs together).

ADLs   *See* Activities of daily living.

Adrenocorticotropic hormone (ACTH)   *See* ACTH.

Advance (medical) directive   Advance directives preserve the person's right to accept or reject a course of medical treatment even after the person becomes mentally or physically incapacitated to the point of being unable to communicate those wishes. Advance directives come in two basic forms: (1) a living will, in which the person outlines specific treatment guidelines that are to be followed by health care providers; (2) a health care proxy (also called a power of attorney for health care decision-making), in which the person designates a trusted individual to make medical decisions in the event that he or she becomes too incapacitated to make such decisions. Advance directive requirements vary greatly from one state to another and should therefore be drawn up in consultation with an attorney who is familiar with the laws of the particular state.

Affective release   Also called pseudo-bulbar affect; a condition in which episodes of laughing and/or crying occur with no apparent precipitating event. The person's actual mood may be unrelated to the emotion being expressed. This condition is thought to be caused by lesions in the limbic system, a group of brain structures involved in emotional feeling and expression.

Afferent pupillary defect   An abnormal reflex response to light that is a sign of nerve fiber damage due to optic neuritis. A pupil normally gets smaller when a light is shined either into that eye (direct response) or the other eye (indirect response). In an afferent pupillary defect (also called Marcus Gunn pupil), there is a relative decrease in the direct response. This is most clearly demonstrated by the "swinging flashlight test." When the flashlight is shined first in the abnormal eye, then in the healthy eye, and then again in the eye with the pupillary defect, the affected pupil becomes larger rather than smaller.

AFO *See* Ankle-foot orthosis.

Ankle-foot orthosis (AFO) An ankle-foot orthosis is a brace, usually plastic, that is worn on the lower leg and foot to support the ankle and correct foot drop. By holding the foot and ankle in the correct position, the AFO promotes correct heel-toe walking. *See* Foot drop.

Antibodies Proteins of the immune system that are soluble (dissolved) in blood serum or other body fluids and which are produced in response to bacteria, viruses, and other types of foreign antigens. *See* Antigen.

Anticholinergic Refers to the action of certain medications commonly used in the management of neurogenic bladder dysfunction. These medications inhibit the transmission of parasympathetic nerve impulses and thereby reduce spasms of smooth muscle in the bladder.

Antigen Any substance that triggers the immune system to produce an antibody; generally refers to infectious or toxic substances. *See* Antibody.

Aspiration Inhalation of food particles or fluids into lungs.

Aspiration pneumonia Inflammation of the lungs due to aspiration.

Assistive devices Any tools that are designed, fabricated, and/or adapted to assist a person in performing a particular task, e.g., cane, walker, shower chair.

Ataxia The incoordination and unsteadiness that result from the brain's failure to regulate the body's posture and the strength and direction of limb movements. Ataxia is most often caused by disease activity in the cerebellum.

Atrophy A wasting or decrease in size of a part of the body because of disease or lack of use.

Autoimmune disease A process in which the body's immune system causes illness by mistakenly attacking healthy cells, organs, or tissues in the body that are essential for good health. Multiple sclerosis is believed to be an autoimmune disease, along with systemic lupus erythematosus, rheumatoid arthritis, scleroderma, and many others. The precise origin and pathophysiologic processes of these diseases are unknown.

Autonomic nervous system The part of the nervous system that regulates involuntary vital functions, including the activity of the cardiac (heart) muscle, smooth muscles (e.g., of the gut), and glands. The autonomic nervous system has two divisions: the sympathetic nervous system accelerates heart rate, constricts blood vessels, and raises blood pressure; the parasympathetic nervous system slows heart rate, increases intestinal and gland activity, and relaxes sphincter muscles.

B-cell   A type of lymphocyte (white blood cell) manufactured in the bone marrow that makes antibodies.

Babinski reflex   A neurological sign in MS in which stroking the outside sole of the foot with a pointed object causes an upward (extensor) movement of the big toe rather than the normal (flexor) bunching and downward movement of the toes. *See* Sign.

Bell's palsy   A paralysis of the facial nerve (usually on one side of the face), which can occur as a consequence of MS, viral infection, or other infections. It has acute onset and can be transient or permanent.

Blood-brain barrier   A semi-permeable cell layer around blood vessels in the brain and spinal cord that prevents large molecules, immune cells, and potentially damaging substances and disease-causing organisms (e.g., viruses) from passing out of the blood stream into the central nervous system (brain and spinal cord). A break in the blood-brain barrier may underlie the disease process in MS.

Brainstem   The part of the central nervous system that houses the nerve centers of the head as well as the centers for respiration and heart control. It extends from the base of the brain to the spinal cord.

Brainstem auditory evoked potential (BAEP)   A test in which the brain's electrical activity in response to auditory stimuli (e.g., clicking sounds) is recorded by an electroencephalograph and analyzed by computer. Demyelination results in a slowing of response time. This test is sometimes useful in the diagnosis of MS because it can confirm the presence of a suspected lesion or identify the presence of an unsuspected lesion that has produced no symptoms. BAEPs have been shown to be less useful in the diagnosis of MS than either visual or somatosensory evoked potentials.

CAT scan   *See* Computerized axial tomography.

Catheter   A hollow, flexible tube, made of plastic or rubber, which can be inserted through the urinary opening into the bladder to drain excess urine that cannot be excreted normally.

Central nervous system   The part of the nervous system that includes the brain, optic nerves, and spinal cord.

Cerebellum   A part of the brain situated above the brainstem that controls balance and coordination of movement.

Cerebrospinal fluid (CSF)   A watery, colorless, clear fluid that bathes and protects the brain and spinal cord. The composition of this fluid can be altered by a variety of diseases. Certain changes in CSF that are characteristic of MS can be detected with a lumbar puncture (spinal tap), a test sometimes used to help make the MS diagnosis. *See* Lumbar puncture.

Cerebrum   The large, upper part of the brain, which acts as a master control system and is responsible for initiating thought and motor activity.

Chronic   Of long duration, not acute; a term often used to describe a disease that shows gradual worsening.

Clinical finding   An observation made during a medical examination indicating change or impairment in a physical or mental function.

Clinical trial   Rigorously controlled studies designed to provide extensive data that will allow for statistically valid evaluation of the safety and efficacy of a particular treatment. *See also* Double-blind clinical study; Placebo.

Clonus   A sign of spasticity in which involuntary shaking or jerking of the leg occurs when the toe is placed on the floor with the knee slightly bent. The shaking is caused by repeated, rhythmic, reflex muscle contractions.

Cognition   High level functions carried out by the human brain, including comprehension and use of speech, visual perception and construction, calculation ability, attention (information processing), memory, and executive functions such as planning, problem-solving, and self-monitoring.

Cognitive impairment   Changes in cognitive function caused by trauma or disease process. Some degree of cognitive impairment occurs in approximately 50–60 percent of people with MS, with memory, information processing, and executive functions being the most commonly affected functions. *See* Cognition.

Cognitive rehabilitation   Techniques designed to improve the functioning of individuals whose cognition is impaired because of physical trauma or disease. Rehabilitation strategies are designed to improve the impaired function via repetitive drills or practice, or to compensate for impaired functions that are not likely to improve. Cognitive rehabilitation is provided by psychologists and neuropsychologists, speech/language pathologists, and occupational therapists. While these three types of specialists use different assessment tools and treatment strategies, they share the common goal of improving the individual's ability to function as independently and safely as possible in the home and work environment.

Combined (bladder) dysfunction   A type of neurogenic bladder dysfunction is MS (also called detrusor-external sphincter dyssynergia—DESD). Simultaneous contractions of the bladder's detrusor muscle and external sphincter cause urine to be trapped in the bladder, resulting in symptoms of urinary urgency, hesitancy, dribbling, and incontinence.

Computerized axial tomography (CAT scan)   A non-invasive diagnostic radiology technique for examining soft tissues of the body. A computer integrates X-ray scanned "slices" of the organ being examined into a cross-sectional picture.

Condom catheter   A tube connected to a thin, flexible sheath that is worn over the penis to allow drainage of urine into a collection system; can be used to manage male urinary incontinence.

Constipation   A condition in which bowel movements happen less frequently than is normal for the particular individual, or the stool is small, hard, and difficult or painful to pass.

Contraction   A shortening of muscle fibers that results in the movement of a joint.

Contracture   A permanent shortening of the muscles and tendons adjacent to a joint, which can result from severe, untreated spasticity and interferes with normal movement around the affected joint. If left untreated, the affected joint can become frozen in a flexed (bent) position.

Coordination   An organized working together of muscles and groups of muscles aimed at bringing about a purposeful movement such as walking or standing.

Corpus callosum   The broad band of nerve fibers tissue that connects the two cerebral hemispheres of the brain.

Cortex   The outer layer of brain tissue.

Corticosteroid   Any of the natural or synthetic hormones associated with the adrenal cortex (which influences or controls many body processes). Corticosteroids include glucocorticoids, which have an anti-inflammatory and immunosuppressive role in the treatment of MS exacerbations. *See also* Glucocorticoids; Immunosuppression; Exacerbation.

Cortisone   A glucocorticoid steroid hormone, produced by the adrenal glands or synthetically, that has anti-inflammatory and immune-system suppressing properties. Prednisone and prednisolone also belong to this group of substances.

Cranial nerves   Nerves that carry sensory, motor, or parasympathetic fibers to the face and neck. Included among this group of twelve nerves are the optic nerve (vision), trigeminal nerve (sensation along the face), vagus nerve (pharynx and vocal cords). Evaluation of cranial nerve function is part of the standard neurologic exam.

Cystoscopy   A diagnostic procedure in which a special viewing device called a cystoscope is inserted into the urethra (a tubular structure that drains urine from the bladder) to examine the inside of the urinary bladder.

Cystostomy   A surgically created opening through the lower abdomen into the urinary bladder. A plastic tube inserted into the opening drains urine from the bladder into a plastic collection bag. This relatively simple procedure is done when a person requires an indwelling catheter to drain excess urine from the bladder but cannot, for some reason, have it pass through the urethral opening.

Decubitus   An ulcer (sore) of the skin resulting from pressure and lack of movement such as occurs when a person is bed- or wheelchair-bound. The ulcers occur most frequently in areas where the bone lies directly under the skin, such as elbow, hip, or over the coccyx (tailbone). A decubitus ulcer may become infected and cause general worsening of the person's health.

Deep tendon reflexes   The involuntary jerks that are normally produced at certain spots on a limb when the tendons are tapped with a hammer. Reflexes are tested as part of the standard neurologic exam.

Dementia   A generally profound and progressive loss of intellectual function, sometimes associated with personality change, that results from loss of brain substance and is sufficient to interfere with a person's normal functional activities.

Demyelination   A loss of myelin in the white matter of the central nervous system (brain, spinal cord).

DESD   *See* Detrusor-external sphincter dyssynergia.

Detrusor muscle   A muscle of the urinary bladder that contracts and causes the bladder to empty.

Detrusor-external sphincter dyssynergia (DESD)   *See* Combined (bladder) dysfunction.

Diplopia   Double vision, or the simultaneous awareness of two images of the same object that results from a failure of the two eyes to work in a coordinated fashion. Covering one eye will erase one of the images.

Disability   As defined by the World Health Organization, a disability (resulting from an impairment) is a restriction or lack of ability to perform an activity in the manner or within the range considered normal for a human being.

Double-blind clinical study   A study in which none of the participants, including experimental subjects, examining doctors, attending nurses, or any other research staff, know who is taking the test drug and who is taking a control or placebo agent. The purpose of this research design is to avoid inadvertent bias of the test results. In all studies, procedures are designed to "break the blind" if medical circumstances require it.

Dysarthria   Poorly articulated speech resulting from dysfunction of the muscles controlling speech, usually caused by damage to the central nervous system or a peripheral motor nerve. The content and meaning of the spoken words remain normal.

Dysesthesia   Distorted or unpleasant sensations experienced by a person when the skin is touched, that are typically caused by abnormalities in the sensory pathways in the brain and spinal cord.

Dysmetria   A disturbance of coordination, caused by lesions in the cerebellum. A tendency to over- or underestimate the extent of motion needed to place an arm or leg in a certain position as, for example, in overreaching for an object.

Dysphagia   Difficulty in swallowing. It is a neurologic or neuromuscular symptom that may result in aspiration (whereby food or saliva enters the airway), slow swallowing (possibly resulting in inadequate nutrition), or both.

Dysphonia   Disorders of voice quality (including poor pitch control, hoarseness, breathiness, and hypernasality) caused by spasticity, weakness, and incoordination of muscles in the mouth and throat.

EAE   *See* Experimental allergic encephalomyelitis.

EEG   *See* Electroencephalography.

Electroencephalography (EEG)   A diagnostic procedure that records, via electrodes attached to various areas of the person's head, electrical activity generated by brain cells.

Electromyography (EMG)   Electromyography is a diagnostic procedure that records muscle electrical potentials through a needle or small plate electrodes. The test can also measure the ability of peripheral nerves to conduct impulses.

EMG   *See* Electromyography.

Etiology   The study of all factors that may be involved in the development of a disease, including the patient's susceptibility, the nature of the disease-causing agent, and the way in which the person's body is invaded by the agent.

Euphoria   Unrealistic cheerfulness and optimism, accompanied by a lessening of critical faculties; generally considered to be a result of damage to the brain.

Evoked potentials (EPs)   EPs are recordings of the nervous system's electrical response to the stimulation of specific sensory pathways (e.g., visual, auditory, general sensory). In tests of evoked potentials, a person's recorded responses are displayed on an oscilloscope and analyzed on a computer that allows comparison with normal response times. Demyelination results in a slowing of response time. EPs can demonstrate lesions along specific nerve pathways whether or not the lesions are producing symptoms, thus making this test useful in confirming the diagnosis of MS.

Exacerbation   The appearance of new symptoms or the aggravation of old ones, lasting at least twenty-four hours (synonymous with attack, relapse, flare-up, or worsening); usually associated with inflammation and demyelination in the brain or spinal cord.

Experimental allergic encephalomyelitis (EAE)   Experimental allergic encephalomyelitis is an autoimmune disease resembling MS that has been induced in some genetically susceptible research animals. Before testing on humans, a potential treatment for MS may first be tested on laboratory animals with EAE in order to determine the treatment's efficacy and safety.

Extensor spasm   A symptom of spasticity in which the legs straighten suddenly into a stiff, extended position. These spasms, which typically last for several minutes, occur most commonly in bed at night or on rising from bed.

Failure to empty (bladder)   A type of neurogenic bladder dysfunction in MS resulting from demyelination in the voiding reflex center of the spinal cord. The bladder tends to overfill and become flaccid, resulting in symptoms of urinary urgency, hesitancy, dribbling, and incontinence.

Failure to store (bladder)   A type of neurogenic bladder dysfunction in MS resulting from demyelination of the pathways between the spinal cord and brain. Typically seen in a small, spastic bladder, storage failure can cause symptoms of urinary urgency, frequency, incontinence, and nocturia.

FDA   *See* Food and Drug Administration.

Finger-to-nose test   As a test of dysmetria and intention tremor, the person is asked, with eyes closed, to touch the tip of the nose with the tip of the index finger. This test is part of the standard neurologic exam.

Flaccid   A decrease in muscle tone resulting in weakened muscles and therefore loose, "floppy" limbs.

Flexor spasm   Involuntary, sometimes painful contractions of the flexor muscles, which pull the legs upward into a clenched position. These spasms, which last two to three seconds, are symptoms of spasticity. They often occur during sleep, but can also occur when the person is in a seated position.

Foley catheter   *See* Indwelling catheter.

Food and Drug Administration (FDA)   The U.S. federal agency that is responsible for enforcing governmental regulations pertaining to the manufacture and sale of food, drugs, and cosmetics. Its role is to prevent the sale of impure or dangerous substances. Any new drug that is proposed for the treatment of MS must be approved by the FDA.

Foot drop   A condition of weakness in the muscles of the foot and ankle, caused by poor nerve conduction, which interferes with a person's ability to flex the ankle and walk with a normal heel-toe pattern. The toes touch the ground before the heel, causing the person to trip or lose balance.

Frontal lobes   The largest lobes of the brain. The anterior (front) part of each of the cerebral hemispheres that make up the cerebrum. The back part of the frontal lobe is the motor cortex, which controls voluntary movement; the area of the frontal lobe that is further forward is concerned with learning, behavior, judgment, and personality.

Gadolinium   A chemical compound that can be administered to a person during magnetic resonance imaging to help distinguish between new lesions and old lesions.

Gastrocolic reflex   A mass peristaltic (coordinated, rhythmic, smooth muscle contraction that acts to force food through the digestive tract) movement of the colon that often occurs fifteen to thirty minutes after ingesting a meal.

Gastrostomy   *See* Percutaneous endoscopic gastrostomy.

Glucocorticoid hormones   Steroid hormones that are produced by the adrenal glands in response to stimulation by adrenocorticotropic hormone (ACTH) from the pituitary. These hormones, which can also be manufactured synthetically (prednisone, prednisolone, methylprednisolone, betamethasone, dexamethasone), serve both an immunosuppressive and an anti-inflammatory role in the treatment of MS exacerbations: they damage or destroy certain types of T-lymphocytes that are involved in the overactive immune response and interfere with the release of certain inflammation-producing enzymes.

Handicap   As defined by the World Health Organization, a handicap is a disadvantage, resulting from an impairment or a disability, that interferes with a person's efforts to fulfill a role that is normal for that person. Handicap is therefore a social concept, representing the social and environmental consequences of a person's impairments and disabilities.

Health care proxy   *See* Advance (medical) directive.

Heel-knee-shin test   A test of coordination in which the person is asked, with eyes closed, to place one heel on the opposite knee and slide it up and down the shin.

Helper T-lymphocytes   White blood cells that are a major contributor to the immune system's inflammatory response against myelin.

Hemiparesis   Weakness of one side of the body, including one arm and one leg.

Hemiplegia   Paralysis of one side of the body, including one arm and one leg.

Hyperbaric oxygen   A procedure in which the person breathes oxygen under greater than atmospheric pressure in a specially constructed chamber. Once thought to be a potential treatment for MS, it has been evaluated in several controlled, double-blind studies and found to be ineffective for this purpose.

Immune system   A complex system of various types of cells that protects the body against disease-producing organisms and other foreign invaders.

Immunocompetent cells   White blood cells (B- and T-lymphocytes and others) that defend against invading agents in the body.

Immunoglobulin   *See* Antibody.

Immunosuppression   In MS, a form of treatment that slows or inhibits the body's natural immune responses, including those directed against the body's own tissues. Examples of immunosuppressive treatments in MS include cyclosporine, methotrexate, and azathioprine.

Impairment   As defined by the World Health Organization, an impairment is any loss or abnormality of psychological, physiological, or anatomical structure or function. It represents a deviation from the person's usual biomedical state. An impairment is thus any loss of function directly resulting from injury or disease.

Incidence   The number of new cases of a disease in a specified population over a defined period of time.

Incontinence   Also called spontaneous voiding; the inability to control passage of urine or bowel movements.

Indwelling catheter   A type of catheter (*see* Catheter) that remains in the bladder on a temporary or permanent basis. It is used only when intermittent catheterization is not possible or is medically contraindicated. The most common type of indwelling catheter is a Foley catheter, which consists of a flexible rubber tube that is inserted in the bladder to allow the urine to flow into an external drainage bag. A small balloon, inflated after insertion, holds the Foley catheter in place.

Inflammation   A tissue's immunologic response to injury, characterized by mobilization of white blood cells and antibodies, swelling, and fluid accumulation.

Intention tremor   Rhythmic shaking that occurs in the course of a purposeful movement, such as reaching to pick something up or bringing an outstretched finger in to touch one's nose.

Interferon   A group of immune system proteins, produced and released by cells infected by a virus, which inhibit viral multiplication and modify the body's immune response. One of the interferons, interferon beta-1b (Betaseron®) was approved by the Food and Drug Administration in 1993 for treatment of relapsing-remitting MS. It was found in a clinical trial to reduce the frequency and severity of exacerbations by approximately 30 percent. A second interferon, interferon beta-1a (Avonex®) has also been shown to reduce the frequency and severity of MS exacerbations in people with relapsing-remitting disease, as well as to reduce the risk of clinically significant disease progression. Avonex® was approved for use in MS in 1996.

Intermittent self-catheterization (ISC)   A procedure in which the person periodically inserts a catheter into the urinary opening to drain urine from the bladder. ISC is used in the management of bladder dysfunction to drain urine that remains after voiding, prevent bladder distention, prevent kidney damage, and restore bladder function.

Internuclear ophthalmoplegia   A disturbance of coordinated eye movements in which the eye turned outward to look toward the side develops nystagmus (rapid, involuntary movements) while the other eye simultaneously fails to turn completely inward. This neurologic sign, of which the person is usually unaware, can be detected during the neurologic exam.

Intrathecal space   The space surrounding the brain and spinal cord that contains cerebrospinal fluid.

Intravenous   Within a vein; often used in the context of an injection into a vein of medication dissolved in a liquid.

Lesion   *See* Plaque.

Leukocyte   White blood cell.

L'Hermitte's sign   An abnormal sensation of electricity or "pins and needles" going down the spine into the arms and legs that occurs when the neck is bent forward so that the chin touches the chest.

Living will   *See* Advance (medical) directive.

Loftstrand crutch   A type of crutch with an attached holder for the forearm that provides extra support.

Lumbar puncture   A diagnostic procedure that uses a hollow needle (canula) to penetrate the spinal canal at the level of third–fourth or fourth–fifth lumbar vertebrae to remove cerebrospinal fluid for analysis. This procedure is used to examine the cerebrospinal fluid for changes in composition that are characteristic of MS (e.g., elevated white cell count, elevated protein content, the presence of oligoclonal bands).

Lymphocyte   A type of white blood cell that is part of the immune system. Lymphocytes can be subdivided into two main groups: B-lymphocytes, which originate in the bone marrow and produce antibodies; T-lymphocytes, which are produced in the bone marrow and mature in the thymus. Helper T-lymphocytes heighten the production of antibodies by B-lymphocytes; suppressor T-lymphocytes suppress B-lymphocyte activity and seem to be in short supply during an MS exacerbation.

Macrophage   A white blood cell with scavenger characteristics that has the ability to ingest and destroy foreign substances such as bacteria and cell debris.

Magnetic resonance imaging (MRI)   A diagnostic procedure that produces visual images of different body parts without the use of X-rays. Nuclei of atoms are influenced by a high frequency electromagnetic impulse inside a strong magnetic field. The nuclei then give off resonating signals that can produce pictures of parts of the body. An important diagnostic tool in MS, MRI makes it possible to visualize and count lesions in the white matter of the brain and spinal cord.

Marcus Gunn pupil   *See* Afferent pupillary defect.

Minimal Record of Disability (MRD)   A standardized method for quantifying the clinical status of a person with MS. The

MRD is made up of five parts: demographic information; the Neurological Functional Systems (developed by John Kurtzke), which assign scores to clinical findings for each of the various neurologic systems in the brain and spinal cord (pyramidal, cerebellar, brainstem, sensory, visual, mental, bowel and bladder); the Disability Status Scale (developed by John Kurtzke), which gives a single composite score for the person's disease; the Incapacity Status Scale, which is an inventory of functional disabilities relating to activities of daily living; the Environmental Status Scale, which provides an assessment of social handicap resulting from chronic illness. The MRD has two main functions: to assist doctors and other professionals in planning and coordinating the care of persons with MS, and to provide a standardized means of recording repeated clinical evaluations of individuals for research purposes.

Monoclonal antibodies   Laboratory-produced antibodies, which can be programmed to react against a specific antigen in order to suppress the immune response.

Motor neurons   Nerve cells of the brain and spinal cord that enable movement of various parts of the body.

Motor point block   *See* Nerve block.

MRI   *See* Magnetic resonance imaging.

Muscle tone   A characteristic of a muscle brought about by the constant flow of nerve stimuli to that muscle, which describes its resistance to stretching. Abnormal muscle tone can be defined as: hypertonus (increased muscle tone, as in spasticity); hypotonus (reduced muscle tone); flaccid (paralysis); atony (loss of muscle tone). Muscle tone is evaluated as part of the standard neurologic exam in MS.

Myelin   A soft, white coating of nerve fibers in the central nervous system, composed of lipids (fats) and protein. Myelin serves as insulation and as an aid to efficient nerve fiber conduction. When myelin is damaged in MS, nerve fiber conduction is faulty or absent. Impaired bodily functions or altered sensations associated with those demyelinated nerve fibers are identified as symptoms of MS in various parts of the body.

Myelin basic protein   Proteins associated with the myelin of the central nervous system that may be found in higher than normal concentrations in the cerebrospinal fluid of individuals with MS and other diseases that damage myelin.

Myelitis   An inflammatory disease of the spinal cord. In transverse myelitis, the inflammation spreads across the tissue of the spinal cord, resulting in a loss of its normal function to transmit nerve impulses up and down, as though the spinal cord had been severed.

Myelogram   An X-ray procedure by which the spinal canal and the spinal cord can be visualized. It is performed in conjunction with a lumbar puncture and injection of a special X-ray contrast material into the spinal canal.

Nerve   A bundle of nerve fibers (axons). The fibers are either afferent (leading toward the brain and serving in the perception of sensory stimuli of the skin, joints, muscles, and inner organs) or efferent (leading away from the brain and mediating contractions of muscles or organs).

Nerve block   A procedure used to relieve otherwise intractable spasticity, including painful flexor spasms. An injection of phenol into the affected nerve interferes with the function of that nerve for up to three months, potentially increasing a person's comfort and mobility.

Nervous system   Includes all of the neural structures in the body: the central nervous system consists of the brain, spinal cord, and optic nerves; the peripheral nervous system consists of the nerve roots, nerve plexi, and nerves throughout the body.

Neurogenic   Related to activity of the nervous system, as in "neurogenic bladder."

Neurogenic bladder   Bladder dysfunction associated with neurologic malfunction in the spinal cord and characterized by a failure to empty, failure to store, or a combination of the two. Symptoms that result from these three types of dysfunction include urinary urgency, frequency, hesitancy, nocturia, and incontinence.

Neurologist   Physician who specializes in the diagnosis and treatment of conditions related to the nervous system.

Neurology   Study of the central, peripheral, and autonomic nervous system.

Neuron   The basic nerve cell of the nervous system. A neuron consists of a nucleus within a cell body and one or more processes (extensions) called dendrites and axons.

Neuropsychologist A psychologist with specialized training in the evaluation of cognitive functions. Neuropsychologists use a battery of standardized tests to assess specific cognitive functions and identify areas of cognitive impairment. They also provide remediation for individuals with MS-related cognitive impairment. *See* Cognition and Cognitive impairment.

Nocturia The need to urinate during the night.

Nystagmus Rapid, involuntary movements of the eyes in the horizontal or, occasionally, the vertical direction.

Occupational therapist (OT) Occupational therapists assess functioning in activities of everyday living, including dressing, bathing, grooming, meal preparation, writing, and driving, which are essential for independent living. In making treatment recommendations, the OT addresses (1) fatigue management, (2) upper body strength, movement, and coordination, (3) adaptations to the home and work environment, including both structural changes and specialized equipment for particular activities, and (4) compensatory strategies for impairments in thinking, sensation, or vision.

Oligoclonal bands A diagnostic sign indicating abnormal levels of certain antibodies in the cerebrospinal fluid; seen in approximately 90 percent of people with multiple sclerosis, but not specific to MS.

Oligodendrocyte A type of cell in the central nervous system that is responsible for making and supporting myelin.

Ophthalmoscope An instrument designed for examination of the interior of the eye.

Optic atrophy A wasting of the optic disc that results from partial or complete degeneration of optic nerve fibers and is associated with a loss of visual acuity.

Optic disc The small blind spot on the surface of the retina where cells of the retina converge to form the optic nerve; the only part of the retina that is insensitive to light.

Optic neuritis Inflammation or demyelination of the optic (visual) nerve with transient or permanent impairment of vision and occasionally pain.

Orthotic Also called orthosis; a mechanical appliance such as a leg brace or splint that is specially designed to control, correct, or compensate for impaired limb function.

Orthotist A person skilled in making mechanical appliances (orthotics) such as leg braces or splints that help to support limb function. *See* Orthotic.

Oscillopsia Continuous, involuntary, and chaotic eye movements that result in a visual disturbance in which objects appear to be jumping or bouncing.

Osteoporosis Decalcification of the bones, which can result from the lack of mobility experienced by wheelchair-bound individuals.

Paralysis Inability to move a part of the body.

Paraparesis A weakness but not total paralysis of the lower extremities (legs).

Paraplegia Paralysis of both lower extremities (legs).

Paresis Partial or incomplete paralysis of a part of the body.

Paresthesia A spontaneously occurring sensation of burning, prickling, tingling, or creeping on the skin that may or may not be associated with any physical findings on neurologic examination.

Paroxysmal spasm A sudden, uncontrolled limb contraction that occurs intermittently, lasts for a few moments, and then subsides.

Paroxysmal symptom Any one of several symptoms that have sudden onset, apparently in response to some kind of movement or sensory stimulation, last for a few moments, and then subside. Paroxysmal symptoms tend to occur frequently in those individuals who have them, and follow a similar pattern from one episode to the next. Examples of paroxysmal symptoms include acute episodes of trigeminal neuralgia (sharp facial pain), tonic seizures (intense spasm of limb or limbs on one side of the body), dysarthria (slurred speech often accompanied by loss of balance and coordination), and various paresthesias (sensory disturbances ranging from tingling to severe pain).

PEG *See* Percutaneous endoscopic gastrostomy.

Percutaneous endoscopic gastrostomy (PEG) A PEG is a tube inserted into the stomach through the abdominal wall to provide food or other nutrients when eating by mouth is not possible. The tube is inserted in a bedside procedure using an endoscope to guide the tube through a small abdominal incision. An endoscope is a lighted instrument that allows the doctor to see inside the stomach.

Percutaneous rhizotomy   An outpatient surgical procedure used in the management of severe, intractable trigeminal neuralgia. The surgeon makes a tiny incision in the side of the person's face and blocks the function of the trigeminal nerve using laser surgery, cryosurgery (freezing), or cauterization.

Periventricular region   The area surrounding the four fluid-filled cavities within the brain. MS plaques are commonly found within this region.

Physiatrist   Physicians who specialize in physical medicine and rehabilitation of physical impairments.

Physical therapist (PT)   Physical therapists are trained to evaluate and improve movement and function of the body, with particular attention to physical mobility, balance, posture, fatigue, and pain. The physical therapy program typically involves (1) educating the person with MS about the physical problems caused by the disease, (2) designing an individualized exercise program to address the problems, and (3) enhancing mobility and energy conservation through the use of a variety of mobility aids and adaptive equipment.

Placebo   An inactive, non-drug compound that is designed to look just like the test drug. It is administered to control group subjects in double-blind clinical trials (in which neither the researchers nor the subjects know who is getting the drug and who is getting the placebo) as a means of assessing the benefits and liabilities of the test drug taken by experimental group subjects.

Placebo effect   An apparently beneficial result of therapy that occurs because of the patient's expectation that the therapy will help.

Plantar reflex   A reflex response obtained by drawing a pointed object along the outer border of the sole of the foot from the heel to the little toe. The normal flexor response is a bunching and downward movement of the toes. An upward movement of the big toe is called an extensor response, or Babinski reflex, which is a sensitive indicator of disease in the brain or spinal cord.

Plaque   An area of inflamed or demyelinated central nervous system tissue.

Plasma cell   A lymphocyte-like cell found in the bone marrow, connective tissue, and blood that is involved in the body's immune system. *See also* Lymphocyte.

Position sense   The ability to tell, with one's eyes closed, where fingers and toes are in space. Position sense is evaluated during the standard neurologic exam in MS.

Post-void residual test (PVR)   The PVR test involves passing a catheter into the bladder following urination in order to drain and measure any urine that is left in the bladder after urination is completed. The PVR is a simple but effective technique for diagnosing bladder dysfunction in MS.

Postural tremor   Rhythmic shaking that occurs when the muscles are tensed to hold an object or stay in a given position.

Power grading   A measurement of muscle strength used to evaluate weakness or paralysis. Power is tested as part of the standard neurologic exam in MS.

Prevalence   The number of all new and old cases of a disease in a defined population at a particular point in time.

Primary progressive MS   A clinical course of MS characterized from the beginning by progressive disease, with no plateaus or remissions, or an occasional plateau and very short-lived, minor improvements.

Prognosis   Prediction of the future course of the disease.

Progressive-relapsing MS   A clinical course of MS that shows disease progression from the beginning, but with clear, acute relapses, with or without full recovery from those relapses along the way.

Prospective memory   The ability to remember an event or commitment scheduled for the future. Thus, a person who agrees to meet or call someone at a given time on the following day must be able to remember the appointment when the time comes. People with MS-related memory impairment frequently report problems with this type of memory for upcoming appointments.

Pseudo-bulbar affect   *See* Affective release.

Pseudo-exacerbation   A temporary aggravation of disease symptoms, resulting from an elevation in body temperature or other stressor (e.g., an infection, severe fatigue, constipation), that disappears once the stressor is removed. A pseudo-exacerbation involves symptom flare-up rather than new disease activity or progression.

Pyramidal tracts   Motor nerve pathways in the brain and spinal cord that connect nerve cells in the brain to the motor cells located in the cranial, thoracic, and lumbar parts of the spinal cord. Damage to these tracts causes spastic paralysis or weakness.

Pyuria   The presence of pus in the urine, causing it to appear cloudy; indicative of bacterial infection in the urinary tract.

Quad cane   A cane that has a broad base on four short "feet," which provide extra stability.

Quadriplegia   The paralysis of both arms and both legs.

Recent memory   The ability to remember events, conversations, content of reading material or television programs from a short time ago, i.e., an hour or two ago or last night. People with MS-related memory impairment typically experience greatest difficulty remembering these types of things in the recent past.

Reflex   An involuntary response of the nervous system to a stimulus, such as the stretch reflex, which is elicited by tapping a tendon with a reflex hammer, resulting in a contraction. Increased, diminished, or absent reflexes can be indicative of neurologic damage, including MS, and are therefore tested as part of the standard neurologic exam.

Relapsing-remitting MS   A clinical course of MS that is characterized by clearly defined, acute attacks with full or partial recovery and no disease progression between attacks.

Remission   A lessening in the severity of symptoms or their temporary disappearance during the course of the illness.

Remote memory   The ability to remember people or events from the distant past. People with MS tend to experience few, if any, problems with their remote memory.

Remyelination   The repair of damaged myelin. Myelin repair occurs spontaneously in MS but very slowly. Research is currently underway to find a way to speed the healing process.

Residual urine   Urine that remains in the bladder following urination.

Retrobulbar neuritis   *See* Optic neuritis.

Romberg's sign   The inability to maintain balance in a standing position with feet and legs drawn together and eyes closed.

Scanning speech   Abnormal speech characterized by staccato-like articulation that sounds clipped because the person unintentionally pauses between syllables and skips some of the sounds.

Sclerosis   Hardening of tissue. In MS, sclerosis is the body's replacement of lost myelin around CNS nerve cells with scar tissue.

Scotoma   A gap or blind spot in the visual field.

Secondary progressive MS   A clinical course of MS that initially is relapsing-remitting and then becomes progressive at a variable rate, possibly with an occasional relapse and minor remission.

Sensory   Related to bodily sensations such as pain, smell, taste, temperature, vision, hearing, acceleration, and position in space.

Sepsis   The presence of sufficient bacteria in the blood to cause illness.

Sign   An objective physical problem or abnormality identified by the physician during the neurologic examination. Neurologic signs may differ significantly from the symptoms reported by the patient because they are identifiable only with specific tests and may cause no overt symptoms. Common neurologic signs in multiple sclerosis include altered eye movements and other changes in the appearance or function of the visual system; altered reflexes; weakness; spasticity; circumscribed sensory changes.

Somatosensory evoked potential   A test that measures the brain's electrical activity in response to repeated (mild) electrical stimulation of different parts of the body. Demyelination results in a slowing of response time. This test is useful in the diagnosis of MS because it can confirm the presence of a suspected lesion (area of demyelination) or identify the presence of an unsuspected lesion that has produced no symptoms.

Spasticity   Abnormal increase in muscle tone, manifested as a spring-like resistance to moving or being moved.

Speech/language pathologist   Speech/language pathologists specialize in the diagnosis and treatment of speech and swallowing disorders. A person with MS may be referred to a speech/language pathologist for help with either one or both of these problems. Because of their expertise with speech and language difficulties, these specialists also provide cognitive remediation for individuals with cognitive impairment.

Sphincter   A circular band of muscle fibers that tightens or closes a natural opening of the body, such as the external anal sphincter, which closes the anus, and the internal and external urinary sphincters, which close the urinary canal.

Sphincterotomy A surgical enlargement of the urinary sphincter in a male whose spasticity is so severe that he cannot empty his bladder. Once the surgery is performed, the man loses urinary control and must wear an external, condom catheter to collect the urine. This procedure is seldom required in MS. It is performed only on males because urinary drainage problems in females might lead to skin breakdown.

Spinal tap *See* Lumbar puncture.

Spirometer An instrument used to assess lung function; it measures the volume and flow rate of inhaled and exhaled air.

Spontaneous voiding *See* Incontinence.

Stance ataxia An inability to stand upright due to disturbed coordination of the involved muscles, which results in swaying and a tendency to fall in one or another direction.

Steroids *See* ACTH; Corticosteroid; Glucocorticoid hormones.

Suppressor T-lymphocytes White blood cells that act as part of the immune system and may be in short supply during an MS exacerbation.

Symptom A subjectively perceived problem or complaint reported by the patient. In multiple sclerosis, common symptoms include visual problems, fatigue, sensory changes, weakness or paralysis of limbs, tremor, lack of coordination, poor balance, bladder or bowel changes, and psychological changes.

T-cell A lymphocyte (white blood cell) that develops in the bone marrow, matures in the thymus, and works as part of the immune system in the body.

Tandem gait A test of balance and coordination that involves alternately placing the heel of one foot directly against the toes of the other foot.

Tenotomy An irreversible surgical procedure performed to cut severely contracted tendons attached to muscles that do not respond to any other type of spasticity control and are causing intractable pain and skin complications related to lack of physical movement.

Titubation A form of tremor, resulting from demyelination in the cerebellum, that manifests itself primarily in the head and neck.

Tonic seizure   An intense spasm that lasts for a few minutes and affects one or both limbs on one side of the body. Like other types of paroxysmal symptoms in MS, these spasms occur abruptly and fairly frequently in those individuals who have them, and are similar from one brief episode to the next. The attacks may be triggered by movement or occur spontaneously. *See* Paroxysmal symptom.

Transcutaneous electric nerve stimulation (TENS)   TENS is a nonaddictive and noninvasive method of pain control that applies electric impulses to nerve endings via electrodes that are attached to a stimulator by flexible wires and placed on the skin. The electric impulses block the transmission of pain signals to the brain.

Transurethral resection   A procedure to remove excess thickened tissue at the point of connection between the bladder and the urethra. This thickened tissue, which occasionally develops with the prolonged use of a Foley catheter, obstructs the flow of urine when the catheter is removed. This procedure is quite uncommon and is done mostly in males.

Transverse myelitis   An acute attack of inflammatory demyelination that involves both sides of the spinal cord. The spinal cord loses its ability to transmit nerve impulses up and down. Paralysis and numbness are experienced in the legs and trunk below the level of the inflammation.

Trigeminal neuralgia   Lightning-like, acute pain in the face caused by demyelination of nerve fibers at the site where the sensory (trigeminal) nerve root for that part of the face enters the brainstem.

Urethra   Duct or tube that drains the urinary bladder.

Urinary frequency   Feeling the urge to urinate even when urination has occurred very recently.

Urinary hesitancy   The inability to void urine spontaneously even though the urge to do so is present.

Urinary incontinence   *See* Incontinence.

Urinary sphincter   The muscle closing the urethra, which in a state of flaccid paralysis causes urinary incontinence and in a state of spastic paralysis results in an inability to urinate.

Urinary urgency   The inability to postpone urination once the need to void has been felt.

Urine culture and sensitivity (C & S)   A diagnostic procedure to test for urinary tract infection and identify the appropriate treatment. Bacteria from a mid-stream urine sample is allowed to grow for three days in a laboratory medium and then tested for sensitivity to a variety of antibiotics.

Urologist   A physician who specializes in the branch of medicine (urology) concerned with the anatomy, physiology, disorders, and care of the male and female urinary tract, as well as the male genital tract.

Urology   A medical specialty that deals with disturbances of the urinary (male and female) and reproductive (male) organs.

Vertigo   A dizzying sensation of the environment spinning, often accompanied by nausea and vomiting.

Vibration sense   The ability to feel vibrations against various parts of the body. Vibration sense is tested (with a tuning fork) as part of the sensory portion of the neurologic exam.

Videofluoroscopy   A radiographic study of a person's swallowing mechanism that is recorded on videotape. Videofluoroscopy shows the physiology of the pharynx, the location of the swallowing difficulty, and confirms whether or not food particles or fluids are being aspirated into the airway.

Visual acuity   Clarity of vision. Acuity is measured as a fraction of normal vision. 20/20 vision indicates an eye that sees at 20 feet what a normal eye should see at 20 feet; 20/400 vision indicates an eye that sees at 20 feet what a normal eye sees at 400 feet.

Visual evoked potential   A test in which the brain's electrical activity in response to visual stimuli (e.g., a flashing checkerboard) is recorded by an electroencephalograph and analyzed by computer. Demyelination results in a slowing of response time. Because this test is able to confirm the presence of a suspected brain lesion (area of demyelination) as well as identify the presence of an unsuspected lesion that has produced no symptoms, it is extremely useful in diagnosing MS. VEPs are abnormal in approximately 90 percent of people with MS.

Vocational rehabilitation (VR)   Vocational rehabilitation is a program of services designed to enable people with disabilities to become or remain employed. Originally mandated by the Rehabilitation Act of 1973, VR programs are carried out by individually created state agencies. In order to be eligible for

VR, a person must have a physical or mental disability that results in a substantial handicap to employment. VR programs typically involve evaluation of the disability and need for adaptive equipment or mobility aids, vocational guidance, training, job-placement, and follow-up.

White matter   The part of the brain that contains myelinated nerve fibers and appears white, in contrast to the cortex of the brain, which contains nerve cell bodies and appears gray.

Medications Commonly Used in Multiple Sclerosis

The information sheets are intended as a guide to the drugs commonly used in the treatment and management of multiple sclerosis. They describe the ways in which each medication is most often prescribed in MS, as well as precautions to be noted and the side effects that may occur with their use. Those side effects that could possibly be confused with symptoms of multiple sclerosis are marked with an asterisk. For a more complete discussion of the possible side effects of each drug and its potential interaction with other medications, refer to the package insert that is available from your pharmacist or to one of the drug references listed in Appendix D.

The information contained in these sheets will help you to be more informed about the medications you are taking and therefore more able to discuss your questions and concerns with your physician. This information should never be used as a substitute for your own physician's instructions and recommendations.

The following guidelines apply to the use of any and all of the medications that you take:

◇ Make sure that your physician knows your medical history, including all medical conditions for which you are currently being treated and any allergies you have.

◇ Tell your physician if you are breast-feeding, currently pregnant, or planning to become pregnant in the near future.

◇ Make a list of all of the drugs you are currently taking—including both prescription and over-the-counter medications—and provide your physician with a copy for your medical chart.

◇ Take your medications only as your physician prescribes them for you. If you have questions about the recommended dosage, ask your physician.

◇ Unless otherwise instructed, store medications in a cool, dry place; exposure to heat or moisture may cause the medication to break down. Liquid medications that are stored in the refrigerator should not be allowed to freeze.

◇ Unless otherwise directed by your physician or pharmacist, the general instructions concerning a missed dose of medication are as follows: if you miss a dose, take it as soon as possible. However, if it is almost time for your next dose, skip the one you missed and go back to the regular dosing schedule. Do not double dose.

◇ Keep all medications out of the reach of children.

Index of Medications

Prescription

Alprostadil
Amantadine
Amitriptyline
Baclofen
Carbamazepine
Ciprofloxacin
Clonazepam
Desmopressin
Diazepam
Fluoxetine
Imipramine
Interferon beta-1a
Interferon beta-1b
Meclizine

Methenamine
Methylprednisolone
Oxybutynin
Papavarine
Paroxetine
Pemoline
Phenazopyridine
Phenytoin
Prednisone
Propantheline bromide
Sertraline
Sulfamethoxazole and
    trimethoprim combination

Non-Prescription
(Over-the-Counter)

Bisacodyl (Dulcolax)—
  tablet or suppository
Docusate (Colace)
Docusate mini enema
  (Therevac Plus)
Glycerin suppository
Magnesium hydroxide
  (Phillips' Milk of Magnesia)

Mineral oil
Psyllium hydrophilic
  mucilloid (Metamucil)
Sodium phosphate
  (Fleet Enema)

Chemical Name: Alprostadil (al-**pross**-ta-dill); also called Prostaglandin E1

Brand Name: Prostin VR (U.S. and Canada)

Generic Available: No

Description: Alprostadil belongs to a group of medicines called vasodilators, which cause blood vessels to expand, thereby increasing blood flow. When alprostadil is injected into the penis, it produces an erection by increasing blood flow to the penis.

Proper Usage

◇ Alprostadil should never be used as a sexual aid by men who are not impotent. If improperly used, this medication can cause permanent damage to the penis.

◇ Alprostadil is available by prescription and should be used only as directed by your physician, who will instruct you in the proper way to give yourself an injection so that it is simple and essentially pain-free.

◇ Alprostadil is sometimes used in combination with a medicine called phentolamine (Regitine—U.S.; Rogitine—Canada).

Precautions

◇ Do not use more of this medicine or use it more often than it has been prescribed for you. Using too much of this medicine will result in a condition called priapism, in which the erection lasts too long and does not resolve when it should. Permanent damage to the penis can occur if blood flow to the penis is cut off for too long a period of time.

Possible Side Effects

◇ Side effects that you should report to your physician so he or she can adjust the dosage or change the medication: pain at the injection site; burning or aching during erection.

◇ Rare side effects that require immediate attention: erection continuing for more than four hours. If you cannot be seen immediately by your physician, you should go to the emergency room for prompt treatment.

Chemical Name: Amantadine (a-**man**-ta-deen)

Brand Name: Symmetrel (U.S. and Canada)

Generic Available: Yes (U.S.)

Description: Amantadine is an antiviral medication used to prevent or treat certain influenza infections; it is also given as an adjunct for the treatment of Parkinson's disease. It has been demonstrated that this medication, through some unknown mechanism, is sometimes effective in relieving fatigue in multiple sclerosis.

Proper Usage

◇ The usual dosage for the management of fatigue in MS is 100 to 200 mg daily, taken in the earlier part of the day in order to avoid sleep disturbance. Doses in excess of 300 mg daily usually cause livedo reticularis, a blotchy discoloration of the skin of the legs.

Precautions

The precautions listed here pertain to the use of this medication as an antiviral or Parkinson's disease treatment. There are no reports at this time concerning the precautions in the use of the drug to treat fatigue in multiple sclerosis.

◇ Drinking alcoholic beverages while taking this medication may cause increased side effects such as circulation problems, dizziness, lightheadedness, fainting, or confusion. Do not drink alcohol while taking this medication.

◇ This medication may cause some people to become dizzy, confused, or lightheaded, or to have blurred vision or trouble concentrating.

◇ Amantadine may cause dryness of the mouth and throat. If your mouth continues to feel dry for more than two weeks, check with your physician or dentist since continuing dryness may increase the risk of dental disease.

◇ This medication may cause purplish red, net-like, blotchy spots on the skin. This problem occurs more often in females and usually occurs on the legs and/or feet after amantadine has been taken regularly for a month or more. The blotchy spots usually go away within two to twelve weeks after you stop taking the medication.

◇ Studies of the effects of amantadine in pregnancy have not been done in humans. Studies in some animals have shown that amantadine is harmful to the fetus and causes birth defects.

◇ Amantadine passes into breast milk. However, the effect of amantadine in newborn babies and infants is not known.

Possible Side Effects

The side effects listed here pertain to the use of amantadine as an antiviral or Parkinson's disease treatment. There are no reports at the present time of the side effects associated with the use of this drug in the treatment of MS-related fatigue.

◇ Side effects that may go away as your body adjusts to the medication and do not require medical attention unless they continue or are bothersome: difficulty concentrating; dizziness; headache; irritability; loss of appetite; nausea; nervousness; purplish red, net-like, blotchy spots on skin; trouble sleeping or nightmares; constipation[*]; dryness of the mouth; vomiting.

◇ Rare side effects that should be reported as soon as possible to your physician: blurred vision[*]; confusion; difficult urination[*]; fainting; hallucinations; convulsions; unusual difficulty in coordination[*]; irritation and swelling of the eye; mental depression; skin rash; swelling of feet or lower legs; unexplained shortness of breath.

[*]Since it may be difficult to distinguish between certain common symptoms of MS and some side effects of amantadine, be sure to consult your health care professional if an abrupt change of this type continues for more than a few days.

Chemical Name: Amitriptyline (a-mee-**trip**-ti-leen)

Brand Name: Elavil (U.S. and Canada)

Generic Available: Yes (U.S. and Canada)

Description: Amitriptyline is a tricyclic antidepressant used to treat mental depression. In multiple sclerosis, it is frequently used to treat painful paresthesias in the arms and legs (e.g., burning sensations, pins and needles, stabbing pains) caused by damage to the pain regulating pathways of the brain and spinal cord.

Note: Other tricyclic antidepressants are also used for the management of neurologic pain symptoms. Clomipramine (Anafranil—U.S. and Canada), desipramine (Norpramin—U.S. and Canada), doxepin (Sinequan—U.S. and Canada), imipramine (Tofranil—U.S. and Canada), nortriptyline (Pamelor— U.S.; Aventyl—Canada), trimipramine (U.S. and Canada). While each of these medications is given in different dosage levels, the precautions and side effects listed for amitriptyline apply to these other tricyclic medications as well.

Precautions

◇ Amitriptyline adds to the effects of alcohol and other central nervous system depressants (e.g., antihistamines, sedatives, tranquilizers, prescription pain medications, seizure medications, muscle relaxants, sleeping medications), possibly causing drowsiness. Be sure that your physician knows if you are taking these or other medications.

◇ This medication causes dryness of the mouth. Because continuing dryness of the mouth may increase the risk of dental disease, alert your dentist that you are taking amitriptyline.

◇ This medication may cause your skin to be more sensitive to sunlight than it is normally. Even brief exposure to sunlight may cause a skin rash, itching, redness or other discoloration of the skin, or severe sunburn.

◇ This medication may affect blood sugar levels of diabetic individuals. If you notice a change in the results of your blood or urine sugar tests, check with your physician.

◇ Do not stop taking this medication without consulting your physician. The physician may want you to reduce the amount you are taking gradually in order to reduce the possibility of withdrawal symptoms such as headache, nausea, and/or an overall feeling of discomfort.

◇ Studies of amitriptyline have not been done in pregnant women. There have been reports of newborns suffering from muscle spasms and heart, breathing, and urinary problems when their mothers had taken tricyclic antidepressants immediately before delivery. Studies in animals have indicated the possibility of unwanted effects in the fetus.

◇ Tricyclics pass into breast milk. Only doxepin (Sinequan) has been reported to cause drowsiness in the nursing baby.

Possible Side Effects

◇ Side effects that may go away as your body adjusts to the medication and do not require medical attention unless they continue for more than two weeks or are bothersome: dryness of mouth; constipation*; increased appetite and weight gain; dizziness; drowsiness*; decreased sexual ability*; headache; nausea; unusual tiredness or weakness*; unpleasant taste; diarrhea; heartburn; increased sweating; vomiting.

◇ Uncommon side effects that should be reported to your physician as soon as possible: blurred vision*; confusion or delirium; difficulty speaking or swallowing*; eye pain*; fainting; hallucinations: loss of balance control*; nervousness or restlessness; problems urinating*; shakiness or trembling; stiffness of arms and legs*.

◇ Rare side effects that should be reported to your physician as soon as possible: anxiety; breast enlargement in males and females; hair loss; inappropriate secretion of milk in females; increased sensitivity to sunlight; irritability; muscle twitching; red or brownish spots on the skin; buzzing or other unexplained sounds in the ears; skin rash, itching; sore throat and fever; swelling of face and tongue; weakness*; yellow skin.

◇ Symptoms of acute overdose: confusion; convulsions; severe drowsiness*; enlarged pupils; unusual heartbeat; fever; hallucinations; restlessness and agitation; shortness of breath; unusual tiredness or weakness; vomiting.

---

*Since it may be difficult to distinguish between certain common symptoms of MS and some side effects of amitriptyline, be sure to consult your health care professional if an abrupt change of this type occurs.

Chemical Name: Baclofen (**bak**-loe-fen)
Brand Name: Lioresal (U.S. and Canada)
Generic Available: Yes (U.S. and Canada)
Description: Baclofen acts on the central nervous system to relieve spasms, cramping, and tightness of muscles caused by spasticity in multiple sclerosis. It is usually administered orally in pill form. Recently, an intrathecal delivery system (via a surgically implanted pump) has been approved for those individuals with significant spasticity who cannot tolerate a sufficiently high dose of the oral form of the medication.

Proper Usage

◇ People with MS are usually started on an initial dose of 5 mg every six to eight hours. If necessary, the amount is increased by 5 mg per dose every five days until symptoms improve. The goal of treatment is to find a dosage level that relieves spasticity without causing excessive weakness or fatigue. The effective dose may vary from 15 mg to 160 mg per day or more.

Precautions

◇ If you are taking more than 30 mg daily, do not stop taking this medication suddenly. Stopping high doses of this medication abruptly can cause convulsions, hallucinations, increases in muscle spasms or cramping, mental changes, or unusual nervousness or restlessness. Consult your physician about how to reduce the dosage gradually before stopping the medication completely.

◇ This drug adds to the effects of alcohol and other CNS depressants (such as antihistamines, sedatives, tranquilizers, prescription pain medications, seizure medications, other muscle relaxants), possibly causing drowsiness. Be sure that your physician knows if you are taking these or other medications.

◇ Studies of birth defects with baclofen have not been done with humans. Studies in animals have shown that baclofen, when given in doses several times higher than the amount given to humans, increases the chance of hernias, incomplete or slow development of bones in the fetus, and lower birth weight.

◇ Baclofen passes into the breast milk of nursing mothers but has not been reported to cause problems in nursing infants.

Possible Side Effects

◇ Side effects that typically go away as your body adjusts to the medication and do not require medical attention unless they continue for several weeks or are bothersome: drowsiness or unusual tiredness[*]; increased weakness[*]; dizziness or lightheadedness; confusion; unusual constipation[*]; new or unusual bladder symptoms[*]; trouble sleeping; unusual unsteadiness or clumsiness[*].

◇ Unusual side effects that require immediate medical attention: fainting; hallucinations; severe mood changes; skin rash or itching.

◇ Symptoms of overdose: sudden onset of blurred or double vision[*]; convulsions; shortness of breath or troubled breathing; vomiting.

---

[*]Since it may be difficult to distinguish between certain common symptoms of MS and some side effects of baclofen, be sure to consult your health care professional if an abrupt change of this type occurs.

Chemical Name: Bisacodyl (bis-a-**koe**-dill)

Brand Name: Dulcolax—tablet or suppository (U.S.); Bisacolax—tablet or suppository (Canada)

Generic Available: Yes (U.S. and Canada)

Description: Bisacodyl is an over-the-counter stimulant laxative that can be used in either oral or suppository form. Stimulant laxatives encourage bowel movements by increasing the muscle contractions in the intestinal wall that propel the stool mass. Although stimulant laxatives are popular for self-treatment, they are more likely to cause side effects than other types of laxatives.

Proper Usage

◇ Laxatives are to be used to provide short-term relief only, unless otherwise directed by the nurse or physician who is helping you to manage your bowel symptoms. A regimen that includes a healthy diet containing roughage (whole grain breads and cereals, bran, fruit, and green, leafy vegetables), six to eight full glasses of liquids each day, and some form of daily exercise is most important in stimulating healthy bowel function.

◇ If your physician has recommended this laxative for management of constipation, follow his or her recommendations for its use. If you are treating yourself for constipation, follow the directions on the package insert.

◇ The tablet form of this laxative is usually taken on an empty stomach in order to speed results. The tablets are coated to allow them to work properly without causing stomach irritation or upset. Do not chew or crush the tablets or take them within an hour of drinking milk or taking an antacid.

◇ A bedtime dose usually produces results the following morning. Be sure to consult your physician if you experience problems or do not get relief within a week.

Precautions

◇ Do not take any laxative if you have signs of appendicitis or inflamed bowel (e.g., stomach or lower abdominal pain, cramping, bloating, soreness, nausea, or vomiting). Check with your physician as soon as possible.

◇ Do not take any laxative for more than one week unless you have been told to do so by your physician. Many people tend to overuse laxatives, which often leads to dependence on the laxative action to produce a bowel movement. Discuss the use of laxatives with your health care professional in order to ensure that the laxative is used effectively as part of a comprehensive, healthy bowel management regimen.

◇ Do not take any laxative within two hours of taking other medication because the desired effectiveness of the other medication may be reduced.

◇ If you are pregnant, discuss with your physician the most appropriate type of laxative for you to use.

◇ Some laxatives pass into breast milk. Although it is unlikely to cause problems for a nursing infant, be sure to let your physician know if you are using a laxative and breast-feeding at the same time.

Possible Side Effects

◇ Side effects that may go away as your body adjusts to the medication and do not require medical attention unless they persist or are bothersome: belching; cramping; diarrhea; nausea.

◇ Unusual side effects that should be reported to your physician as soon as possible: confusion; irregular heartbeat; muscle cramps; skin rash, unusual tiredness or weakness.

Chemical Name: Carbamazepine (kar-ba-**maz**-e-peen)
Brand Name: Tegretol (U.S. and Canada)
Generic Available: Yes (U.S.)
Description: Carbamazepine is used to relieve shock-like pain, such as the facial pain caused by trigeminal neuralgia (tic douloureux).

Proper Usage

◇ It is very important that you take this medicine exactly as directed by your physician in order to obtain the best results and lessen the chance of serious side effects.

◇ Carbamazepine is not an ordinary pain reliever. It should be used only when your physician prescribes it for certain types of pain. Do not take this medication for other aches or pains.

◇ If you miss a dose of this medication, take it as soon as possible. If it is almost time for your next dose, skip the missed dose and go back to your regular dosing schedule. Do not double dose. If you miss more than one dose in a day, check with your physician.

◇ It is very important that your physician check your progress at regular intervals. Your physician may want to have certain tests done to see if you are receiving the correct amount of medication or to check for certain side effects of which you might be unaware.

Precautions

◇ Carbamazepine adds to the effects of alcohol and other central nervous system depressants that may cause drowsiness (e.g., antihistamines, sedatives, tranquilizers, prescription pain medications, seizure medications, muscle relaxants). Be sure that your physician knows if you are taking these or other medications.

◇ Some people who take carbamazepine may become more sensitive to sunlight than they are normally. Exposure to sunlight, even for brief periods of time, may cause a skin rash, itching, redness or other discoloration of the skin, or severe sunburn.

◇ Oral contraceptives (birth control pills) that contain estrogen may not work properly while you are taking carbamazepine. You should use an additional or alternative form of birth control while taking this drug.

◇ Carbamazepine affects the urine sugar levels of diabetic patients. If you notice a change in the results of your urine sugar tests, check with your physician.

◇ Before having any medical tests or any kind of surgical, dental, or emergency treatment, be sure to let the health care professional know that you are taking this medication.

◇ Carbamazepine has not been studied in pregnant women. There have been reports of babies having low birth weight, small head size, skull and facial defects, underdeveloped fingernails, and delays in growth when their mothers had taken carbamazepine in high doses during pregnancy. Studies in animals have shown that carbamazepine causes birth defects when given in large doses.

◇ Carbamazepine passes into breast milk, and the baby may receive enough of it to cause unwanted effects. In animal studies, carbamazepine has affected the growth and appearance of nursing babies.

Possible Side Effects

◇ Side effects that typically go away as your body adjusts to the medication and do not require medical attention unless they continue for several weeks or are bothersome: clumsiness or unsteadiness*; mild dizziness*; mild drowsiness*; lightheadedness; mild nausea or vomiting; aching joints or muscles; constipation*; diarrhea; dryness of mouth; skin sensitivity to sunlight; irritation of mouth or tongue; loss or appetite; loss of hair; muscle or abdominal cramps; sexual problems in males*.

◇ Check with your physician as soon as possible if any of the following side effects occur: blurred or double vision*; confusion; agitation; severe diarrhea, nausea, or vomiting; skin rash or hives; unusual drowsiness; chest pain; difficulty speaking or slurred speech*; fainting; frequent urination*; unusual heartbeat; mental depression or other mood or emotional changes; unusual numbness, tingling, pain, or weakness in hands or feet*; ringing or buzzing in ears; sudden decrease in urination; swelling of face, hands, feet, or lower legs; trembling; uncontrolled body movements; visual hallucinations.

◇ Check with your physician immediately if any of the following occur: black tarry stools or blood in urine or stools; bone or joint pain; cough or hoarseness; darkening of urine; nosebleeds or other unusual bleeding or bruising; painful or difficult urination; tenderness, swelling, or bluish color in leg or foot; pale stools; pinpoint red spots on skin; shortness of breath or cough; sores, ulcers, or white spots on lips or in the mouth; sore throat, chills, and fever; swollen glands; unusual tiredness or weakness[*]; wheezing, tightness in chest; yellow eyes or skin.

◇ Symptoms of overdose that require immediate attention: unusual clumsiness or unsteadiness[*]; severe dizziness or fainting; fast or irregular heartbeat; unusually high or low blood pressure; irregular or shallow breathing; severe nausea or vomiting; trembling, twitching, and abnormal body movements.

[*]Since it may be difficult to distinguish between certain common symptoms of MS and some side effects of carbamazepine, be sure to consult your health care professional if an abrupt change of this type occurs.

Chemical Name: Ciprofloxacin (sip-roe-**flox**-a-sin) combination
Brand Name: Cipro (U.S. and Canada)
Generic Available: No
Description: Ciprofloxacin is one of a group of antibiotics (fluoroquinolones) used to kill bacterial infection in many parts of the body. It is used in multiple sclerosis primarily to treat urinary tract infections.

Proper Usage

◇ This medication is best taken with a full glass (eight ounces) of water. Additional water should be taken each day to help prevent some unwanted effects.

◇ Ciprofloxacin may be taken with meals or on an empty stomach.

◇ Finish the full course of treatment prescribed by your physician. Even if your symptoms disappear after a few days, stopping this medication prematurely may result in a return of the symptoms.

◇ This medication works most effectively when it is maintained at a constant level in your blood or urine. To help keep the amount constant, do not miss a dose. It is best to take the doses at evenly spaced times during the day and night.

Precautions

◇ This medication may cause some people to become dizzy, lightheaded, drowsy, or less alert.

◇ If you are taking antacids that contain aluminum or magnesium, be sure to take them at least two hours before or after you take ciprofloxacin. These antacids may prevent the ciprofloxacin from working properly.

◇ This medication may cause your skin to become more sensitive to sunlight. Stay out of direct sunlight during the midday hours, wear protective clothing, and apply a sun block product that has a skin protection factor (SPF) of at least 15.

◇ Studies of birth defects have not been done in humans. This medication is not recommended during pregnancy since antibiotics of this type have been reported to cause bone development problems in young animals.

◇ Some of the antibiotics in this group are known to pass into human breast milk. Since they have been reported to cause bone development problems in young animals, breast-feeding is not recommended during treatment with this medication.

Possible Side Effects

◇ Side effects that may go away as your body adjusts to the medication and do not require medical attention unless they continue or are bothersome: abdominal or stomach pain; diarrhea; dizziness; drowsiness*; headache; light-headedness; nausea or vomiting; nervousness; trouble sleeping.

◇ Rare side effects that should be reported to your physician immediately: agitation; confusion; fever; hallucinations; peeling of the skin; shakiness or tremors*; shortness of breath; skin rash; itching; swelling of face or neck.

---

*Since it may be difficult to distinguish between certain common symptoms of MS and some side effects of ciprofloxacin, be sure to consult your health care professional if an abrupt change of this type occurs.

Chemical Name: Clonazepam (kloe-**na**-ze-pam)

Brand Name: Klonopin (U.S.); Rivotril; Syn-Clonazepam (Canada)

Generic Available: No

Description: Clonazepam is a benzodiazepine that belongs to the group of medications called central nervous system depressants, which slow down the nervous system. Although clonazepam is used for a variety of medical conditions, it is used in multiple sclerosis primarily for the treatment of tremor, pain, and spasticity.

Proper Usage

◇ Keep this medication out of the reach of children. An overdose of this medication may be especially dangerous for children.

Precautions

◇ During the first few months taking clonazepam, your physician should check your progress at regular visits to make sure that this medicine does not cause unwanted effects.

◇ Take this medication only as directed by your physician; do not increase the dose without a prescription to do so.

◇ Clonazepam adds to the effects of alcohol and other central nervous system depressants (e.g., antihistamines, sedatives, tranquilizers, prescription pain medications, seizure medications, muscle relaxants, sleeping medications). Consult your physician before taking any of these CNS depressants while you are taking clonazepam. Taking an overdose of this medication or taking it with alcohol or other CNS depressants may lead to unconsciousness and possibly death.

◇ Stopping this medication suddenly may cause withdrawal side effects. Reduce the amount gradually before stopping completely.

◇ Clonazepam frequently causes people to become drowsy, dizzy, lightheaded, clumsy, or unsteady. Even if taken at bedtime, it may cause some people to feel drowsy or less alert on awakening.

◇ Studies in animals have shown that clonazepam can cause birth defects or other problems, including death of the animal fetus.

◇ Overuse of clonazepam during pregnancy may cause the baby to become dependent on it, leading to withdrawal side effects after birth. The use of clonazepam, especially during the last weeks of pregnancy, may cause breathing problems, muscle weakness, difficulty in feeding, and body temperature problems in the newborn infant.

◇ Clonazepam may pass into breast milk and cause drowsiness, slow heartbeat, shortness of breath, or troubled breathing in nursing babies.

Possible Side Effects

◇ Side effects that may go away during treatment as your body adjusts to the medication and do not require medical attention unless they continue for several weeks or are bothersome: drowsiness or tiredness; clumsiness or unsteadiness*; dizziness or lightheadedness; slurred speech*; abdominal cramps or pain; blurred vision or other changes in vision*; changes in sexual drive or performance*; gastrointestinal changes, including constipation* or diarrhea; dryness of mouth; fast or pounding heartbeat; muscle spasm*; trouble with urination*; trembling.

◇ Unusual side effects that should be discussed as soon as possible with your physician: behavior problems, including difficulty concentrating and outbursts of anger; confusion or mental depression; convulsions; hallucinations; low blood pressure; muscle weakness; skin rash or itching; sore throat, fever, chills; unusual bleeding or bruising; unusual excitement or irritability.

◇ Symptoms of overdose that require immediate emergency help: continuing confusion; severe drowsiness; shakiness; slowed heartbeat; shortness of breath; slow reflexes; continuing slurred speech*; staggering*; unusual severe weakness*.

---

*Since it may be difficult to distinguish between certain common symptoms of MS and some side effects of clonazepam, be sure to consult your health care professional if an abrupt change of this type occurs.

Chemical Name: Desmopressin (des-moe-**press**-in)

Brand Name: DDAVP Nasal Spray (U.S. and Canada)

Generic Available: No

Description: Desmopressin is a hormone used as a nasal spray. The hormone works on the kidneys to control frequent urination.

Proper Usage

◇ Keep this medication in the refrigerator but do not allow it to freeze.

Precautions

◇ Let your physician know if you have heart disease, blood vessel disease, or high blood pressure. Desmopressin can cause an increase in blood pressure.

◇ Studies have not been done in pregnant women. It has been used before and during pregnancy to treat diabetes mellitus and has not been shown to cause birth defects.

◇ Desmopressin passes into breast milk but has not been reported to cause problems in nursing infants.

Possible Side Effects

◇ Side effects that typically go away as your body adjusts to the medication and do not require medical attention unless they continue for several weeks or are bothersome: runny or stuffy nose; abdominal or stomach cramps; flushing of the skin; headache; nausea; pain in the vulva.

◇ Unusual side effects that require immediate medical attention: confusion; convulsions; unusual drowsiness[*]; continuing headache; rapid weight gain; markedly decreased urination.

[*]Since it may be difficult to distinguish between certain common symptoms of MS and some side effects of desmopressin, be sure to consult your health care professional if an abrupt change of this type occurs.

Chemical Name: Diazepam (dye-**az**-e-pam)
Brand Name: Valium (U.S. and Canada)
Generic Available: Yes (U.S.)
Description: Diazepam is a benzodiazepine that belongs to the group of medicines called central nervous system depressants, which slow down the nervous system. Although diazepam is used for a variety of medical conditions, it is used in multiple sclerosis primarily for the relief of muscle spasms and spasticity.

Proper Usage

◇ Keep this medication out of the reach of children. An overdose of this medication may be especially dangerous for children.

Precautions

◇ Your physician should check your progress at regular visits to make sure that this medication does not cause unwanted effects.

◇ Take diazepam only as directed by your physician; do not increase the dose without a prescription to do so.

◇ Diazepam adds to the effects of alcohol and other central nervous system depressants (e.g., antihistamines, sedatives, tranquilizers, prescription pain medications, seizure medications, muscle relaxants, sleeping medications). Consult your physician before taking any of these CNS depressants while you are taking diazepam. Taking an overdose of this medication or taking it with alcohol or other CNS depressants may lead to unconsciousness and possibly death.

◇ Stopping this medication suddenly may cause withdrawal side effects. Reduce the amount gradually before stopping completely.

◇ Diazepam may cause some people to become drowsy, dizzy, lightheaded, clumsy, or unsteady. Even if taken at bedtime, it may cause some people to feel drowsy or less alert on awakening.

◇ The use of diazepam during the first three months of pregnancy has been reported to increase the chance of birth defects.

◇ Overuse of diazepam during pregnancy may cause the baby to become dependent on the medicine, leading to withdrawal side effects after birth. The use of diazepam, especially during the last weeks of pregnancy, may cause breathing problems, muscle weakness, difficulty in feeding, and body temperature problems in the newborn infant. When diazepam is given in high doses (especially by injection) within fifteen hours before delivery, it may cause breathing problems, muscle weakness, difficulty in feeding, and body temperature problems in the newborn infant.

◇ Diazepam may pass into breast milk and cause drowsiness, slow heartbeat, shortness of breath, or troubled breathing in nursing babies.

Possible Side Effects

◇ Side effects that may go away during treatment as your body adjusts to the medication and do not require medical attention unless they continue for several weeks or are bothersome: clumsiness or unsteadiness*; dizziness or lightheadedness; slurred speech*; abdominal cramps or pain; blurred vision or other changes in vision*; changes in sexual drive or performance*; constipation*; diarrhea; dryness of mouth; fast or pounding heartbeat; muscle spasm*; trouble with urination*; trembling*; unusual tiredness or weakness*.

◇ Unusual side effects that should be discussed with your physician as soon as possible: behavior problems, including difficulty concentrating and outbursts of anger; confusion or mental depression; convulsions; hallucinations; low blood pressure; muscle weakness*; skin rash or itching; sore throat, fever, chills; unusual bleeding or bruising; unusual excitement or irritability.

◇ Symptoms of overdose that require immediate emergency help: continuing confusion; unusually severe drowsiness; shakiness; slowed heartbeat; shortness of breath; slow reflexes; continuing slurred speech; staggering; unusually severe weakness*.

---

*Since it may be difficult to distinguish between certain common symptoms of MS and some side effects of desmopressin, be sure to consult your health care professional if an abrupt change of this type occurs.

Chemical Name: Docusate (**doe**-koo-sate)

Brand Name: Colace (U.S. and Canada)

Generic Available: Yes (U.S. and Canada)

Description: Docusate is an over-the-counter stool softener (emollient) that helps liquids to mix into dry, hardened stool, making the stool easier to pass.

Proper Usage

◇ Laxatives are to be used to provide short-term relief only, unless otherwise directed by the nurse or physician who is helping you to manage your bowel symptoms. A regimen that includes a healthy diet containing roughage (whole grain breads and cereals, bran, fruit, and green, leafy vegetables), six to eight full glasses of liquids each day, and some form of daily exercise is most important in stimulating healthy bowel function.

◇ If your physician has recommended this laxative for management of constipation, follow his or her recommendations for its use. If you are treating yourself for constipation, follow the directions on the package insert.

◇ Results usually occur one to two days after the first dose; some individuals may not get results for three to five days. Be sure to consult your physician if you experience problems or do not get relief within a week.

Precautions

◇ Do not take any type of laxative if you have signs of appendicitis or inflamed bowel (e.g., stomach or lower abdominal pain, cramping, bloating, soreness, nausea, or vomiting). Check with your physician as soon as possible.

◇ Do not take any laxative for more than one week unless you have been told to do so by your physician. Many people tend to overuse laxatives, which often leads to dependence on the laxative action to produce a bowel movement. Discuss the use of laxatives with your health care professional in order to ensure that the laxative is used effectively as part of a comprehensive, healthy bowel management regimen.

◇ Do not take mineral oil within two hours of taking docusate. The docusate may increase the amount of mineral oil that is absorbed by the body.

◇ Do not take any laxative within two hours of taking another medication because the desired effectiveness of the other medication may be reduced.

◇ If you are pregnant, discuss with your physician the most appropriate type of laxative for you to use.

◇ Some laxatives pass into breast milk. Although it is unlikely to cause problems for a nursing infant, be sure to let your physician know if you are using a laxative and breast-feeding at the same time.

Possible Side Effects

◇ Side effects that may go away as your body adjusts to the medication and do not require medical attention unless they persist or are bothersome: stomach and/or intestinal cramping.

◇ Unusual side effect that should be reported to your physician as soon as possible: skin rash.

Chemical Name: Docusate (**doe**-koo-sate) mini enema
Brand Name: Therevac Plus (U.S.)
Generic Available: No
Description: Therevac Plus is an over-the counter stool softener
    (emollient) that comes in a plastic, single-dose, two-inch
    ampule for insertion into the rectum. It works to produce
    bowel movements in a short time by helping liquids to mix
    into dry, hardened stool, making the stool easier to pass. The
    small size of this enema makes it easy to use without compro-
    mising its effectiveness.

Proper Usage

◇ Laxatives are to be used to provide short-term relief only,
    unless otherwise directed by the nurse or physician who is
    helping you to manage your bowel symptoms. A regimen
    that includes a healthy diet containing roughage (whole
    grain breads and cereals, bran, fruit, and green, leafy veg-
    etables), 6 to 8 full glasses of liquids each day, and some
    form of daily exercise, is most important in stimulating
    healthy bowel function.

◇ If your physician has recommended this laxative for man-
    agement of constipation, follow his or her recommenda-
    tions for its use. If you are treating yourself for constipa-
    tion, follow the directions on the package insert.

◇ Results usually occur fifteen minutes to one hour after
    insertion. Be sure to consult your physician if you experi-
    ence problems or do not get relief within a day or two.

Precautions

◇ Do not use any type of laxative if you have signs of appen-
    dicitis or inflamed bowel (e.g., stomach or lower abdomi-
    nal pain, cramping, bloating, soreness, nausea, or vomit-
    ing). Check with your physician as soon as possible.

◇ Do not take any laxative for more than one week unless you
    have been told to do so by your physician. Many people
    tend to overuse laxatives, which often leads to dependence
    on the laxative action to produce a bowel movement.
    Discuss the use of laxatives with your health care profes-
    sional in order to ensure that the laxative is used effective-

ly as part of a comprehensive, healthy bowel management regimen.

◇ If you are pregnant, discuss with your physician the most appropriate type of laxative for you to use.

Possible Side Effects

◇ Side effect that may go away as your body adjusts to the medication and does not require medical attention unless it persists or is bothersome: skin irritation surrounding the rectal area.

◇ Less common side effects that should be reported to your physician: rectal bleeding, blistering, burning, itching, or pain.

Chemical Name: Fluoxetine (floo-**ox**-uh-teen)

Brand Name: Prozac (U.S. and Canada)

Generic Available: No

Description: Fluoxetine is used to treat mental depression. It is also used occasionally to treat MS fatigue.

Proper Usage

◇ This medication should be taken in the morning when used to treat depression because it can interfere with sleep. If it upsets your stomach, you may take it with food.

Precautions

◇ It may take four to six weeks for you to feel the beneficial effects of this medication.

◇ Your physician should monitor your progress at regularly scheduled visits in order to adjust the dose and help reduce any side effects.

◇ There have been suggestions that the use of fluoxetine may be related to increased thoughts about suicide in a very small number of individuals. More study is needed to determine if the medicine causes this effect. If you have concerns about this, be sure to discuss them with your physician.

◇ Fluoxetine adds to the effects of alcohol and other central nervous system depressants (e.g., antihistamines, sedatives, tranquilizers, sleeping medicine, prescription pain medicine, barbiturates, seizure medication, muscle relaxants). Be sure that your physician knows if you are taking these or any other medications.

◇ This medication affects the blood sugar levels of diabetic individuals. Check with your physician if you notice any changes in your blood or urine sugar tests.

◇ Dizziness or lightheadedness may occur, especially when you get up from a lying or sitting position. Change positions slowly to help alleviate this problem. If the problem continues or gets worse, consult your physician.

◇ Fluoxetine may cause dryness of the mouth. If your mouth continues to feel dry for more than two weeks, check with your physician or dentist. Continuing dryness of the mouth may increase the chance of dental disease.

◇ Studies have not been done in pregnant women. Fluoxetine has not been shown to cause birth defects or other problems in animal studies.

◇ Fluoxetine passes into breast milk and may cause unwanted effects, such as vomiting, watery stools, crying, and sleep problems in nursing babies. You may want to discuss alternative medications with your physician.

Possible Side Effects

◇ Side effects that may go away as your body adjusts to the medication and do not require medical attention unless they continue for several weeks or are bothersome: decreased sexual drive or ability*; anxiety and nervousness; diarrhea; drowsiness*; headache; trouble sleeping; abnormal dreams; change in vision*; chest pain; decreased appetite; decrease in concentration; dizziness; dry mouth; fast or irregular heartbeat; frequent urination*; menstrual pain; tiredness or weakness*; tremor*; vomiting.

◇ Unusual side effects that should be discussed with your physician as soon as possible: chills or fever; joint or muscle pain; skin rash; hives or itching; trouble breathing.

◇ Symptoms of overdose that require immediate medical attention: agitation and restlessness; convulsions; severe nausea and vomiting; unusual excitement.

---

*Since it may be difficult to distinguish between certain common symptoms of MS and some side effects of fluoxetine, be sure to consult your health care professional if an abrupt change of this type occurs.

Chemical Name: Glycerin (**gli**-ser-in)

Brand Name: Sani-Supp suppository (U.S.)

Generic Available: Yes (U.S. and Canada)

Description: A glycerin suppository is a hyperosmotic laxative that draws water into the bowel from surrounding body tissues. This water helps to soften the stool mass and promote bowel action.

Proper Usage

◇ Laxatives are to be used to provide short-term relief only, unless otherwise directed by the nurse or physician who is helping you to manage your bowel symptoms. A regimen that includes a healthy diet containing roughage (whole grain breads and cereals, bran, fruit, and green, leafy vegetables), six to eight full glasses of liquids each day, and some form of daily exercise is most important in stimulating healthy bowel function.

◇ If your physician has recommended this laxative for management of constipation, follow his or her recommendations for its use. If you are treating yourself for constipation, follow the directions on the package insert.

◇ If the suppository is too soft to insert, refrigerate it for thirty minutes or hold it under cold water before removing the foil wrapper.

◇ Glycerin suppositories often produce results within fifteen minutes to one hour. Be sure to consult your physician if you experience problems or do not get relief within a week.

Precautions

◇ Do not take any type of laxative if you have signs of appendicitis or inflamed bowel (e.g., stomach or lower abdominal pain, cramping, bloating, soreness, nausea, or vomiting). Check with your physician as soon as possible.

◇ Do not take any laxative for more than one week unless you have been told to do so by your physician. Many people tend to overuse laxatives, which often leads to dependence on the laxative action to produce a bowel movement. Discuss the use of laxatives with your health care professional in order to ensure that the laxative is used effectively as part of a comprehensive, healthy bowel management regimen.

◇ If you are pregnant, discuss with your physician the most appropriate type of laxative for you to use.

◇ Use only water to moisten the suppository prior to insertion in the rectum. Do not lubricate the suppository with mineral oil or petroleum jelly, which might affect the way the suppository works.

Possible Side Effects

◇ Side effects that may go away as your body adjusts to the medication and do not require medical attention unless they persist or are bothersome: skin irritation around the rectal area.

◇ Less common side effects that should be reported to your physician as soon as possible: rectal bleeding; blistering, or itching.

Chemical Name: Imipramine (im-**ip**-ra-meen)
Brand Name: Tofranil (U.S. and Canada)
Generic Available: Yes (U.S. and Canada)
Description: Imipramine is a tricyclic antidepressant used to treat mental depression. Its primary use in multiple sclerosis is to treat bladder symptoms, including urinary frequency and incontinence. Imipramine is also prescribed occasionally for the management of neurologic pain in MS.

Proper Usage

◇ To lessen stomach upset, take this medication with food, even for a daily bedtime dose, unless your physician has told you to take it on an empty stomach.

Precautions

◇ Imipramine adds to the effects of alcohol and other central nervous system depressants (e.g., antihistamines, sedatives, tranquilizers, prescription pain medications, seizure medications, muscle relaxants, sleeping medications), possibly causing drowsiness. Be sure that your physician knows if you are taking these or any other medications.

◇ This medication causes dryness of the mouth. Because continuing dryness of the mouth can increase the risk of dental disease, alert your dentist if you are taking imipramine.

◇ Imipramine may cause your skin to be more sensitive to sunlight than it is normally. Even brief exposure to sunlight may cause a skin rash, itching, redness or other discoloration of the skin, or severe sunburn. Stay out of the sun during the midday hours. Wear protective clothing and a sun block that has a skin protection factor (SPF) of at least 15.

◇ This medication may affect blood sugar levels of diabetic individuals. If you notice a change in the results of your blood or urine sugar tests, check with your physician.

◇ Do not stop taking imipramine without consulting your physician. The physician may want you to reduce the amount you are taking gradually in order to reduce the possibility of withdrawal symptoms such as headache, nausea, and/or an overall feeling of discomfort.

◇ Studies of imipramine have not been done in pregnant women. There have been reports of newborns suffering

from muscle spasms and heart, breathing, and urinary problems when their mothers had taken tricyclic antidepressants immediately before delivery. Studies in animals have
indicated the possibility of unwanted effects in the fetus.

◇ Imipramine passes into breast milk but has not been
reported to have any effect on the nursing infant.

Possible Side Effects

◇ Side effects that may go away as your body adjusts to the
medication and do not require medical attention unless
they continue for more than two weeks or are bothersome:
dizziness; drowsiness*; headache; decreased sexual
ability*; increased appetite; nausea; unusual tiredness or
weakness*; unpleasant taste; diarrhea; heartburn; increased
sweating; vomiting.

◇ Uncommon side effects that should be reported to your
physician as soon as possible: blurred vision*; confusion or
delirium; constipation*; difficulty speaking or swallowing;
eye pain*; fainting; fast or irregular heartbeat; hallucinations; loss of balance control*; nervousness or restlessness;
problems urinating*; shakiness or trembling; stiffness of
arms and legs*.

◇ Rare side effects that should be reported to your physician
as soon as possible: anxiety; breast enlargement in males
and females; hair loss; inappropriate secretion of milk in
females; increased sensitivity to sunlight; irritability; muscle twitching; red or brownish spots on the skin; buzzing or
other unexplained sounds in the ears; skin rash; itching;
sore throat and fever; swelling of face and tongue; weakness*; yellow skin.

◇ Symptoms of acute overdose: confusion; convulsions;
severe drowsiness*; enlarged pupils; unusual heartbeat;
fever; hallucinations; restlessness and agitation; shortness
of breath; unusual tiredness or weakness*; vomiting.

---

*Since it may be difficult to distinguish between certain common
symptoms of MS and some side effects of imipramine, be sure to consult your health care professional if an abrupt change of this type
occurs.

Chemical Name: Interferon beta-1a

Brand Name: Avonex (U.S.—approval in Canada is pending)

Generic Available: No

Description: Avonex is a medication manufactured by a biotechnological process from one of the naturally occurring interferons (a type of protein). It is made up of exactly the same amino acids (major components of proteins) as the natural interferon beta found in the human body. In a clinical trial of 380 ambulatory patients with relapsing-remitting MS, those taking the currently recommended dose of the medication had a reduced risk of disability progression, experienced fewer exacerbations, and showed a reduction in number and size of active lesions in the brain (as shown on MRI) when compared with the group taking a placebo.

Proper Usage

◇ Avonex is given as a once-a-week intramuscular (IM) injection, usually in the large muscles of the thigh, upper arm, or hip. If your physician decides that you or a care partner can safely administer the injection, you will be taught how to reconstitute the medication (mix the sterile powder with the sterile water that is packaged with it) and instructed in safe and proper IM injection procedures. If you are unable to self-inject, and have no family member or friend available to do the injections, the injections will be given by your physician or nurse. Do not attempt to mix the medication or inject yourself until you are sure that you understand the procedures.

◇ Avonex must be kept cold. Be sure to store it in a refrigerator both before and after the medication is mixed for injection. Do not expose the medication to high temperatures (in a glove compartment or on a window sill, for example) and do not allow it to freeze. Once the medication has been mixed for use, it is recommended that you administer the injection as soon as possible; the reconstituted powder should not be used once it has been stored in the refrigerator longer than six hours.

◇ Do not reuse needles or syringes. Dispose of the syringes as directed by your physician and keep them out of the reach of children.

◇ Since flu-like symptoms are a fairly common side effect during the initial weeks of treatment, it is recommended

that the injection be given at bedtime. Taking acetaminophen (Tylenol®) or ibuprofen (Advil®) immediately
prior to each injection and during the 24 hours following
the injection will also help to relieve the flu-like symptoms.

Precautions

◇ Avonex should not be used during pregnancy or by any
woman who is trying to become pregnant. Women taking
Avonex should use birth control measures at all times. If
you want to become pregnant while being treated with
Avonex, discuss the matter with your physician. If you
become pregnant while using Avonex, stop the treatment
and contact your physician.

◇ There was no increase in depression reported by people
receiving Avonex in the clinical trial. However, since
depression and suicidal thoughts are known to occur with
some frequency in MS, and depression and suicidal
thoughts have been reported with high doses of various
interferon products, it is recommended that individuals
with a history of severe depressive disorder be closely
monitored while taking Avonex.

◇ Prior to starting treatment with Avonex, alert your physician if you have any prior history of a seizure disorder.

◇ Prior to starting treatment with Avonex, alert your physician if you have any history of cardiac disease, including
angina, congestive heart failure, or arrhythmia.

Possible Side Effects

◇ Common side effects include flu-like symptoms (fatigue,
chills, fever, muscle aches, and sweating). Most of these
symptoms will tend to disappear after the initial few weeks
of treatment. If they continue, become more severe, or
cause you significant discomfort, be sure to talk them over
with your physician.

◇ Symptoms of depression, including ongoing sadness, anxiety, loss of interest in daily activities, irritability, low self-
esteem, guilt, poor concentration, indecisiveness, confusion, and eating and sleep disturbances, should be reported promptly to your doctor.

Avonex Support Line: 800-456-2255

Chemical Name: Interferon beta-1b

Brand Name: Betaseron (U.S. and Canada)

Generic Available: No

Description: Betaseron is a medication manufactured by a biotechnological process from one of the naturally occurring interferons (a type of protein). In a clinical trial of 372 ambulatory patients with relapsing-remitting MS, those taking the currently recommended dose of the medication experienced fewer exacerbations, a longer time between exacerbations, and exacerbations that were generally less severe than those of patients taking a lower dose of the medication or a placebo. Additionally, patients on interferon beta-1b had no increase in total lesion area, as shown on MRI, in contrast to the placebo group, which had a significant increase.

Proper Usage

◇ Betaseron is injected subcutaneously (between the fat layer just under the skin and the muscles beneath) every other day. The physician or nurse will instruct you in the preparation of the medication for injection and the injection procedure itself, using a specially designed set of training materials. Do not attempt to inject yourself until you are sure that you understand the procedures.

◇ Betaseron must be kept cold. Be sure to store it in a refrigerator before and after the medication is mixed for injection.

◇ Do not reuse needles or syringes. Dispose of the syringes as directed by your physician and keep them out of the reach of children.

◇ Since flu-like symptoms are a common side effect associated with at least the initial weeks of taking Betaseron, it is recommended that the medication be taken at bedtime. Taking acetaminophen (Tylenol®) or ibuprofen (Advil®) thirty minutes before each injection will also help to relieve the flu-like symptoms.

◇ Because injection site reactions (swelling, redness, discoloration, or pain) are relatively common, it is recommended that the sites be rotated according to a schedule provided for you by your physician.

Precautions

◇ Betaseron should not be used during pregnancy or by any woman who is trying to become pregnant. Women taking Betaseron should use birth control measures at all times.

◇ During the clinical trial of interferon beta-1b, there were four suicide attempts and one completed suicide among those taking interferon beta-1b. Although there is no evidence that the suicide attempts were related to the medication itself, it is recommended that individuals with a history of severe depressive disorder be closely monitored while taking Betaseron.

Possible Side Effects

◇ Common side effects include flu-like symptoms (fatigue, chills, fever, muscle aches, and sweating) and injection site reactions (swelling, redness, discoloration, and pain). Most of these symptoms tend to disappear over time. If they continue, become more severe, or cause significant discomfort, be sure to talk them over with your physician. Contact your physician if the injection sites become inflamed, hardened, or lumpy, and do not inject into any area that has become hardened or lumpy.

◇ Depression, including suicide attempts, has been reported by patients taking Betaseron. Common symptoms of depression are sadness, anxiety, loss of interest in daily activities, irritability, low self-esteem, guilt, poor concentration, indecisiveness, confusion, and eating and sleep disturbances. If you experience any of these symptoms for longer than a day or two, contact your physician promptly.

Betaseron Customer Service: 800-788-1467

Chemical Name: Magnesium hydroxide (mag-**nee**-zhum hye-**drox**-ide)

Brand Name: Phillips' Milk of Magnesia (available in granule form in Canada, in wafer form in the U.S., and in powder or effervescent powder in the U.S. and Canada) is one of several brands of bulk-forming laxative that are available over-the-counter.

Generic Available: No

Description: Magnesium hydroxide is an over-the-counter hyperosmotic laxative of the saline type that encourages bowel movements by drawing water into the bowel from surrounding body tissue. Saline hyperosmotic laxatives (often called "salts") are used for rapid emptying of the lower intestine and bowel. They are not to be used for the long-term management of constipation.

Proper Usage

◇ Laxatives are to be used to provide short-term relief only, unless otherwise directed by the nurse or physician who is helping you to manage your bowel symptoms. A regimen that includes a healthy diet containing roughage (whole grain breads and cereals, bran, fruit, and green, leafy vegetables), six to eight full glasses of liquids each day, and some form of daily exercise is most important in stimulating healthy bowel function.

◇ If your physician has recommended this laxative for management of constipation, follow his or her recommendations for its use. If you are treating yourself for constipation, follow the directions on the package insert. Results are often obtained ninety minutes to three hours after taking a hyperosmotic laxative. Be sure to consult your physician if you experience problems or do not get relief within a week.

◇ Each dose should be taken with eight ounces or more of cold water or fruit juice. A second glass of water or juice with each dose is often recommended to prevent dehydration. If concerns about loss of bladder control keep you from drinking this amount of water, talk it over with the nurse or physician who is helping you manage your bowel and bladder symptoms.

Precautions

◇ Do not take any type of laxative if you have signs of appendicitis or inflamed bowel (e.g., stomach or lower abdominal pain, cramping, bloating, soreness, nausea, or vomiting). Check with your physician as soon as possible.

◇ Do not take any laxative for more than one week unless you have been told to do so by your physician. Many people tend to overuse laxatives, which often leads to dependence on the laxative action to produce a bowel movement. Discuss the use of laxatives with your health care professional in order to ensure that the laxative is used effectively as part of a comprehensive, healthy bowel management regimen.

◇ Do not take any laxative within two hours of taking another medication because the desired effectiveness of the other medication may be reduced.

◇ Although laxatives are commonly used during pregnancy, some types are better than others. If you are pregnant, consult your physician about the best laxative for you to use.

◇ Some laxatives pass into breast milk. Although it is unlikely to cause problems for a nursing infant, be sure to let your physician know if you are using a laxative and breast-feeding at the same time.

Possible Side Effects

◇ Side effects that may go away as your body adjusts to the medication and do not require medical attention unless they continue or are bothersome: cramping; diarrhea; gas; increased thirst.

◇ Unusual side effects that should be reported to your physician as soon as possible: confusion; dizziness; irregular heartbeat; muscle cramps, unusual tiredness or weakness*.

---

*Since it may be difficult to distinguish between certain common symptoms of MS and some side effects of magnesium hydroxide, be sure to consult your health care professional if an abrupt change of this type occurs.

Chemical Name: Meclizine (**mek**-li-zeen)
Brand Name: Antivert (U.S.); Bonamine (Canada)
Generic Available: Yes (U.S.)
Description: Meclizine is used to prevent and treat nausea, vomiting, and dizziness.

Precautions

◇ This drug adds to the effects of alcohol and other central nervous system depressants (e.g., antihistamines, sedatives, tranquilizers, prescriptions pain medications, seizure medications, muscle relaxants, sleeping medications), possibly causing drowsiness. Be sure that your physician knows if you are taking these or any other medications.

◇ Meclizine may cause dryness of the mouth. If dryness continues for more than two weeks, speak to your physician or dentist since continuing dryness of the mouth may increase the risk of dental disease.

◇ This medication has not been shown to cause birth defects or other problems in humans. Studies in animals have shown that meclizine given in doses many times the usual human dose causes birth defects such as cleft palate.

◇ Although meclizine passes into breast milk, it has not been reported to cause problems in nursing babies. However, since this medication tends to decrease bodily secretions, it is possible that the flow of breast milk may be reduced in some women.

Possible Side Effects

◇ Side effects that typically go away as your body adjusts to the medication and do not require medical attention unless they continue for more than two weeks or are bothersome: drowsiness[*]; blurred vision[*]; constipation[*]; difficult or painful urination; dizziness; dryness of mouth, nose, and throat; fast heartbeat; headache; loss of appetite; nervousness or restlessness; trouble sleeping; skin rash; upset stomach.

---

[*]Since it may be difficult to distinguish between certain common symptoms of MS and some side effects of meclizine, be sure to consult your health care professional if an abrupt change of this type occurs.

Chemical Name: Methenamine (meth-**en**-a-meen)

Brand Name: Hiprex; Mandelamine (U.S.); Hip-Rex; Mandelamine (Canada)

Generic Available: No

Description: Methenamine is an anti-infective medication that is used to help prevent infections of the urinary tract. It is usually prescribed on a long-term basis for individuals with a history of repeated or chronic urinary tract infections.

Proper Usage

◇ Before you start taking this medication, check your urine with phenaphthazine paper or another test to see if it is acidic. Your urine must be acidic (pH 5.5 or below) for this medicine to work properly. Consult your health care professional about possible changes in your diet if necessary to increase the acidity of your urine (e.g., avoiding citrus fruits and juices, milk and other dairy products, antacids; eating more protein and foods such as cranberries and cranberry juice with added vitamin C, prunes, or plums).

Precautions

◇ The effects of methenamine in pregnancy have not been studied in either humans or animals. Individual case reports have not shown that this medication causes birth defects or other problems in humans.

◇ Methenamine passes into breast milk but has not been reported to cause problems in nursing infants.

Possible Side Effects

◇ Side effects that typically go away as your body adjusts to the medication and do not require medical attention unless they continue or are bothersome: nausea; vomiting.

◇ Unusual side effects that should be reported immediately to your physician: skin rash.

Chemical Name: Methylprednisolone (meth-ill-pred-**niss**-oh-lone)

Brand Name: Depo-Medrol (U.S. and Canada)

Generic Available: Yes (U.S. and Canada)

Description: Methylprednisolone is one of a group of corticosteroids (cortisone-like medications) that are used to relieve inflammation in different parts of the body. Corticosteroids are used in MS for the management of acute exacerbations because they have the capacity to close the damaged blood-brain barrier and reduce inflammation in the central nervous system. Although methylprednisolone is among the most commonly used corticosteroids in MS, it is only one of several possibilities. Other commonly used corticosteroids include dexamethazone, prednisone, betamethasone, and prednisolone. The following information pertains to all of the various corticosteroids.

Proper Usage

◇ Most neurologists treating MS believe that high-dose corticosteroids given intravenously are the most effective treatment for an exacerbation, although the exact protocol for the drug's use may differ somewhat from one treating physician to another. Patients generally receive a four-day course of treatment (either in the hospital or as an outpatient), with doses of the medication spread throughout the day. This high-dose, intravenous steroid treatment is then typically followed by a gradually tapering dose of an oral corticosteroid (see Prednisone).

Precautions

◇ Since corticosteroids can stimulate the appetite and increase water retention, it is advisable to follow a low-salt and/or potassium-rich diet and watch your caloric intake. Your physician will make specific dietary recommendations for you.

◇ Corticosteroids can lower your resistance to infection and make any infection that you get more difficult to treat. Contact your physician if you notice any sign of infection, such as sore throat, fever, coughing, or sneezing.

◇ Avoid close contact with anyone who has chicken pox or measles. Tell your physician right away if you think you have been exposed to either of these illnesses. Do not have any immunizations after you stop taking this medication until you have consulted your physician. People living in your home should not have the oral polio vaccine while you are being treated with corticosteroids since they might pass the polio virus on to you.

◇ Corticosteroids may affect the blood sugar levels of diabetic patients. If you notice a change in your blood or urine sugar tests, be sure to speak to your physician.

◇ The risk of birth defects for women taking corticosteroids is not known. Overuse of corticosteroids during pregnancy may slow the growth of the infant after birth. Animal studies have demonstrated that corticosteroids cause birth defects.

◇ Corticosteroids pass into breast milk and may slow the infant's growth. If you are nursing or plan to nurse, be sure to discuss this with your physician. It may be necessary for you to stop nursing while taking this medication.

◇ Corticosteroids may produce mood changes and/or mood swings of varying intensity. These mood alterations can vary from relatively mild to extremely intense, and can vary in a single individual from one course of treatment to another. Neither the patient nor the physician can predict with any certainty whether the corticosteroids are likely to precipitate these mood alterations. If you have a history of mood disorders (depression or bipolar disorder, for example), be sure to share this information with your physician. If you begin to experience mood changes or swings that feel unmanageable, contact your physician so that a decision can be made about whether or not you need an additional medication to help you until the mood alterations subside.

Possible Side Effects

◇ Side effects that may go away as your body adjusts to the medication and do not require medical attention unless they continue or are bothersome: increased appetite; indigestion; nervousness or restlessness; trouble sleeping; headache; increased sweating; unusual increase in hair growth on body or face.

◇ Less common side effects that should be reported as soon as possible to your physician: severe mood changes or mood swings; decreased or blurred vision*; frequent urination*.

◇ Additional side effects that can result from the prolonged use of corticosteroids and should be reported to your physician: acne or other skin problems; swelling of the face; swelling of the feet or lower legs; rapid weight gain; pain in the hips or other joints (caused by bone cell degeneration); bloody or black, tarry stools; elevated blood pressure; markedly increased thirst (with increased urination indicative of diabetes mellitus); menstrual irregularities; unusual bruising of the skin; thin, shiny skin; hair loss; muscle cramps or pain. Once you stop this medication after taking it for a long period of time, it may take several months for your body to readjust.

*Since it may be difficult to distinguish between certain common symptoms of MS and some side effects of methylprednisolone, be sure to consult your health care professional if an abrupt change of this type occurs.

Chemical Name: Mineral oil

Mineral oil is available in a variety of brands in the U.S. and
 Canada.

Generic Available: Yes

Description: Mineral oil is a lubricant laxative that is taken by
 mouth. It encourages bowel movements by coating the bowel
 and the stool with a waterproof film that helps to retain moisture in the stool.

Proper Usage

◇ Laxatives are to be used to provide short-term relief only,
 unless otherwise directed by the nurse or physician who is
 helping you to manage your bowel symptoms. A regimen
 that includes a healthy diet containing roughage (whole
 grain breads and cereals, bran, fruit, and green, leafy vegetables), six to eight full glasses of liquids each day, and
 some form of daily exercise is most important in stimulating healthy bowel function.

◇ If your physician has recommended this type of laxative
 for management of constipation, follow his or her recommendations for its use. If you are treating yourself for constipation, follow the directions on the package insert.
 Mineral oil is usually taken at bedtime because it takes six
 to eight hours to produce results. Be sure to consult your
 physician if you experience problems or do not get relief
 within a week.

◇ Mineral oil should not be taken within two hours of meal-
 time because the mineral oil may interfere with food digestion and the absorption of important nutrients.

◇ Mineral oil should not be taken within two hours of taking
 a stool softener (see Docusate) because the stool softener
 may increase the amount of mineral oil that is absorbed by
 the body.

Precautions

◇ Do not take any type of laxative if you have signs of appendicitis or inflamed bowel (e.g., stomach or lower abdominal pain, cramping, bloating, soreness, nausea, or vomiting). Check with your physician as soon as possible.

◇ Do not take any laxative for more than one week unless you have been told to do so by your physician. Many people tend to overuse laxative products, which often leads to dependence on the laxative action to produce a bowel movement. Discuss the use of laxatives with your health care professional in order to ensure that the laxative is used effectively as part of a comprehensive, healthy bowel management regimen.

◇ Mineral oil should not be used very often or for long periods of time. Its gradual build-up in body tissues can cause problems, and may interfere with the body's absorption of important nutrients and vitamins A, D, E, and K.

◇ Do not take any laxative within two hours of taking another medication because the desired effectiveness of the other medication may be reduced.

◇ Mineral oil should not be used during pregnancy because it may interfere with absorption of nutrients in the mother and, if used for prolonged periods, cause severe bleeding in the newborn infant.

◇ Be sure to let your physician know if you are using a laxative and breast-feeding at the same time.

Possible Side Effects

◇ Uncommon side effect that usually does not need medical attention: skin irritation around the rectal area.

Chemical Name: Oxybutynin (ox-i-**byoo**-ti-nin)

Brand Name: Ditropan (U.S. and Canada)

Generic Available: Yes (U.S.)

Description: Oxybutynin is an antispasmodic that helps decrease muscle spasms of the bladder and the frequent urge to urinate caused by these spasms.

Proper Usage

◇ This medication is usually taken with water on an empty stomach, but your physician may want you to take it with food or milk to lessen stomach upset.

Precautions

◇ This medication adds to the effects of alcohol and other central nervous system depressants (such as antihistamines, sedatives, tranquilizers, prescription pain medications, seizure medications, muscle relaxants). Be sure that your physician knows if you are taking these or any other medications.

◇ This medication may cause your eyes to become more sensitive to light.

◇ Oxybutynin may cause drying of the mouth. Since continuing dryness of the mouth can increase the risk of dental disease, alert your dentist if you are taking oxybutynin.

◇ Oxybutynin has not been studied in pregnant women. It has not been shown to cause birth defects or other problems in animal studies.

◇ This medication has not been reported to cause problems in nursing babies. However, since it tends to decrease body secretions, oxybutynin may reduce the flow of breast milk.

Possible Side Effects

◇ Side effects that typically go away as your body adjusts to the medication and do not require medical attention unless they continue for a few weeks or are bothersome: constipation[*]; decreased sweating; unusual drowsiness[*]; dryness of mouth, nose, throat; blurred vision[*]; decreased flow of breast milk; decreased sexual ability[*]; difficulty swallowing[*]; headache; increased light sensitivity; nausea or vomiting; trouble sleeping; unusual tiredness or weakness[*].

◇ Less common side effects that should be reported to your physician immediately: difficulty in urination[*].

---

[*]Since it may be difficult to distinguish between certain common symptoms of MS and some side effects of oxybutynin, be sure to consult your health care professional if an abrupt change of this type occurs.

Chemical Name: Papaverine (pa-**pav**-er-een)
Brand Name: None
Generic Available: Yes (U.S. and Canada)
Description: Papaverine belongs to a group of medicines called vasodilators, which cause blood vessels to expand, thereby increasing blood flow. Papaverine is used in MS to treat erectile dysfunction. When papaverine is injected into the penis, it produces an erection by increasing blood flow to the penis.

Proper Usage

◇ Papaverine should never be used as a sexual aid by men who are not impotent. If improperly used, this medication can cause permanent damage to the penis.

◇ Papaverine is available by prescription and should be used only as directed by your physician, who will instruct you in the proper way to give yourself an injection so that it is simple and essentially pain-free.

Precautions

◇ Do not use more of this medication or use it more often than it has been prescribed for you. Using too much of this medicine will result in a condition called priapism, in which the erection lasts too long and does not resolve when it should. Permanent damage to the penis can occur if blood flow to the penis is cut off for too long a period of time.

◇ Examine your penis regularly for possible lumps near the injection sites or for curvature of the penis. These may be signs that unwanted tissue is growing (called fibrosis), which should be examined by your physician.

Possible Side Effects

◇ Side effects that you should report to your physician so that he or she can adjust the dosage or change the medication: bruising at the injection site; mild burning along the penis; difficulty ejaculating; swelling at the injection site.

◇ Rare side effects that require immediate treatment: erection continuing for more than four hours. If you cannot be seen immediately by your physician, you should go to the emergency room for prompt treatment.

Chemical Name: Paroxetine (pa-**rox**-uh-teen)
Brand Name: Paxil (U.S. and Canada)
Generic Available: No
Description: Paroxetine is used to treat mental depression.

Proper Usage

◇ Paroxetine may be taken with or without food, on an empty or full stomach.

Precautions

◇ It may take up to four weeks or longer for you to feel the beneficial effects of this medication.

◇ Your physician should monitor your progress at regularly scheduled visits in order to adjust the dose and help reduce any side effects.

◇ This medication could add to the effects of alcohol and other central nervous system depressants (e.g., antihistamines, sedatives, tranquilizers, sleeping medicine, prescription pain medicine, barbiturates, seizure medication, muscle relaxants). Be sure that your physician knows if you are taking these or any other medications.

◇ Paroxetine may cause dryness of the mouth. If your mouth continues to feel dry for more than two weeks, check with your physician or dentist. Continuing dryness of the mouth may increase the risk of dental disease.

◇ This medication may cause you to become drowsy.

◇ Studies have not been done in pregnant women. Studies in animals have shown that paroxetine may cause miscarriages and decreased survival rates when given in doses that are many times higher than the human dose.

◇ Paroxetine passes into breast milk but has not been shown to cause any problems in nursing infants.

Possible Side Effects

◇ Side effects that typically go away as your body adjusts to the medication and do not require medical attention unless they continue for several weeks or are bothersome: decrease in sexual drive or ability[*]; headache; nausea; problems urinating[*]; decreased or increased appetite; unusual tiredness or weakness[*]; tremor[*]; trouble sleeping;

anxiety; agitation; nervousness or restlessness; changes in vision, including blurred vision[*]; fast or irregular heartbeat; tingling, burning, or prickly sensations[*]; vomiting.

◇ Unusual side effects that should be discussed with your physician as soon as possible: agitation; lightheadedness or fainting; muscle pain or weakness; skin rash; mood or behavior changes.

---

[*]Since it may be difficult to distinguish between certain common symptoms of MS and some side effects of paroxetine, be sure to consult your health care professional if an abrupt change of this type occurs.

Chemical Name: Pemoline (**pem**-oh-leen)

Brand Name: Cylert (U.S. and Canada)

Generic Available: No

Description: Pemoline is a mild central nervous system stimulant that has been used primarily to treat children with attention deficit hyperactivity disorder and adults with narcolepsy. It is used in multiple sclerosis to relieve certain types of fatigue.

Proper Usage

◇ The usual starting dose for the treatment of fatigue in MS is 18.75 mg each morning for one week. If necessary, in order to manage the fatigue, the dosage can be gradually increased in increments of 18.75 mg and spread out over the early part of the day. In order to maximize the medication's effectiveness and minimize sleep disturbance, it should all be taken before mid-afternoon. The maximum dose of this medication is not known. Some individuals feel jittery or uncomfortable taking more than the minimum dose; others tolerate higher doses without discomfort. Typically, the drug is not prescribed at levels over 100–140 mgs per day for MS-related fatigue.

Precautions

◇ Pemoline can increase hypertension. It should not be taken if you have angina and/or known coronary artery disease.

◇ If you are taking pemoline in large doses for a long time, do not stop taking it without consulting your physician. Your physician may want you to reduce the amount you are taking gradually.

◇ This drug may interact with the effects of alcohol and other central nervous system depressants (e.g., antihistamines, sedatives, tranquilizers, prescription pain medications, seizure medications, muscle relaxants, sleeping medications). Be sure your physician knows if you are taking these or any other medications.

◇ Pemoline may cause some people to become dizzy or less alert than they are normally.

◇ If you have been using this medicine for a long time and think you may have become mentally or physically dependent on it, check with your physician. Some signs of dependence on pemoline are a strong desire or need to continue taking the medicine; a need to increase the dose to receive the effects of the medicine; withdrawal side effects such as mental depression, unusual behavior, unusual tiredness* or weakness* after the medication is stopped.

◇ Pemoline has not been shown to cause birth defects or other problems in humans. Studies in animals given large doses of pemoline have shown that it causes an increase in stillbirths and decreased survival of the offspring.

◇ It is not known if pemoline is excreted in breast milk.

Possible Side Effects

Side effects of this medication have not been studied in adults. Side effects that have been reported by some adults in clinical practice include insomnia; elevated heart rate; nervousness; agitation; loss of appetite and weight loss; gastrointestinal upset, including constipation and diarrhea; hallucinations.

---

*Since it may be difficult to distinguish between certain common symptoms of MS and some side effects of pemoline, be sure to consult your health care professional if an abrupt change of this type occurs.

Chemical Name: Phenazopyridine (fen-az-oh-**peer**-i-deen)
Brand Name: Pyridium (U.S. and Canada)
Generic Available: Yes (U.S.)
Description: Phenazopyridine is used to relieve the pain, burning, and discomfort caused by urinary tract infections. It is not an antibiotic and will not cure the infection itself. This medication is available in the U.S. only with a prescription; it is available in Canada without a prescription. The medication comes in tablet form.

Precautions

◇ The medication causes the urine to turn reddish orange. This effect is harmless and goes away after you stop taking phenazopyridine.

◇ It is best not to wear soft contact lenses while taking this medication; phenazopyridine may cause permanent discoloration or staining of soft lenses.

◇ Check with your physician if symptoms such as bloody urine, difficult or painful urination, frequent urge to urinate, or sudden decrease in the amount of urine appear or become worse while you are taking this medication.

◇ Phenazopyridine has not been studied in pregnant women. It has not been shown to cause birth defects in animal studies.

◇ It is not known whether this medication passes into breast milk. It has not been reported to cause problems in nursing babies.

Possible Side Effects

◇ Uncommon side effects that typically go away as your body adjusts to the medication and do not require medical attention unless they continue or are bothersome: dizziness; headache; indigestion; stomach cramps or pain.

◇ Unusual side effects that should be reported to your physician: blue or blue-purple color of skin; fever and confusion; shortness of breath; skin rash; sudden decrease in amount of urine; swelling of face, fingers, feet and/or lower legs; unusual weakness or tiredness[*]; weight gain; yellow eyes or skin.

[*]Since it may be difficult to distinguish between certain common symptoms of MS and some side effects of phenazopyridine, be sure to consult your health care professional if an abrupt change of this type occurs.

Chemical Name: Phenytoin (**fen**-i-toyn)

Brand Name: Dilantin (U.S. and Canada)

Generic Available: Yes (U.S.)

Description: Phenytoin is one of a group of hydantoin anticonvulsants that are used most commonly in the management of seizures in epilepsy. It is used in MS to manage painful dysesthesias (most commonly trigeminal neuralgia) caused by abnormalities in the sensory pathways in the brain and spinal cord.

Precautions

◇ This drug may interact with the effects of alcohol and other central nervous system depressants (e.g., antihistamines, sedatives, tranquilizers, certain prescription pain medications, seizure medications, muscle relaxants, sleeping medications). Be sure your physician knows if you are taking these or any other medications.

◇ Oral contraceptives (birth control pills) that contain estrogen may not be as effective if taken in conjunction with phenytoin. Consult with your physician about using a different or additional form of birth control to avoid unplanned pregnancies.

◇ This medication may affect the blood sugar levels of diabetic individuals. Check with your physician if you notice any change in the results of your blood or urine sugar level tests while taking phenytoin.

◇ Antacids or medicines for diarrhea can reduce the effectiveness of phenytoin. Do not take any of these medications within two to three hours of the phenytoin.

◇ Before having any type of dental treatment or surgery, be sure to inform your physician or dentist if you are taking phenytoin. Medications commonly used during surgical and dental treatments can increase the side effects of phenytoin.

◇ There have been reports of increased birth defects when hydantoin anticonvulsants were used for seizure control during pregnancy. It is not definitely known whether these medications were the cause of the problem. Be sure to tell your physician if you are pregnant or considering becoming pregnant.

◇ Phenytoin passes into breast milk in small amounts.

Possible Side Effects

◇ Side effects that may go away as your body adjusts to the medication and do not require medical attention unless they continue or are bothersome: constipation*; mild dizziness*; mild drowsiness*.

◇ Side effects that should be reported to your physician: bleeding or enlarged gums; confusion; enlarged glands in the neck or underarms; mood or mental changes*; muscle weakness or pain*; skin rash or itching; slurred speech or stuttering; trembling; unusual nervousness or irritability.

◇ Symptoms of overdose that require immediate attention: sudden blurred or double vision*; sudden severe clumsiness or unsteadiness*; sudden severe dizziness or drowsiness*; staggering walk*; severe confusion or disorientation.

---

*Since it may be difficult to distinguish between certain common symptoms of MS and some side effects of phenytoin, be sure to consult your health care professional if an abrupt change of this type occurs.

Chemical Name: Prednisone (**pred**-ni-sone)

Brand Name: Deltasone (U.S. and Canada)

Generic Available: Yes (U.S. and Canada)

Description: Prednisone is one of a group of corticosteroids (cortisone-like medicines) that are used to relieve inflammation in different parts of the body. Corticosteroids are used in MS for the management of acute exacerbations because they have the capacity to close the damaged blood-brain barrier and reduce inflammation in the central nervous system. Although prednisone is among the most commonly used corticosteroids in MS, it is only one of several different possibilities. Other commonly used corticosteroids include dexamethasone; prednisone; betamethasone; and prednisolone. The following information pertains to all of the various corticosteroids.

Proper Usage

◇ Most neurologists treating MS believe that high-dose corticosteroids given intravenously are the most effective treatment for an MS exacerbation, although the exact protocol for the drug's use may differ somewhat from one treating physician to another. Patients generally receive a four-day course of treatment (either in the hospital or as an outpatient), with doses of the medication spread throughout the day (see Methylprednisolone). The high-dose, intravenous dose is typically followed by a gradually tapering dose of an oral corticosteroid (usually ranging in length from ten days to five or six weeks). Prednisone is commonly used for this oral taper. Oral prednisone may also be used instead of the high-dose, intravenous treatment if the intravenous treatment is not desired or is medically contraindicated.

Precautions

◇ This medication can cause indigestion and stomach discomfort. Always take it with a meal and/or a glass or milk. Your physician may prescribe an antacid for you to take with this medication.

◇ Take this medication exactly as prescribed by your physician. Do not stop taking it abruptly; your physician will give you a schedule that gradually tapers the dose before you stop it completely.

◇ Since corticosteroids can stimulate the appetite and increase water retention, it is advisable to follow a low-salt and/or a potassium-rich diet and watch your caloric intake.

◇ Corticosteroids can lower your resistance to infection and make any infection that you get more difficult to treat. Contact your physician if you notice any sign of infection, such as sore throat, fever, coughing, or sneezing.

◇ Avoid close contact with anyone who has chicken pox or measles. Tell your physician immediately if you think you have been exposed to either of these illnesses. Do not have any immunizations after you stop taking this medication until you have consulted your physician. People living in your home should not have the oral polio vaccine while you are being treated with corticosteroids since they might pass the polio virus on to you.

◇ Corticosteroids may affect the blood sugar levels of diabetic patients. If you notice a change in your blood or urine sugar tests, be sure to discuss it with your physician.

◇ The risk of birth defects in women taking corticosteroids during pregnancy has not been studied. Overuse of corticosteroids during pregnancy may slow the growth of the infant after birth. Animal studies have demonstrated that corticosteroids cause birth defects.

◇ Corticosteroids pass into breast milk and may slow the infant's growth. If you are nursing or plan to nurse, be sure to discuss this with your physician. It may be necessary for you to stop nursing while taking this medication.

◇ Corticosteroids can produce mood changes and/or mood swings of varying intensity. These mood alterations can vary from relatively mild to extremely intense, and can vary in a single individual from one course of treatment to another. Neither the patient nor the physician can predict with any certainty whether the corticosteroids are likely to precipitate these mood alterations. If you have a history of mood disorders (depression or bipolar disorder, for example), be sure to share this information with your physician. If you begin to experience unmanageable mood changes or swings while taking corticosteroids, contact your physician so that a decision can be made whether or not you need an additional medication to help you until the mood alterations subside.

Possible Side Effects

◇ Side effects that may go away as your body adjusts to the medication and do not require medical attention unless they continue or are bothersome: increased appetite; indigestion; nervousness or restlessness; trouble sleeping; headache; increased sweating; unusual increase in hair growth on body or face.

◇ Less common side effects that should be reported as soon as possible to your physician: severe mood changes or mood swings; decreased or blurred vision[*]; frequent urination[*].

◇ Additional side effects that can result from the prolonged use of corticosteroids and should be reported to your physician: acne or other skin problems; swelling of the face; swelling of the feet or lower legs; rapid weight gain; pain in the hips or other joints (caused by bone cell degeneration); bloody or black, tarry stools; elevated blood pressure; markedly increased thirst (with increased urination indicative of diabetes mellitus); menstrual irregularities; unusual bruising of the skin; thin, shiny skin; hair loss; muscle cramps or pain. Once you stop this medication after taking it for a long period of time, it may take several months for your body to readjust.

---

[*]Since it may be difficult to distinguish between certain common symptoms of MS and some side effects of prednisone, be sure to consult your health care professional if an abrupt change of this type occurs.

Chemical Name: Propantheline (proe-**pan**-the-leen) bromide
Brand Name: Pro-Banthine (U.S. and Canada)
Generic Available: Yes (U.S.)
Description: Propantheline is one of a group of antispasmod-
   ic/anticholinergic medications used to relieve cramps or
   spasms of the stomach, intestines, and bladder. Propantheline
   is used in the management of neurogenic bladder symptoms
   to control urination.

Proper Usage

◇ Take this medicine thirty minutes to one hour before meals
   unless otherwise directed by your physician.

Precautions

◇ Do not stop this medication abruptly. Stop gradually to
   avoid possible vomiting, sweating, and dizziness.

◇ Anticholinergic medications such as propantheline can
   cause blurred vision and light sensitivity. Make sure you
   know how you react to this medication before driving.

◇ Anticholinergic medications may cause dryness of the
   mouth. If your mouth continues to feel dry for more than
   two weeks, check with your dentist. Continuing dryness of
   the mouth may increase the chance of dental disease.

◇ No studies of the effects of this drug in pregnancy have
   been done in either humans or animals.

◇ Anticholinergic medications have not been reported to
   cause problems in nursing babies. The flow of breast milk
   may be reduced in some women.

◇ Be sure that your physician knows if you are taking a tricyclic antidepressant or any other anticholinergic medication. Taking propantheline with any of these may
   increase the anticholinergic effects, resulting in urinary
   retention.

Possible Side Effects

◇ Side effects that typically go away as your body adjusts to
   the medication and do not require medical attention unless
   they continue for several weeks or are bothersome: constipation[*]; decreased sweating; dryness of mouth, nose, and

throat; bloated feeling; blurred vision[*]; difficulty swallowing.

◇ Unusual side effects that require immediate medical attention: inability to urinate; confusion; dizziness[*]; eye pain[*]; skin rash or hives.

◇ Symptoms of overdose that require immediate emergency attention: unusual blurred vision[*]; unusual clumsiness or unsteadiness[*]; unusual dizziness; unusually severe drowsiness[*]; seizures; hallucinations; confusion; shortness of breath; unusual slurred speech[*]; nervousness; unusual warmth, dryness, and flushing of skin.

[*]Since it may be difficult to distinguish between certain common symptoms of MS and some side effects of propantheline, be sure to consult your health care professional if an abrupt change of this type occurs.

Chemical Name: Psyllium hydrophilic mucilloid (**sill**-i-yum hye-droe-**fill**-ik **myoo**-sill-oid)

Brand Name: Metamucil (available in granule form in Canada, in wafer form in the U.S., and in powder or effervescent powder in the U.S. and Canada) is one of several available brands of bulk-forming laxative.

Generic Available: No

Description: Psyllium hydrophilic mucilloid is a bulk-forming oral laxative. This type of laxative is not digested by the body; it absorbs liquids from the intestines and swells to form a soft, bulky stool. The bowel is then stimulated normally by the presence of the bulky stool.

Proper Usage

◇ Laxatives are to be used to provide short-term relief only, unless otherwise directed by the nurse or physician who is helping you to manage your bowel symptoms. A regimen that includes a healthy diet containing roughage (whole grain breads and cereals, bran, fruit, and green, leafy vegetables), six to eight full glasses of liquids each day, and some form of daily exercise is most important in stimulating healthy bowel function.

◇ If your physician has recommended this laxative for management of constipation, follow his or her recommendations for its use. If you are treating yourself for constipation, follow the directions on the package insert. Results are often obtained in twelve hours but may take as long as two or three days. Be sure to consult your physician if you experience problems or do not get relief within a week.

◇ In order for this type of bulk-forming laxative to work effectively without causing intestinal blockage, it is advisable to drink six to eight glasses (eight ounces) of water each day. Each dose of the laxative should be taken with eight ounces of cold water or fruit juice. If concerns about loss of bladder control keep you from drinking this amount of water, discuss it with the nurse or physician who is helping you manage your bowel and bladder symptoms.

Precautions

◇ Do not take any type of laxative if you have signs of appendicitis or inflamed bowel (e.g., stomach or lower abdominal pain, cramping, bloating, soreness, nausea, or vomiting). Check with your physician as soon as possible.

◇ Do not take any laxative for more than one week unless you have been told to do so by your physician. Many people tend to overuse laxatives, which often leads to dependence on the laxative action to produce a bowel movement. Discuss the use of laxatives with your health care professional in order to ensure that the laxative is used effectively as part of a comprehensive, healthy bowel management regimen.

◇ Do not take any laxative within two hours of taking another medication because the desired effectiveness of the other medication may be reduced.

◇ Bulk-forming laxatives are commonly used during pregnancy. Some of them contain a large amount of sodium or sugars, which may have possible unwanted effects such as increasing blood pressure or causing fluid retention. Look for those that contain lower sodium and sugar.

◇ Some laxatives pass into breast milk. Although it is unlikely to cause problems for a nursing infant, be sure to let your physician know if you are using a laxative and breast-feeding at the same time.

Possible Side Effects:

◇ Check with your physician as soon as possible if you experience any of the following: difficulty breathing; intestinal blockage; skin rash or itching; swallowing difficulty (feelings of lump in the throat).

Chemical Name: Sertraline (**ser**-tra-leen)
Brand Name: Zoloft (U.S. and Canada)
Generic Available: No
Description: Sertraline is used to treat mental depression.

Proper Usage

This medication should always be taken at the same time in relation to meals and snacks to make sure that it is absorbed in the same way. Because sertraline may be given to different individuals at different times of the day, you and your physician should discuss what to do about any missed doses.

Precautions

◇ It may take four to six weeks for you to feel the beneficial effects of this medication.

◇ Your physician should monitor your progress at regularly scheduled visits in order to adjust the dose and help reduce any side effects.

◇ This medication could add to the effects of alcohol and other central nervous system depressants (e.g., antihistamines, sedatives, tranquilizers, sleeping medicine, prescription pain medicine, barbiturates, seizure medication, muscle relaxants). Be sure that your physician knows if you are taking these or any other medications.

◇ Sertraline may cause dryness of the mouth. If your mouth continues to feel dry for more than two weeks, check with your physician or dentist. Continuing dryness of the mouth may increase the risk of dental disease.

◇ This medication may cause drowsiness.

◇ Studies have not been done in pregnant women. Studies in animals have shown that sertraline may cause delayed development and decreased survival rates of offspring when given in doses many times the usual human dose.

◇ It is not known if sertraline passes into breast milk.

Possible Side Effects

◇ Side effects that typically go away as your body adjusts to the medication and do not require medical attention unless they continue for several weeks or are bothersome: decreased appetite or weight loss; decrease sexual drive or ability[*]; drowsiness[*]; dryness of mouth; headache; nausea; stomach or abdominal cramps; tiredness or weakness[*]; tremor[*]; trouble sleeping; anxiety; agitation; nervousness or restlessness; changes in vision including blurred vision[*]; constipation[*]; fast or irregular heartbeat; flushing of skin; increased appetite; vomiting.

◇ Unusual side effects that should be discussed with your physician as soon as possible: fast talking and excited feelings or actions that are out of control; fever; skin rash; hives; itching.

---

[*]Since it may be difficult to distinguish between certain common symptoms of MS and some side effects of sertraline, be sure to consult your health care professional if an abrupt change of this type occurs.

Chemical Name: Sodium phosphate
Brand Name: Fleet Enema (U.S. and Canada)
Generic Available: No
Description: Sodium phosphate enemas are available over-the-counter.

Proper Usage

◇ Rectal enemas are to be used to provide short-term relief only, unless otherwise directed by the nurse or physician who is helping you to manage your bowel symptoms. A regimen that includes a healthy diet containing roughage (whole grain breads and cereals, bran, fruit, and green, leafy vegetables), six to eight full glasses of liquids each day, and some form of daily exercise is most important in stimulating healthy bowel function.

◇ If your physician has recommended this rectal laxative for management of constipation, follow his or her recommendations for its use. If you are treating yourself for constipation, follow the directions on the package insert.

◇ Results usually occur within two to five minutes. Be sure to consult your physician if you notice rectal bleeding, blistering, pain, burning, itching, or other signs of irritation that was not present before you began using a sodium phosphate enema.

Precautions

◇ Do not use any type of laxative if you have signs of appendicitis or inflamed bowel (e.g., stomach or lower abdominal pain, cramping, bloating, soreness, nausea, or vomiting). Check with your physician as soon as possible.

◇ Do not use any laxative for more than one week unless you have been told to do so by your physician. Many people tend to overuse laxatives, which often leads to dependence on the laxative action to produce a bowel movement. Discuss the use of laxatives with your health care professional in order to ensure that the laxative is used effectively as part of a comprehensive, healthy bowel management regimen.

◇ If you are pregnant, discuss with your physician the most appropriate type of laxative for you to use.

Possible Side Effects

◇ Side effect that may go away as your body adjusts to the medication and does not require medical attention unless it persists or is bothersome: skin irritation in the rectal area.

◇ Unusual side effects that should be reported to your physician as soon as possible: rectal bleeding, blistering, burning, itching.

Chemical Name: Sulfamethoxazole (sul-fa-meth-**ox**-a-zole) and trimethoprim (try-**meth**-oh-prim) combination
Brand Name: Bactrim; Septra (U.S. and Canada)
Generic Available: Yes (U.S.)
Description: Sulfamethoxazole and trimethoprim combination is used in multiple sclerosis to treat (and sometimes to prevent) urinary tract infections.

Proper Usage

◇ This medication is best taken with a full glass (eight ounces) of water. Additional water should be taken each day to help prevent unwanted effects.

◇ Finish the full course of treatment prescribed by your physician. Even if your symptoms disappear after a few days, stopping this medication prematurely may result in a return of the symptoms.

◇ This medication works most effectively when it is maintained at a constant level in your blood or urine. To help keep the amount constant, do not miss any doses. It is best to take the doses at evenly spaced times during the day and night. For maximum effectiveness, four doses per day would be spaced at six-hour intervals.

Precautions

◇ This medication may cause dizziness.

◇ If taken for a long time, sulfamethoxazole and trimethoprim combination may cause blood problems. It is very important that your physician monitor your progress at regular visits.

◇ This medication can cause changes in the blood, possibly resulting in a greater chance of certain infections, slow healing, and bleeding of the gums. Be careful with the use of your toothbrush, dental floss, and toothpicks. Delay dental work until your blood counts are completely normal. Check with your dentist if you have questions about oral hygiene during treatment.

◇ This medication may cause your skin to become more sensitive to sunlight. Stay out of direct sunlight during the midday hours, wear protective clothing, and apply a sun block product that has a skin protection factor (SPF) of at least 15.

◇ Sulfamethoxazole and trimethoprim combination has not been reported to cause birth defects or other problems in humans. Studies in mice, rats, and rabbits have shown that some sulfonamides cause birth defects, including cleft palate and bone problems. Studies in rabbits have also shown that trimethoprim causes birth defects, as well as a decrease in the number of successful pregnancies.

◇ Sulfamethoxazole and trimethoprim pass into breast milk. This medication is not recommended for use during breast-feeding. It may cause liver problems, anemia, and other problems in nursing babies.

Possible Side Effects

◇ Side effects that may go away as your body adjusts to the medication and do not require medical attention unless they continue or are bothersome: diarrhea; dizziness; headache; loss of appetite; nausea or vomiting.

◇ Less common side effects that should be reported to your physician immediately: itching; skin rash; aching of muscles and joints; difficulty in swallowing; pale skin; redness, blistering, peeling, or loosening of skin; sore throat and fever; unusual bleeding or bruising; unusual tiredness or weakness[*]; yellow eyes or skin.

[*]Since it may be difficult to distinguish between the tiredness that is common in MS (especially in the prewsence of an infection) and this side effect of sulfamethoxazole and trimethoprim combination, be sure to consult yourphysicianl if an abrupt change of this type occurs.

Appendix C

Additional Readings

NOTE: The Information Resource Center and Library of the National Multiple Sclerosis Society (1-800-344-4867) has a complete collection of booklets and articles about all aspects of MS research, treatments, and management. Operators are available to answer your questions and send you information on any MS-related topics that are of interest to you.

Bondo BE. (1995). *Tax Options and Strategies: A State-by-State Guide for Persons with Disabilities, Senior Citizens, Veterans, and Their Families.* New York: Demos Vermande.

Burnfield A. (1985). *Multiple Sclerosis: A Personal Exploration.* New York: Demos.

Enders A, Hall M. (1990). *Assistive Technology Sourcebook.* Washington, D.C.: Resna Press.

Garee B (ed.) (1989). *Parenting: Tips from Parents (Who Happen to Have a Disability) on Raising Children.* Bloomington, IL: Accent Press.

Giffels JJ. (1996). *Clinical Trials: What You Should Know Before Volunteering to Be a Research Subject.* New York: Demos Vermande.

Halligan F. (1995). *The Art of Coping.* New York: Crossroad.

Hecker H. (1995). *Travel for the Disabled: A Handbook of Travel Resources and 500 Worldwide Access Guides*. Vancouver, WA: Twin Peaks Press.

James JL. (1993). *One Particular Harbor: The Outrageous True Adventures of One Woman with Multiple Sclerosis Living in the Alaskan Wilderness*. Chicago: Noble Press.

Kalb RC, Scheinberg LC. (1992). *Multiple Sclerosis and the Family*. New York: Demos Vermande.

Kraft GH, Catanzaro M. (1996). *Living with Multiple Sclerosis: A Wellness Approach*. New York: Demos Vermande.

Kroll K, Klein EL. (1995). *Enabling Romance: A Guide to Love, Sex, and Relationships for the Disabled*. Bethesda, MD: Woodbine House.

Lechtenberg R. (1995). *Multiple Sclerosis Fact Book*. Philadelphia: Davis.

LeMaistre J. (1994). *Beyond Rage: Mastering Unavoidable Health Changes*. Dillon, CO: Alpine Guild.

Lunt S. (1982). *A Handbook for the Disabled: Ideas and Inventions for Easier Living*. New York: Charles Scribner's Sons.

MacFarlane EB, Burstein P. (1994). *Legwork: An Inspiring Journey Through a Chronic Illness*. New York: Charles Scribner's Sons.

Mackenzie L (ed.) (1991). *The Complete Directory for the Disabled*. Lakeville, CT: Grey House Publishing, Inc.

Mendelsohn SB. (1996). *Tax Options and Strategies for People with Disabilities (2nd edition)*. New York: Demos Vermande.

Pitzele SK. (1986). *We Are Not Alone: Learning to Live with Chronic Illness*. New York: Workman.

Pitzele SK. (1988). *One More Day: Daily Meditations for the Chronically Ill*. Minneapolis: Hazelden.

Rao S (ed.) (1990). *Neurobehavioral Aspects of Multiple Sclerosis*. New York: Oxford.

Register C. (1987). *Living with Chronic Illness: Days of Patience and Passion*. New York: Free Press.

Resources for Rehabilitation (1993a). *Meeting the Needs of Employees with Disabilities*. Lexington, MA: Resources for Rehabilitation.

Resources for Rehabilitation (1993b). *Resources for People with Disabilities and Chronic Conditions*. Lexington, MA: Resources for Rehabilitation.

Resources for Rehabilitation (1994). *A Woman's Guide to Coping with Disability*. Lexington, MA: Resources for Rehabilitation.

Resources for Rehabilitation (1996). *Living with Low Vision: A Resource Guide for People with Sight Loss*. Lexington, MA: Resources for Rahabilitation.

Rogers J, Matsumura M. (1990). *Mother to Be: A Guide to Pregnancy and Birth for Women with Disabilities*. New York: Demos Vermande.

Rosner LJ, Ross S. (1987). *Multiple Sclerosis: New Hope and Practical Guidelines for People with MS and Their Families*. New York: Prentice Hall.

Russell LM, Grant AE, Joseph SM, Fee RW. (1993). *Planning for the Future: Providing a Meaningful Life for a Child with a Disability After Your Death (2nd edition)*. Evanston, IL: American Publishing.

Schapiro RT. (1991). *Multiple Sclerosis: A Rehabilitation Approach*. New York: Demos Vermande.

Schapiro RT. (1994). *Symptom Management in Multiple Sclerosis (2nd edition)*. New York: Demos Vermande.

Scheinberg LC, Holland N (eds.). (1987). *Multiple Sclerosis: A Guide for Patients and Their Families*. New York: Raven Press.

Shrout RN. (1991). *Resource Directory for the Disabled*. New York: Oxford.

Shuman R, Schwartz J. (1988). *Understanding Multiple Sclerosis*. Riverside, NJ: Macmillan.

Sibley WA. (1996). *Therapeutic Claims in Multiple Sclerosis (4th edition)*. New York: Demos Vermande.

Stolman MD. (1994). *A Guide to Legal Rights for People With Disabilities*. New York: Demos Vermande.

Strong M. (1988). *For the Well Spouse of the Chronically Ill*. Mainstay, NY: Little, Brown.

Webster B. (1989). *All of a Piece: A Life with Multiple Sclerosis*. Baltimore: Johns Hopkins.

Wolf J. (1987). *Mastering Multiple Sclerosis: A Guide to Management*. Rutland, VT: Academy Books.

Wolf J, Miles M, Pickett K. (1993). *Vignettes: Stories from Lives with Multiple Sclerosis*. Rutland, VT: Academy Books.

Wolf J. (1991). *Fall Down Seven Times, Get Up Eight*. Rutland, VT: Academy Books.

Wright LM, Leahey M. (1987). *Families and Chronic Illness*. Philadelphia: Spring House.

Younger V, Sardegna J. (1994). *A Guide to Independence for the Visually Impaired and Their Families*. New York: Demos Vermande.

Zola IK. (1982). *Missing Pieces: A Chronicle of Living with a Disability*. Philadelphia: Temple University Press.

National Multiple Sclerosis Society Publications (212-986-3240; 800-344-4867)

Booklets:

○ *Living with MS*—Debra Frankel, M.S., O.T.R., with Hettie Jones

○ *What Everyone Should Know About Multiple Sclerosis*

○ *Things I Wish Someone Had Told Me: Practical Thoughts for People Newly Diagnosed with Multiple Sclerosis*—Suzanne Rogers

○ *Research Directions in Multiple Sclerosis*—Stephen C. Reingold, Ph.D.

○ *ADA and People with MS*—Laura Cooper, Esq., Nancy Law, L.S.W., with Jane Sarnoff

○ *Enhancing Productivity On Your Job: The Win-Win Approach*—Richard T. Roessler, Ph.D., and Phillip Rumrill, Ph.D.

○ *The Rehab Outlook*—Lisa J. Bain and Randall T. Schapiro, M.D.

○ *Food for Thought: MS and Nutrition*—Jane Sarnoff, with Daniel Kosich, Ph.D.

○ *Multiple Sclerosis and Your Emotions*—Mary Eve Sanford, Ph.D., and Jack H. Petajan, M.D.

○ *At Home with MS: Adapting Your Environment*—Jane E. Harmon, O.T.R.

- ✪ *Solving Cognitive Problems*—Nicholas G. LaRocca, Ph.D., with Martha King
- ✪ *Understanding Bladder Problems in MS*—Nancy J. Holland, Ed.D. and Michele G. Madonna, R.N., M.A.
- ✪ *Understanding Bowel Problems in MS*—Nancy J. Holland, Ed.D., with Robin Frames
- ✪ *Moving with Multiple Sclerosis*—Iris Kimberg, M.S., O.T.R., R.P.T.
- ✪ *PLAINTALK: A Booklet About MS for Families*—Debra Frankel, M.S., O.T.R. and Sarah Minden, M.D.
- ✪ *Someone You Know Has MS: A Book for Families*—Cyrisse Jaffee, Debra Frankel, Barbara LaRoche, and Patricia Dick
- ✪ *When a Parent Has MS: A Teenager's Guide*—Pamela Cavallo, M.S.W., with Martha Jablow
- ✪ *Taking Care: A Guide for Well Partners*—Nancy J. Holland, Ed.D., R.N., with Jane Sarnoff
- ✪ *Taming Stress in Multiple Sclerosis*—Frederick Foley, Ph.D., with Jane Sarnoff

Other MS Society Publications:
- ✪ *Facts and Issues* (reprints of articles that originally appeared in the National MS Society magazine, *Inside MS*, covering such topics as diagnosis, pregnancy, pain, sexuality, hiring home help, gait problems, genes and MS susceptibility, fatigue, etc.)
- ✪ *Inside MS*—a 32-page magazine for people living with MS published three times yearly
- ✪ *Inside MS Bulletin*—an 8-page newsletter for donors and friends (published three times a year)
- ✪ Monograph Series (1995)

Families Affected by Multiple Sclerosis: Disease Impacts and Coping Strategies—Rosalind C. Kalb, Ph.D.

Long-Term Care and Multiple Sclerosis—Debra Frankel, M.S., O.T.R.

Employment and Multiple Sclerosis—Nicholas G. LaRocca, Ph.D.

Economic Costs of Multiple Sclerosis: How Much and Who Pays—Carol Harvey, Ph.D.

Utilization and Perceptions of Healthcare Services by People with MS—Leon Sternfeld, M.D., Ph.D., M.P.H.

Canadian Multiple Sclerosis Society Publication (416-922-6065)

✪ *Coping with Fatigue in MS Takes Understanding and Planning*—Alexander Burnfield, M.B., M.R.C. Psych.

Eastern Paralyzed Veterans Association Publications (800-444-0120)

✪ *Understanding the Americans with Disabilities Act* (English and Spanish)

✪ *The ADA: Resource Information Guide* (bibliography of books and videotapes)

✪ *Air Carrier Access* (defines the Air Carrier Access Act and gives information about air travel for wheelchair users)

✪ *Accessible Building Design* (a description of the essential components of an accessible building, including dimensions)

✪ *Planning for Access: A Guide for Planning and Modifying Your Home*

✪ *Programs of EPVA* (a summary of fifteen programs designed to improve the lives of spinal cord injured veterans and people with disabilities)

General Publications

✪ *Access to Travel*—A quarterly magazine published by the Society for the Advancement of Travel for the Handicapped—SATH—a nonprofit organization that works to create a barrier-free environment throughout the travel and tourism industry (347 Fifth Avenue, Suite 610, New York, NY 10016; 212-447-7284)

- *An Approach to Barrier Free Design*—A magazine available from A Positive Approach, Inc., a nonprofit organization that services individuals with disabilities (P.O. Box 910, Millville, NJ 08322; 609-451-4777)

- *Handicapped Americans Reports*—a biweekly newsletter that reports disability-related events and issues, published by Capital Publications, Inc. (1300 N. 17th Street, Arlington, VA 22209; 703-528-1100)

- *Mainstream*—A monthly magazine available from Exploding Myths, Inc. (2973 Beech Street, San Diego, CA 92101; 619-234-3138)

- *MessageS*—A newsletter sponsored by an unrestricted grant from Berlex Laboratories) available at no cost from Phase Five Communications (114 Fifth Avenue, NY, NY 10011; FAX 212-866-3271)

- *Multiple Sclerosis Quarterly Report*—A quarterly publication with articles on medical management, living with MS, and summaries of research on the cause and treatment of MS, available on a subscription basis from Demos Vermande (386 Park Avenue South, Suite 201, New York, NY 10016; 800-532-8663)

- *New Mobility*—A monthly magazine available from Miramar Communications (23815 Stuart Ranch Road, P.O. Box 8987, Malibu, CA 90265; 800-543-4116)

- *A Positive Approach*—A magazine available from A Positive Approach, Inc., a nonprofit organization that services individuals with disabilities (P.O. Box 910, Millville, NJ 08322; 609-451-4777)

- *Real Living with MS*—A monthly newsletter available by subscription from the Cobb Group (9420 Bunsen Parkway, Louisville, KY 40220; 800-223-8720)

- *Take Care*—A quarterly newsletter for caregivers published by the National Family Caregivers Association (9621 East Bexhill Drive, Kensington, MD 20895; 301-942-6430)

- *The Very Special Traveler*—A bimonthly newsletter for people with disabilities who travel, published by Beverly Nelson (The Very Special Traveler, P.O. Box 756, New Windsor, MD 21776-9016; 410-635-2881)

✪ *'We're Accessible': News for Disabled Travelers*—A newsletter from British Colombia for world travelers with disabilities (Lynne Atkinson, 32-1675 Cypress St., Vancouver, B.C. V6J3L4; 604-731-2197)

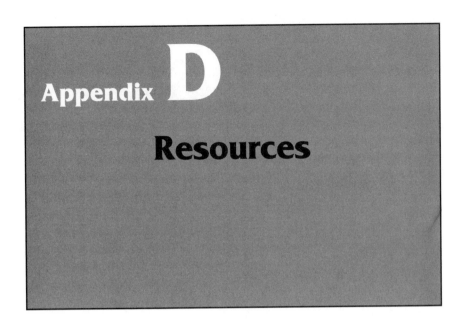

Appendix D

Resources

There is a vast array of resources available to help you in your efforts to meet the challenges of multiple sclerosis. This list is by no means a complete one; it is designed as a starting point in your efforts to identify the resources you need. Each resource that you investigate will lead you to others and they, in turn, will lead you to even more.

Information Sources

Accent on Living (P.O. Box 700, Bloomington, IL 61702; tel: 309-379-2961). A computerized retrieval system of information for the disabled about problems relating to activities of daily living and home management. There is a small charge for a basic search and photocopies, but disabled persons unable to pay are never denied services.

Easter Seals/March of Dimes National Council (90 Eglinton Avenue East, Suite 511, Toronto, Ontario M4P 2Y3, Canada; tel: 416-932-8382). The Council is a federation of regional and provincial groups serving individuals with disabilities through-out Canada. It operates an information service and publishes a newsletter and a quarterly journal.

Clearinghouse on Disability Information, Communications and Information Services, Office of Special Education and Rehabilitative Services, U.S. Department of Education, Switzer Building, 330 C Street, S.W., Washington, D.C. 20202; tel: 202-205-8241. Created by the Rehabilitation Act of 1973, the Clearinghouse responds to inquiries about federal laws, services, and programs for individuals of all ages with disabilities. Their quarterly magazine, "OSERS News in Print," is available free of charge.

Disability Rights Education and Defense Fund, Inc. (DREDF) (2212 Sixth Street, Berkeley, CA 94710; tel: 610-644-2555; 800-466-4232). DREDF is a national law and policy center dedicated to furthering the civil rights of people with disabilities. The Center provides assistance, information, and referrals on disability rights laws; legal representation in cases involving civil rights; and education/training for legislators, policy makers, and law students.

HealthTalk Interactive (800-335-2500). An MS education network available twenty-four hours a day, providing various kinds of information, including answers to commonly asked questions, a replay of a recent "Living with MS" live broadcast, and presentations on various aspects of symptom management.

Information Center and Library, National Multiple Sclerosis Society (733 Third Avenue, New York, NY 10017; tel: 800-FIGHT MS). The Center will answer questions and send you publications of the Society as well as copies of published articles on any topics related to MS.

Inglis House (2600 Belmont Avenue, Philadelphia, PA 19131; tel: 215-878-5600). A national information exchange network specializing in long-term facilities for mentally alert persons with physical disabilities.

National Health Information Center (P.O. Box 1133, Washington, D.C. 20013; tel: 800-336-4797). The Center maintains a library and a database of health-related organizations. It also provides referrals related to health issues for consumers and professionals.

President's Committee on Employment of People with Disabilities (1331 F Street, N.W., Washington, D.C. 20004-1107; tel: 202-376-6200). The Committee publishes employment-related brochures for individuals with disabilities and their employers, and provides the Job Accommodation Network (tel: 800-526-7234).

Electronic Information Sources

One of the most flexible ways to obtain information on multiple sclerosis is by using a computer and a modem. It is possible to dial a number of services that provide access to information about MS. These include the "big three" online services— America OnLine, CompuServe, and Prodigy (see below for customer service numbers). If you are not currently a subscriber and would like information on how to join, call one or more of these numbers. If you are a subscriber, you can access information about MS by entering one of the commands listed below.

Some of these sources of information are available only if you are a subscriber to the service. However, there are also many sources of information available free through the Internet on the World Wide Web. For example, the National Multiple Sclerosis Society has a home page on the World Wide Web at: http://www.nmss.org/. The other sources of MS information on the World Wide Web are too numerous to list. If you are an experienced "net surfer," switch to your favorite search facility and enter the key words "MS" or "multiple sclerosis." This will generally give you a listing of dozens of web sites that pertain to MS. Keep in mind, however, that the World Wide Web is a free and open medium; while many of the web sites have excellent and useful information, others may contain highly unusual and inaccurate information.

◇ *America OnLine*: 800-827-6364 (GO TO NMSS).
◇ *CompuServe*: 800-487-6227 (GO MULTSCLER).
◇ *Prodigy*: 800-776-3449 (JUMP MS FORUM).

On the Internet: Access USENET NEWSGROUP-ALT.SUPPORT.MULT-SCLEROSIS.

Resource Materials

*Assistive Technology Sourceboo*k. (Written by A. Enders and M. Hall, published by Resna Press, Washington, D.C. 1990).

The Complete Directory for People with Disabilities. (Edited by L. Mackenzie, published by Grey House Publishing Inc., Lakeville, CT).

Complete Drug Reference. (Compiled by United States Pharmacopoeia, published by Consumer Report Books, A division of Consumers Union, Yonkers, NY.). This comprehensive, readable, and easy-to-use drug reference includes almost every prescription and non-prescription medication available in the United States and Canada. A new edition is published yearly.

Complete Guide to Prescription and Non-Prescription Drugs. (Written by H. Winter Griffith, M.D., published by The Body Press/Perigee, 200 Madison Avenue, New York, NY 10016, 1995).

Directory of National Information Sources on Disabilities. (Published by the National Institute on Disability and Rehabilitation Research, Washington, D.C. 1994-1995. Vols. I and II).

Exceptional Parent: Parenting Your Child or Young Adult with a Disability. A magazine for families and professionals. (Exceptional Parent, P.O. Box 3000, Dept. EP, Denville, NJ 07834; tel: 800-247-8080). A monthly magazine that celebrated its 25th anniversary by producing the 1996 Resource Guide, which includes ten directories with more than one thousand resources in the United States and Canada. This is a very useful directory for adults with disabilities as well.

Guide to Catalogs for People with Disabilities, Their Families and Their Friends. (EKA Publications, Inc., 9151 Hampton Overlook, Capital Heights, MD 20743; tel: 800-386-5367).

Living with Low Vision: A Resource Guide for People with Sight Loss. (Resources for Rehabilitation, 33 Bedford Street, Suite 19A, Lexington, MA 02173; tel: 617-862-6455). The only large print comprehensive guide to services and products designed to assist individuals with vision loss throughout North America.

Parenting with a Disability. (Through the Looking Glass, 2198 Sixth Street, Suite 100, Berkeley, CA 94710; tel: 510-848-1112; 800-644-2666).

Resources for People with Disabilities and Chronic Conditions. (Resources for Rehabilitation, 33 Bedford Street, Suite 19A, Lexington, MA 02173; tel: 617-862-6455). A comprehensive resource guide covering a variety of disabling conditions as well as general information on rehabilitation services, assistive technology for independent living, and laws that affect people with disabilities.

Resource Directory for the Disabled. (Written by R.N. Shrout, published by Facts-on-File, 460 Park Avenue South, New York, NY 10016; 1991). A resource directory that includes associations and organizations, government agencies, libraries and research centers, publications, and products of all types for disabled individuals.

Agencies and Organizations

American Self-Help Clearinghouse (Northwest Covenant Medical Center, Denville, NJ 07834; tel: 201-625-7101). The Clearinghouse makes referrals to national self-help organizations as well as individual self-help groups for various problems. They also provide referrals to local self-help clearinghouses.

Beach Center on Families and Disabilities (c/o Life Span Institute, University of Kansas, 3111 Haworth Hall, Lawrence, KS 66045; tel: 913-864-7600). The federally funded Center conducts research and training about the functioning of families in which one member is disabled. They have a publications catalog relating to family coping, professional roles, and service delivery. They offer a free newsletter, "Families and Disability."

Consortium of Multiple Sclerosis Centers (CMSC) (c/o Gimbel MS Center at Holy Name Hospital, 718 Teaneck Road, Teaneck, NJ 07666; tel: 201-837-0727). The CMSC is made up of numerous MS centers throughout the United States and Canada. The Consortium's mission is to disseminate information to clinicians, increase resources and opportunities for research, and advance the standard of care for multiple sclerosis. The CMSC is a multidisciplinary organization, bringing together health care professionals from many fields involved in MS patient care.

Department of Veterans Affairs (VA) (810 Vermont Avenue, N.W., Washington, D.C. 20420; tel: 202-273-5400). The VA provides a wide range of benefits and services to those who have served in the armed forces, their dependents, beneficiaries of deceased veterans, and dependent children of veterans with severe disabilities.

Equal Employment Opportunity Commission (EEOC) (Office of Communication and Legislative Affairs, 1801 L Street, N.W., 10th Floor, Washington, D.C. 20507; tel: 800-669-3362 (to order publications); 800-669-4000 (to speak to an investigator; 202-663-4900). The EEOC is responsible for monitoring the section of the ADA on employment regulations. Copies of the regulations are available.

Eastern Paralyzed Veterans Association (EPVA) (75-20 Astoria Boulevard, Jackson Heights, NY 11370; tel: 718-803-EPVA). EPVA is a private, nonprofit organization dedicated to serving the needs of its members as well as other people with disabilities. While offering a wide range of benefits to member veterans with spinal cord dysfunction (including hospital liaison, sports and recreation, wheelchair repair, adaptive architectural consultations, research and educational services, communications, and library and information services, they will also provide brochures and information on a variety of subjects, free of charge to the general public (see Appendix C).

Handicapped Organized Women (HOW) (P.O. Box 35481, Charlotte, NC 28235; tel: 704-376-4735). HOW strives to build self-esteem and confidence among disabled women by encouraging volunteer community involvement. HOW seeks to train disabled women for leadership positions and works in conjunction with the National Organization of Women (NOW).

Multiple Sclerosis Society of Canada (250 Bloor Street East, Suite 1000, Toronto, Ontario M4W 3P9, Canada; tel: 416-922-6065; in Canada: 800-268-7582). A national organization that funds research, promotes public education, and produces publications in both English and French. They provide an "ASK MS Information System" database of articles on a wide variety of topics including treatment, research, and social services. Regional divisions and chapters are located throughout Canada.

Health Resource Center for Women with Disabilities (Rehabilitation Institute of Chicago, 345 East Superior Street, Chicago, IL 60611; tel: 312-908-7997). The Center is a project run by and for women with disabilities. It publishes a free newsletter, "Resourceful Women," and offers support groups and educational seminars addressing issues from a disabled woman's perspective. Among its many educational resources, the Center has developed a video on mothering with a disability.

National Council on Disability (NCD) (1331 F Street, N.W., Suite 1050, Washington, D.C. 20004; tel: 202-272-2004). The Council is an independent federal agency whose role is to study and make recommendations about public policy for people with disabilities. Publishes a free newsletter, "Focus."

National Family Caregivers Association (NFCA) (9621 East Bexhill Drive, Kensington, MD 20895; tel: 301-942-6430). NFCA is dedicated to improving the quality of life of America's 18,000,000 caregivers. It publishes a quarterly newsletter and has a resource guide, an information clearinghouse, and a toll-free hotline: 800-896-3650.

National Multiple Sclerosis Society (NMSS) (733 Third Avenue, New York, NY 10017; tel: 800-FIGHT MS). The NMSS is a nonprofit organization that supports national and international research into the prevention, cure, and treatment of MS. The Society's goals include provision of nationwide services to assist people with MS and their families, and provision of information to those with MS, their families, professionals, and the public. The programs and services of the Society promote knowledge, health, and independence while providing education and emotional support:

◇ Referral to neurologists, physical therapists, and other medical/rehabilitation professionals knowledgeable about MS.

◇ National information line (recording) through the Society's Information Resource Center (IRC) at 800-FIGHT MS. Following selection of the IRC option, a recorded voice requests the topic of interest and mailing information.

◇ Toll-free access to your local chapter by selecting the appropriate option at 800-FIGHT MS.

◇ Internet web site with updated information about treatments, current research, and programs (http://www, nmss.org); local home page in many areas.

◇ Knowledge Is Power educational program (serial mailings) for people *newly diagnosed* with MS and their families, available through most chapters.

◇ Moving Forward group educational program for people *newly diagnosed* with MS and their families, available through most chapters.

◇ Educational programs on various topics throughout the year.

◇ Annual national teleconference at over 500 sites throughout the United States on three Saturdays in May; call your chapter for the location nearest you.

◇ Swimming and other exercise programs sponsored or cosponsored by some chapters, or referral to existing programs in the community.

◇ Wellness programs in some chapters.

National Park Service, U.S. Department of the Interior (P.O. Box 37127, Washington, D.C. 20013-7127). The service will provide you with a listing of national parks and numbers for you to call to obtain up-to-date accessibility information for the individual parks.

Office on the Americans with Disabilities Act (Department of Justice, Civil Rights Division, P.O. Box 66118, Washington, D.C. 20035; tel: 202-514-0301). This office is responsible for enforcing the ADA. To order copies of its regulations, call 202-514-6193.

Paralyzed Veterans of America (PVA) (801 Eighteenth Street N.W., Washington, D.C. 20006; tel: 800-424-8200). PVA is a national information and advocacy agency working to restore function and quality of life for veterans with spinal cord dysfunction. It supports and funds education and research and has a national advocacy program that focuses on accessibility issues. PVA publishes brochures on many issues related to rehabilitation.

Social Security Administration (6401 Security Boulevard, Baltimore, MD 21235; tel: 800-772-1213). To apply for social security benefits based on disability, call this office or visit your local social security branch office. The Office of Disability within the Social Security Administration publishes a free brochure entitled "Social Security Regulations: Rules for Determining Disability and Blindness."

Through the Looking Glass: National Research and Training Center on Families of Adults with Disabilities (2198 Sixth Street, Suite 100, Berkeley, CA 94710; tel: 510-848-4445; 800-644-2666).

Well Spouse Foundation (610 Lexington Avenue, New York, NY 10022-6005; tel: 212-644-1241; 800-838-0879). An emotional support network for people married to or living with a chronically ill partner. Advocacy for home health and long-term care and a newsletter are among the services offered.

Assistive Technology

Access to Recreation: Adaptive Recreation Equipment for the Physically Challenged (2509 E. Thousand Oaks Boulevard, Suite 430, Thousand Oaks, CA 91362; tel: 800-634-4351). Products include exercise equipment and assistive devices for sports, environmental access, games, crafts, and hobbies.

adaptABILITY (Department 2082, 75 Mill Street, Colchester, CT 06415; tel: 800-243-9232). A free catalog of assistive devices and self-care equipment designed to enhance independence.

Adaptive Parenting: Idea Book I (Though the Looking Glass, 2198 Sixth Street, Suite 100, Berkeley, CA 94710; tel: 510-848-1112; 800-644-2666).

American Automobile Association (1712 G Street N.W., Washington, D.C. 20015). The AAA will provide a list of automobile hand-control manufacturers.

AT&T Special Needs Center (2001 Route 46, Parsippany, NJ 07054; tel: 800-233-1222). A catalog of special telephone equipment for individuals with physical disabilities.

Enrichments (P.O. Box 5050, Bolingbrook, IL 60440; tel: 800-323-5547). A free catalog of assistive devices and self-care equipment designed to enhance independence.

Life Enhancement Technologies, LLC (2682 Middlefield Road, Bldg. L, Redwood City, CA 94063; tel: 800-779-6953). The company manufactures a variety of cooling suits that can be used in management of heat-related symptoms in MS.

Medic Alert Foundation International (P.O. Box 1009, Turlock, CA 95380; tel: 800-344-3226; 209-668-3333). A medical identification tag worn to identify a person's medical condition, medications, and any other important information that might be needed in case of an emergency. A file of the person's health data is maintained in a central database to be accessed by a physician or other emergency personnel who need to know the person's pertinent medical information.

National Rehabilitation Information Center (NARIC) (8455 Colesville Road, Silver Spring, MD 20910; tel: 800-346-2742;

301-588-9284; fax: 301-587-1967). NARIC is a library and information center on disability and rehabilitation, funded by the National Institute on Disability and Rehabilitation Research (NIDRR). NARIC operates two databases—ABLEDATA and REHABDATA. NARIC collects and disseminates the results of federally funded research projects and has a collection that includes commercially published books, journal articles, and audiovisual materials. NARIC is committed to serving both professionals and consumers who are interested in disability and rehabilitation. Information specialists can answer simple information requests and provide referrals immediately and at no cost. More complex database searches are available at nominal cost.

◇ ABLEDATA (8455 Colesville Road, Suite 935, Silver Spring, MD 20910; tel: 301-588-9284; 800-227-0216; fax: 301-589-3563). ABLEDATA is a national database of information on assistive technology designed to enable persons with disabilities to identify and locate the devices that will assist them in their home, work, and leisure activities. Information specialists are available to answer questions during regular business hours. ABLE INFORM BBS is available twenty-four hours a day to customers with a computer, modem, and telecommunications software.

◇ REHABDATA (8455 Colesville Road, Suite 935, Silver Spring, MD 20910; tel: 301-588-9284; 800-346-2742). REHABDATA is a database containing bibliographic records with abstracts and summaries of the materials contained in the NARIC (National Rehabilitation Information Information Center) library of disability rehabilitation materials. Information specialists are available to conduct a database search on any rehabilitation related topic.

RESNA: Rehabilitation, Engineering, and Assistive Technology Society of North America (1700 North Moore Street, Suite 1540, Arlington, VA 22209-1903; tel: 703-524-6686, P.O. Box 969, Etobicoke Station U, Etobicoke, Ontario M82 5P9. RESNA is an international association for the advancement of rehabilitation technology. Their objectives are to improve the quality of life for the disabled through the application of science and technology and to influence policy relating to the delivery of technology to disabled persons. They will respond by mail to specific questions about modifying existing equipment and designing new devices.

Sears Home Health Care Catalog (P.O. Box 3123, Naperville, IL 60566; tel: 800-326-1750). The catalog includes medical equipment such as hospital beds, commodes, and wheelchairs, as well as adaptive clothing.

Sentry Detection Corporation (exclusive Westinghouse distributor) (tel: 800-695-0110). The company will install a Life Alert system (separately or as part of a total home security system) that allows a disabled person to get immediate assistance in the event of an emergency.

Steele, Inc. (26112 Iowa Avenue, N.E., P.O. Box 7304, Kingston, WA 98346; tel: 360-297-4555). The company manufactures the Steele Vest® for cooling. It can be used for the management of heat-related symptoms in MS.

Environmental Adaptations

A Consumer's Guide to Home Adaptation (Adaptive Environments Center, 374 Congress Street, Suite 301, Boston, MA 02210; tel: 617-695-1225). A workbook for planning adaptive home modifications such as lowering kitchen countertops and widening doorways.

"Adapting the Home for the Physically Challenged" (A/V Health Services, P.O. Box 1622, West Sacramento, CA 95691; tel: 540-389-4339). A 22-minute videotape that describes home modifications for individuals who use walkers or wheelchairs. Ramp construction and room modification specifications are included.

American Institute of Architects (AIA) (1735 New York Avenue, N.W., Washington, D.C. 20006; tel: 202-626-7300; publications catalog and orders: 800-365-2724). This organization will make referrals to architects who are familiar with the design requirements of people with disabilities.

Financing Home Accessibility Modifications (Center for Universal Design, North Carolina State University, Box 8613, Raleigh, NC 27695; tel: 919-515-3082). This publication identifies state and local sources of financial assistance for homeowners (or tenants) who need to make modifications in their homes.

GE Answer Center (9500 Williamsburg Plaza, Louisville, KY 40222; tel: 800-626-2000). The Center, which is open twenty-four hours a day, seven days a week, offers assistance to individuals with disabilities as well as the general public. They offer two free brochures, "Appliance Help for Those with Special Needs," and "Basic Kitchen Planning for the Physically Handicapped."

National Association of Home Builders (NAHB) (NAHB Research Center, Economics and Policy Analysis Division, 400 Prince George's Boulevard, Upper Marlboro, MD 20774; tel: 301-249-4000). The Research Center produces publications and provides training on housing and special needs. A publication entitled "Homes for a Lifetime" includes an accessibility checklist, financing options, and recommendations for working with builders and remodelers.

National Kitchen and Bath Association (687 Willow Grove Street, Hackettstown, NJ 07840; tel: 908-852-0033). The Association produces a technical manual of barrier-free planning and has directories of certified designers and planners.

Travel

Directory of Travel Agencies for the Disabled. (Written by Helen Hecker, published by Twin Peaks Press, P.O. Box 129, Vancouver, WA 98666-0129). This directory lists travel agents who specialize in arranging travel plans for people with disabilities.

The Disability Bookshop (P.O. Box 129, Vancouver, WA 98666; tel: 800-637-2256). The Disability Bookshop has an extensive list of books for disabled travelers, dealing with such topics as accessibility, travel agencies, accessible van rentals, medical resources, air travel, and guides to national parks.

Information for Handicapped Travelers (available free of charge from the National Library Service for the Blind and Physically Handicapped, 1291 Taylor Street, N.W., Washington, D.C. 20542; tel: 800-424-8567; 202-707-5100). A booklet providing information about travel agents, transportation, and information centers for individuals with disabilities.

Society for the Advancement of Travel for the Handicapped (SATH) (347 Fifth Avenue, Suite 610, New York, NY 10016; tel: 212-447-7284). SATH is a nonprofit organization that acts as a clearinghouse for accessible tourism information and is in contact with organizations in many countries to promote the development of facilities for disabled people. SATH publishes a quarterly magazine, "Access to Travel."

Travel for the Disabled: A Handbook of Travel Resources and 500 Worldwide Access Guides. (Written by Helen Hecker, published by Twin Peaks Press, P.O. Box 129, Vancouver, WA 98666; tel: 800-637-2256). The handbook provides information for disabled travelers about accessibility.

Travel Information Service (Moss Rehabilitation Hospital, 1200 West Tabor Road, Philadelphia, PA 19141; tel: 215-456-9900). The Service provides information and referrals for people with disabilities.

Travelin' Talk (P.O. Box 3534, Clarksville, TN 37043; tel: 615-552-6670). A network of more than one thousand people and organizations around the world who are willing to provide assistance to travelers with disabilities and share their knowledge about the areas in which they live. Travelin' Talk publishes a newsletter by the same name and has an extensive resource directory.

The Wheelchair Traveler (Accent on Living, P.O. Box 700, Bloomington, IL 61702; tel: 309-378-2961). A directory that provides ratings of hotels and motels in the United States.

Wilderness Inquiry (1313 5th Street, S.E., Box 84, Minneapolis, MN 55414; tel: 800-728-0719; 612-379-3858). Wilderness Inquiry sponsors trips into the wilderness for people with disabilities or chronic conditions.

Visual Impairment

Canadian National Institute for the Blind (CNIB) (1929 Bayview Avenue, Toronto, Ontario M4G 3E8, Canada; tel: 416-480-7580). The Institute provides counseling and rehabilitation services for Canadians with any degree of functional visual impairment. They offer public information literature and operate resource and technology centers. The national office has a list of provincial and local CNIB offices.

The Lighthouse Low Vision Products Consumer Catalog (36-20 Northern Boulevard, Long Island City, NY 11101; tel: 800-829-0500). This large-print catalog offers a wide range of products designed to help people with impaired vision.

The Library of Congress, Division for the Blind and Physically Handicapped (1291 Taylor Street, N.W., Washington, D.C. 20542; tel: 800-424-8567; 800-424-9100; for application: 202-287-5100. The Library Service provides free talking book equipment on loan as well as a full range of recorded books for individuals with disabilities or visual impairment. It also provides a variety of free library services through one hundred forty cooperating libraries.

Living with Low Vision: A Resource Guide for People with Sight Loss. (Published by Resources for Rehabilitation, 33 Bedford Street, Suite 19A, Lexington, MA 02173; tel: 617-862-6455). A comprehensive directory designed to help individuals with impaired vision to locate the products and services they need in order to remain independent.

Publishing Companies Specializing in Health and Disability Issues

Demos Vermande (386 Park Avenue South, Suite 201, New York, NY 10016; tel: 800-532-8663).

Resources for Rehabilitation (33 Bedford Street, Suite 19A, Lexington, MA 02173; tel: 617-862-6455).

Twin Peaks Press (P.O. Box 129, Vancouver, WA 98666; tel: 800-637-2256).

Woodbine House (Publishers of the Special-Needs Collection) (6510 Bells Mill Road, Bethesda, MD 20817; tel: 301-897-3570; 800-843-7323).

Appendix E

Professional Biographies of the Authors

Kathy Birk, M.D.

While majoring in biology and women's studies at Washington University in St. Louis, Kathy Birk started a women's health clinic and directed a conference on women and health. Dr. Birk went on to receive her medical degree from the University of Missouri and completed her residency in obstetrics and gynecology. During her residency, Dr. Birk cared for two patients with MS who were concerned that becoming pregnant might worsen their disease. Finding that there was little written about this topic in the medical literature, she decided to pursue the answer in her own research.

Dr. Birk's study was unable to identify any hormone or protein in the blood of pregnant women that could explain why women with MS tend to have fewer exacerbations during pregnancy. Dr. Birk did conclude, however, that having MS was not sufficient reason for women to avoid becoming pregnant; bearing a child did not seem to make the disease worse. Ten years later, the blood samples from the women in this study are being examined to identify a possible genetic explanation for disease improvement during pregnancy.

Dr. Birk's interest and involvement in MS research grew initially out of her experience with her grandmother's multiple sclerosis. Barbara Birk, to whom Dr. Birk dedicates this chapter, lived most of her life with the disease.

Angela Chan, B.P.T.

Angela Chan received her degree in physical therapy from McGill University. Since 1981 Ms. Chan has been the physical therapist for the Multiple Sclerosis Clinic at St. Michael's Hospital in Toronto, Canada, giving individuals with MS recommendations to improve their physical well-being and mobility.

In addition to providing clinical care to individuals with MS, Ms. Chan has extensive experience teaching about MS care to physical therapy students, health care practitioners, and various chapters of the MS Society of Canada. She holds the title of Lecturer in the Department of Physical Therapy at the University of Toronto.

Ms. Chan is an active member of the Consortium of Multiple Sclerosis Centers. She served as Co-Chair and subsequently Chairperson of the Consortium's Clinical Care Committee from 1992 to 1994. Ms. Chan was senior author of the paper entitled "Balance and Spasticity: What We Know and What We Believe," published in a special issue of the *Journal of Neurologic Rehabilitation* in 1994, devoted to the outcome of a two-year research project spearheaded by the Consortium.

Laura Cooper, Esq.

Laura Cooper graduated from the University of Washington Law School in 1986. She has been a practicing attorney for the past ten years, two as counsel to the Chairman of the Interstate Commerce Commission in Washington, D.C., and the latter four as national Independent Living & Legal Consultant to the National Multiple Sclerosis Society. She is a nationally recognized expert in disability law.

Ms. Cooper was teaching science on an Indian reservation when she first experienced gait problems, vertigo, numbness, and tingling. The severity of her MS forced her to leave her job at the age of twenty-two. She enrolled in a couple of graduate school courses, paid her tuition with savings, and received support from the Department of Vocational Rehabilitation for wheel-chair assistance. Her failing health put her in and out of hospitals and eventually, at age twenty-three, into a nursing home.

Three months later, Ms. Cooper found an ad in a newspaper for a wheelchair-accessible apartment complex. She negotiated for herself the space, some furniture, a hospital bed, and a commode, which she ordered on an old Visa card. She later used her Social Security payment to help pay the rent. Her parents helped her by purchasing a lift-equipped van.

Ms. Cooper applied to law school and received a full tuition scholarship to Gonzaga University in Spokane, Washington. While in law school, she experienced several exacerbations that left her temporarily blind and quadriplegic. She transferred to the University of Washington to finish her degree, following which she was named one of the twenty outstanding young American lawyers "who make a difference" by the American Bar Association.

During her search for employment, Ms. Cooper received more than 400 rejections, until one law firm was willing to look at her abilities instead of her disabilities. Following her most recent exacerbation, Ms. Cooper has been consulting on a number of projects involving disability rights.

Robert Enteen, Ph.D.

Robert Enteen, who received his doctorate in sociology from New York University, is Director of Health Research and Policy Programs at the National Multiple Sclerosis Society. He created and oversees the Society's grant, contract, and dissertation fellowship programs in health services, psychosocial, and policy research.

A former health services researcher, Dr. Enteen worked for several years as the director of a national demonstration project that produced the nation's first labor union program to promote and protect employment for job-seekers and employees with disabilities.

In 1992 Dr. Enteen authored *Health Insurance: How to Get It, Keep It, or Improve What You've Got*. A second edition of the book was published in 1996 by Demos Vermande. He is a member of the editorial board and columnist for *MS Management*, the journal of the International Federation of Multiple Sclerosis Societies.

Dr. Enteen hosts a weekly talk show, "Disability and Health Today," which he created in 1995 for the public radio satellite system. The show is the first nationally syndicated program emphasizing disability and chronic disease issues.

Jill Fischer, Ph.D.

Jill Fischer is the Director of the Psychology Program at the Cleveland Clinic Foundation's Mellen Center for MS Treatment and Research. She received her doctorate from the University of Wisconsin-Madison in 1985 and since then has developed an active program of psychological services and research within the interdisciplinary Mellen Center. She has published a number of scientific articles and book chapters related to this work.

Dr. Fischer's current interests include the assessment of individuals whose cognitive function has changed as a result of MS, the development of interventions for individuals with MS-related cognitive deficits, and the refinement of methods for monitoring cognitive function over time. She is Principal Investigator on two studies (a three-year National Multiple Sclerosis Society-funded study of interventions for MS-related cognitive dysfunction, and a Pharmacia/Upjohn-funded multicenter study of neuropsychological outcomes in the current Linomide® clinical trial), and Co-Investigator on a third study (a National Multiple Sclerosis Society-funded study to develop an MS Quality of Life Inventory). She was Neuropsychology Principal Investigator on the recently completed National Institute of Neurologic Diseases and Stroke (NINDS)-funded multicenter trial of Avonex® for relapsing MS and on the National Multiple Sclerosis Society-funded trial of oral methotrexate in chronic progressive MS.

Dr. Fischer served as President of the Consortium of Multiple Sclerosis Centers (CMSC) from 1992 to 1993, and currently serves as a member of the CMSC's Board of Trustees, the National Multiple Sclerosis Society's Clinical Outcomes Assessment Task Force, and the Executive Board of the American Psychological Association's Division 40 (Clinical Neuropsychology).

Frederick Foley, Ph.D.

Frederick Foley is Associate Professor of Psychology and the Director of Clinical Training for the Ph.D. program in Clinical Health Psychology at Ferkauf Graduate School of Psychology and the Albert Einstein College of Medicine of Yeshiva University. Since receiving his doctorate in clinical psychology from Fordham University, he has been actively involved in MS research, education, and clinical work, and has published numerous scientific articles and book chapters related to psychological factors in MS.

Dr. Foley is also on the staff of the Medical Rehabilitation Research and Training Center for Multiple Sclerosis at St. Agnes Hospital, White Plains, New York. He has conducted studies on the efficacy of psychotherapy in MS and on the relationship between psychological factors and immune regulation in MS. One study, entitled "Psychoimmunologic Dysregulation in Multiple Sclerosis," won the 1989 Dorfman Award from the Academy of Psychosomatic Medicine.

Dr. Foley's current interests include investigating methods of enhancing intimacy, communication, and sexuality in couples in which one partner has MS. He is also developing the Multiple Sclerosis Intimacy and Sexuality Questionnaire, which attempts to measure these factors in MS.

June Halper, MSN, RN.CS, ANP

June Halper is a certified adult nurse practitioner who has specialized in multiple sclerosis since 1978. She originally became interested in MS while working as a public health nurse. While pursuing her undergraduate degree in nursing, Ms. Halper worked for a chapter of the National Multiple Sclerosis Society developing a variety of service programs, including support groups, home outreach programs, home care and respite services, local and regional educational conferences, and a student internship program. In 1985 she obtained funding for the first in-home respite program for MS.

Ms. Halper founded the Gimbel MS Center in Teaneck, New Jersey, in 1985 and has been Executive Director for the past three years. The Center was named the administrative seat for the Consortium of Multiple Sclerosis Centers in 1993, with Ms. Halper serving as the Consortium's Administrative Director since that time. While serving as Administrative Director, Ms. Halper and Dr. Jack Burks organized the Consortium's 1993 *What Do We Know About MS* Conference. As an outgrowth of this conference, specialty groups in MS care summarized the current knowledge and clinical practices in their individual fields and identified future research priorities.

Ms. Halper spearheaded the development of a national task force on disabled women's health issues. She is particularly interested in hormonal influences in MS and has conducted research into the effect of the menstrual cycle in MS, the health of bottle-feeding vs. breast-feeding mothers, and menopause and MS. Ms. Halper participated in a national teleconference sponsored by the National MS Society in 1995 on symptom management in MS, and a national conference on women and MS in Washington, D.C., in 1996.

Ms. Halper is a member of her local MS chapter's Professional Advisory Committee and currently serves as President of the Consortium of Multiple Sclerosis Centers.

Robert M. Herndon, M.D.

Robert Herndon received his medical degree from the University of Tennessee Medical School and did his internship and neurology residency at Wayne State University. He began his basic research in MS in 1968 while on the faculty of the Stanford University Medical School. He discovered free myelin fragments in the spinal fluid of people with MS while carrying out electron microscopic studies on spinal fluid. In 1969 Dr. Herndon joined the faculty at Johns Hopkins Medical School, where he worked with viruses that cause myelin destruction. While at Johns Hopkins, he became director of the multiple sclerosis clinic and began his clinical research in MS.

In 1977 Dr. Herndon became director of the Center for Brain Research and Professor of Brain Research and Neurology at the University of Rochester. While there, he served as director of the Rochester Area Multiple Sclerosis Society Clinic. In 1988 he became Professor of Neurology at Oregon Health Sciences University and Chief of Neurology at Good Samaritan Hospital in Portland.

From 1969 to 1991, Dr. Herndon was involved in research on regeneration of myelin and myelin-forming cells in experimental animals. This work played an important role in our understanding of the process of myelin regeneration in MS.

In 1981 Dr. Herndon began a collaborative effort with Drs. Lawrence Jacobs and Andre Salazar to work on the treatment of MS with interferons. This led to the initial trial of intraspinal interferon in MS and then to the more recent intramuscular interferon beta-1a (Avonex®) trial.

Dr. Herndon serves on the Medical Advisory Board of the National and International MS Societies. He is also past president of the Consortium of Multiple Sclerosis Centers.

Jean Hietpas, OTR, LCSW

Jean Hietpas is currently a Clinical Specialist in Occupational Therapy at the Department of Rehabilitative Services of the University of California in San Francisco. Following her training at the University of Wisconsin-Milwaukee in both occupational therapy and clinical social work, Ms. Hietpas remained at the University to teach courses in occupational therapy. She served as Program Director of the Mental Health and Alcohol and Drug Abuse Clinic at de Paul Rehabilitation Hospital in Milwaukee from 1986 to 1987, and then became Clinical Director of Drug and Alcohol Programs at Elmbrook Memorial Hospital in Milwaukee.

Ms. Hietpas is a contributing author of several publications, including a chapter on multiple sclerosis in *Occupational Therapy Practice Skills for Physical Dysfunction (4th edition)*.

Nancy J. Holland, Ed.D., R.N.

Nancy Holland is Vice President of Client & Community Services, National Multiple Sclerosis Society. In this capacity she directs program development throughout the Society's ninety chapters in the areas of MS knowledge, health, and independence. Dr. Holland earned her doctorate in higher and adult education from Teachers College, Columbia University, in 1992. She also holds undergraduate and graduate degrees in nursing. Her career in the field of MS began in 1974 at the first comprehensive care center for people with MS in the country. Her roles in this setting included clinician, clinical coordinator, director of training, co-therapist for MS groups, and research associate. Dr. Holland was also recipient of a Career Development Award from the National Institute on Disability and Rehabilitation Research.

Dr. Holland has authored over thirty MS-related publications covering topics such as rehabilitation, coping, management of bladder, bowel, and sexual dysfunction, employment, and overall adaptation to the many challenges of MS. She is associate editor of *Multiple Sclerosis: A Guide for Patients and Their Families*.

Rosalind C. Kalb, Ph.D.

Rosalind Kalb is a clinical psychologist and Assistant Professor of Medicine at the Medical Rehabilitation Research and Training Center for Multiple Sclerosis at St. Agnes Hospital and New York Medical College. After receiving her doctorate from Fordham University, she began her career in MS, providing individual, group, and family therapy at the MS Care Center at the Albert Einstein College of Medicine. Following the MS Center's relocation to New York Medical College, Dr. Kalb added a variety of other clinical and research activities to her work in MS, including groups for well spouses and couples living with MS, and neuropsychological evaluation and cognitive rehabilitation for research and treatment purposes.

Dr. Kalb has authored or edited a number of publications about multiple sclerosis. Along with Dr. Labe Scheinberg, she edited *Multiple Sclerosis and the Family*, which was published in 1992 by Demos Vermande. She is the author of *Families Affected by Multiple Sclerosis: Disease Impacts and Coping Strategies*, a monograph published in 1995 by the National Multiple Sclerosis Society.

With funding from the National MS Society, Dr. Kalb is investigating "The Impact of Multiple Sclerosis in Childhood and Adolescence." The study is evaluating the effects of early-onset MS on intellectual function and academic performance, as well as a variety of psychosocial variables. She is also conducting a study with Dr. Nicholas LaRocca and Dr. Charles Smith, funded by the National Institute on Disability and Rehabilitation Research, entitled "The Psychosocial Impact of Parental Multiple Sclerosis on Children and Adolescents."

Donna C. Kulha

Donna Kulha is a Donor Recruitment Specialist for the American Red Cross Blood Services, New England Region. Prior to her move to the American Red Cross, Ms. Kulha served as Program Manager for the Massachusetts Chapter of the National Multiple Sclerosis Society. In this capacity she worked with individuals with MS, family members, and health care providers, providing referral and supportive services, and networking with community agencies.

During her fifteen years with the National MS Society, Ms. Kulha managed several demonstration projects related to employment and chronic diseases. She served as coordinator for Project Alliance, a three-year U.S. Department of Education, Rehabilitation Services Administration grant awarded to the National MS Society. The project was designed to gather information and provide interventions to maximize job retention and enhance job satisfaction and career mobility for people with disabling chronic illnesses.

Nicholas G. LaRocca, Ph.D.

Nicholas LaRocca, Director of Research of the Medical Rehabilitation Research and Training Center for Multiple Sclerosis at St. Agnes Hospital and New York Medical College, received his doctorate in clinical psychology from Fordham University. He has extensive experience in both psychosocial research and psychological treatment in multiple sclerosis. Dr. LaRocca has designed, administered, and analyzed a number of clinical studies in MS, including neurogenic bladder dysfunction, comparison of inpatient and outpatient rehabilitation, and the role of stressful life events in MS. He was Principal Investigator of a study entitled "The Rehabilitation of Memory in Multiple Sclerosis," funded by the National MS Society. Currently, Dr. LaRocca is Principal Investigator of a project funded by the National Institute on Disability and Rehabilitation Research entitled "The Comprehensive Rehabilitation of Cognitive Dysfunction in Multiple Sclerosis." He also served as Principal Investigator of an MS Society-funded "Program to Facilitate Retention of Employment Among Persons with Multiple Sclerosis," and is currently Co-Principal Investigator for the National MS Society-funded project entitled "Development of a Multiple Sclerosis Quality of Life Measurement."

Dr. LaRocca has published numerous articles and chapters on psychosocial issues in MS. In 1995 he wrote a monograph entitled *Employment and Multiple Sclerosis*, which was published by the National MS Society. Dr. LaRocca was an invited speaker for the 1992 audioteleconference of the National MS Society entitled "Multiple Sclerosis: Understanding Your Mind and Emotions."

Dr. LaRocca served as Chairman of the Research Committee of the Consortium of Multiple Sclerosis Centers and is currently the Consortium's President-Elect.

Jeri Logemann, Ph.D.

Jeri Logemann is the Ralph and Jean Sundin Professor of Communication Sciences and Disorders, and Chairperson of the Department, at Northwestern University. She is also Professor of Otolaryngology and Maxillofacial Surgery, and Neurology, at the University's Medical School, as well as Professor of the Cleft Palate Team at the University's Dental School.

Dr. Logemann's research interests include the management of voice disorders, normal swallowing physiology, and the assessment and treatment of speech and swallowing dysfunction in cancer patients and neurologically impaired individuals. She has completed several studies of swallowing disorders resulting from multiple sclerosis, and has worked with other speech-language pathologists to identify research priorities for MS-related speech and swallowing problems.

Dr. Logemann is co-author of the *Fisher-Logemann Test of Articulation Competence*, author of *Evaluation and Treatment of Swallowing Disorders* and *Manual for the Videofluorographic Study of Swallowing*. In 1994 she served as President of the American Speech-Language-Hearing Association (ASHA).

Aaron Miller, M.D.

Aaron Miller received his medical degree from New York University School of Medicine in 1968. Following his residency in neurology at the Albert Einstein College of Medicine, he received additional post-doctoral training in neurovirology and immunology at Johns Hopkins University School of Hygiene and Public Health and at Albert Einstein. Dr. Miller is currently Director of the Division of Neurology at Maimonides Medical Center in Brooklyn, New York, where he also serves as Director of the MS Care Center. He is Professor of Clinical Neurology at the State University of New York-Health Sciences Center at Brooklyn.

Dr. Miller serves as chairman of the Professional Education Committee of the National MS Society, as well as chairman of the Professional Advisory Committee of the New York City Chapter of the NMSS. He is also past president of the Consortium of Multiple Sclerosis Centers. Dr. Miller developed and has for eight years directed a popular seminar at the annual meeting of the American Academy of Neurology entitled "MS: Patient Management."

Dr. Miller has participated in numerous clinical trials of new treatments for MS and is the author of many articles and chapters on MS and other neurologic subjects.

Deborah M. Miller, Ph.D., LISW

Deborah Miller is Director of Comprehensive Care at the Mellen Center for MS Treatment and Research of The Cleveland Clinic Foundation. In this capacity, her responsibilities include program development and evaluation, providing clinical care, conducting psychosocial research, and assuring integration of the Center's clinical, research, and operational activities.

A social worker with fifteen years of experience in the area of chronic disability, she has been a member of the Mellen Center's interdisciplinary care team since 1985. Her practice interests focus on marital and family adjustment to the consequences of MS. Her research interests include quality of life assessment, family health and response to caregiving, causes and interventions for abuse and neglect, and clinical care outcomes.

Using her clinical experience, Dr. Miller has developed and facilitated group treatment programs for school-age children and teenagers whose parents have MS, and for adults who have parenting concerns related to MS.

Dr. Miller has extensive affiliations with the National Multiple Sclerosis Society, including consultant to the Office of Client and Community Services, Chair of the National Panel of Professional Advisors, and member of the committee to establish guidelines for known and suspected abuse. She is a member of the Northeast Ohio Chapter's Patient Services Committee and won that Chapter's "Health Care Professional" award in 1991.

Randall T. Schapiro, M.D.

Randall Schapiro received his medical degree in internal medicine and his residency training in neurology from the University of Minnesota. He then joined the faculty of the University and directed the multiple sclerosis program. He left the full-time faculty in 1977 to found the Fairview MS Center in Minneapolis.

Although Dr. Schapiro has done extensive research and publishing in the management of MS and has participated in numerous clinical trials, he prefers to be known as a clinician and teacher. The majority of his time is spent in patient care and lecturing to MS audiences and health care professionals about the clinical management of MS.

Dr. Schapiro has won numerous awards for his work in MS. He is a member of numerous professional organizations and served as Past President of the Consortium of Multiple Sclerosis Centers. Dr. Schapiro is the author of two classic volumes in MS, *Multiple Sclerosis: A Rehabilitation Approach to Management* and *Symptom Management in Multiple Sclerosis (2nd edition)*, published by Demos Vermande.

Charles R. Smith, M.D.

Charles Smith has been Director of the Medical Rehabilitation Research and Training Center for Multiple Sclerosis at St. Agnes Hospital and New York Medical College since 1989. He has also served since 1991 as Chairman of the Department of Neurology at Bronx Lebanon Hospital Center, Bronx, New York. Following his medical training at the University of Toronto, Dr. Smith completed a two-year fellowship in the Department of Immunology at the Albert Einstein College of Medicine, working on mechanisms of viral persistence in neural cell culture.

In his long association with the Research and Training Center, Dr. Smith has devoted his professional time primarily to the clinical management of MS, with particular interest in the management of fatigue. He served as Principal Investigator of a Social Security Research Demonstration Grant entitled "The Objective Measurement of Fatigue in Multiple Sclerosis." He also directed a study entitled "The Effects of Baclofen on Ambulation Proficiency in Individuals with Spasticity Associated with Multiple Sclerosis," funded by the National MS Society.

Pam Sorensen, M.A., C.C.C.-SLP

Pam Sorensen has served as Director of Speech/Language Pathology and Coordinator of the COPE Program at the Rocky Mountain Multiple Sclerosis Center in Englewood, Colorado, since 1988. She has also acted as speech/language pathology consultant for the Jimmie Heuga Center medical programs since 1992.

After receiving her master's degree from the University of Denver, Ms. Sorensen worked at Good Samaritan Hospital in Phoenix, and subsequently joined the staff of Spalding

Rehabilitation Hospital in Denver. In these settings, she provided evaluation and treatment of speech, voice, swallowing, cognitive-language, and communication disorders due to stroke, head injury, and neurosurgery.

Ms. Sorensen has served on the Patient Care, Research, and Nominating Committees of the Consortium of Multiple Sclerosis Centers. She was also appointed liaison for the National MS Society's Employment Committee. She presently sits on the editorial advisory board for *Real Living with MS*, a monthly publication of the Cobb Group. Since 1989 Ms. Sorensen has given many local and national presentations on the subject of cognitive-communication disorders in MS. She is an author of several articles about MS care, including "Communication Disorders and Dysphagia" in the *Journal of Neurologic Rehabilitation* (1994).

Michael A. Werner, M.D.

Michael Werner is on the faculty of the New York Medical College in the Department of Urology and serves as Regional Medical Advisor for New York and Connecticut for the Impotence Institute of America.

Following his residency in urology at Mount Sinai Medical Center in New York, Dr. Werner received his specialized fellowship training in male infertility and male sexual dysfunction at Boston University Medical Center. Dr. Werner has authored many chapters and articles for professional journals on male infertility and sexual dysfunction. One of his areas of particular interest is ejaculatory dysfunction. Dr. Werner works with many men with MS to maximize their fertility and sexual function.

Index